T0177673

What Is Enough?

What Is Enough?

Sufficiency, Justice, and Health

Edited by

CARINA FOURIE

ANNETTE RID

Oxford University Press is a department of the University of Oxford. It furthers
the University's objective of excellence in research, scholarship, and education
by publishing worldwide. Oxford is a registered trade mark of Oxford University
Press in the UK and certain other countries.

Published in the United States of America by Oxford University Press
198 Madison Avenue, New York, NY 10016, United States of America.

© Oxford University Press 2017

Library of Congress Cataloging-in-Publication Data
Names: Fourie, Carina, editor. | Rid, Annette, editor.
Title: What is enough? : sufficiency, justice, and health / edited by Carina Fourie
and Annette Rid.
Description: Oxford ; New York : Oxford University Press, [2016] | Includes
bibliographical references and index.
Identifiers: LCCN 2016006945 | ISBN 9780199385263 (hardcover : alk. paper) |
ISBN 9780199385287 (ebook (updf)) | ISBN 9780199385294 (ebook (epub)) |
ISBN 9780199385270 (online content)
Subjects: | MESH: Health Care Rationing—ethics | Health Care
Rationing—economics | Health Services Needs and Demand | Social Justice | Health Policy
Classification: LCC RA418 | NLM WA 525 | DDC 362.1—dc23 LC record available
at http://lccn.loc.gov/2016006945

9 8 7 6 5 4 3 2 1

Printed by Sheridan Books, Inc., United States of America

Contents

Acknowledgments   vii

Contributors   ix

Introduction—CARINA FOURIE AND ANNETTE RID   1

PART I: *Groundwork*

1. The Sufficiency View: A Primer—CARINA FOURIE   11
2. Sufficiency, Health, and Health Care Justice: The State of
   the Debate—ANNETTE RID   30

PART II: *The Sufficiency View*

3. Axiological Sufficientarianism—IWAO HIROSE   51
4. Sufficiency, Priority, and Aggregation—ROBERT HUSEBY   69
5. Some Questions (and Answers) for Sufficientarians—LIAM SHIELDS   85
6. Essentially Enough: Elements of a Plausible Account
   of Sufficientarianism—DAVID V. AXELSEN AND LASSE NIELSEN   101

PART III: *Sufficiency, Health, and Health Care Justice*

7. Intergenerational Justice, Sufficiency, and Health—AXEL GOSSERIES   121
8. Basic Human Functional Capabilities as the Currency
   of Sufficientarian Distribution in Health Care—EFRAT RAM-TIKTIN   144

9. Disability, Disease, and Health Sufficiency—SEAN AAS
   AND DAVID WASSERMAN   164

10. Sufficiency of Capabilities, Social Equality, and Two-Tiered Health Care
    Systems—CARINA FOURIE   185

11. Determining a Basic Minimum of Accessible Health Care:
    A Comparative Assessment of the Well-Being Sufficiency
    Approach—PAUL T. MENZEL   205

12. Just Caring: The Insufficiency of the Sufficiency Principle
    in Health Care—LEONARD M. FLECK   223

PART IV: *Implementing Sufficiency in Health Care Policy and Economics*

13. Defining Health Care Benefit Packages: How Sufficientarian
    Is Current Practice?—DIMITRA PANTELI
    AND EWOUT VAN GINNEKEN   247

14. Sufficiency, Comprehensiveness of Health Care Coverage,
    and Cost-Sharing Arrangements in the Realpolitik of Health
    Policy—GOVIND PERSAD AND HARALD SCHMIDT   267

15. Applying the Capability Approach in Health Economic
    Evaluations: A Sufficient Solution—PAUL MARK MITCHELL,
    TRACY E. ROBERTS, PELHAM M. BARTON, AND JOANNA COAST   281

Bibliography   303

Index   329

Acknowledgments

KNOWLEDGE AND INSIGHT are typically the result of collaborative, rather than individual, effort, and they require dedication and tenacity from everyone engaged. Both observations have particular salience for this book. It started with the idea for a workshop on "The Relevance of Sufficiency for Just Health Care" in the spring of 2010, when we first met at the University of Zurich. The workshop was eventually held in the summer of 2012 and now, around 6 years after everything started, we are the pleased editors of this volume. Along the way, we have also become friends.

We have many people to thank. First and foremost, we express our gratitude to the contributors for their excellent work and patience in engaging with our comments and suggestions. We have bombarded them with ideas and requests for clarification, and we can only hope they appreciate that we were motivated by trying to make this the best volume we could.

The workshop on sufficientarianism at the Ethics Centre, University of Zurich, showed us that an edited volume on the subject would help fill significant gaps in the philosophical and bioethical literature. We thank all workshop participants for their contributions; Anton Leist for co-organizing the workshop; and Lisa Brun, who mastered the event's logistics for us.

Throughout the years, we have had the good fortune of developing the book while being surrounded by many wonderful colleagues. We worked for 2 years together at the Institute of Biomedical Ethics (IBME), University of Zurich, and particularly thank Jan-Christoph Heilinger, Agomoni Ganguli Mitra, and Verina Wild for providing us with a stimulating and fun environment in which to work. Thanks are also due to Nikola Biller-Andorno, the director of the IBME, for her support.

Carina is especially grateful to all her colleagues at the Ethics Centre of the University of Zurich and, later, at the Department of Philosophy at the University of Washington for their support and for the marvelous working environments in which this volume was edited. Although it is difficult to single people out because so many have been helpful, particular mention must go to Peter Schaber and Sebastian Muders at the University of Zurich. Carina is also very grateful to Sabine Hohl of the University of Graz and Fabian Schuppert of Queen's University Belfast for consistently providing constructive feedback and comments.

Annette thanks her colleagues at the Department of Global Health & Social Medicine at King's College London, and the Department of Bioethics, National Institutes of Health (NIH) Clinical Center, for their fantastic support throughout the years. Special thanks are due to Franklin Miller, Joseph Millum, Seema Shah, David Wendler, and the late Alan Wertheimer at NIH, as well as Danielle Bromwich (now at the University of Massachusetts, Boston) and Silvia Camporesi, Barbara Prainsack and Sridhar Venkatapuram at King's College London. In addition, Katharina Kieslich, Peter Littlejohns, Catherine Max, Benedict Rumbold, Albert Weale, and James Wilson have been providing a wonderful forum for discussion as part of the Social Values and Health Priority Setting Group that runs between King's College London and University College London. Annette is also deeply grateful to Thomas Rid for his unfailing encouragement and support.

When our ideas for the book started to take shape, we received many helpful comments on our initial book proposal from Robert Goodin, Australian National University, with whom Annette spent a terrific year at the NIH, and from two anonymous reviewers for Oxford University Press. Our final plan for the book looked very different, and indeed significantly better, than the prior drafts. Our thanks also go to Lucy Randall and Peter Ohlin at Oxford University Press for their capable and steady editorial support; to Rose Mortimer, then an inspiring student in the Postgraduate Programme in Bioethics & Society at King's College London for last-minute help with editing and formatting manuscripts; to Elin Simonson for compiling the book's index; and to Daniel Hays for his diligent copyediting; and to Joseph Lurdu Antoine for his attention to detail in seeing the book through to production. An anonymous reviewer for Oxford University Press also provided excellent feedback to help us make final revisions to the volume.

Finally, this project would not have been possible without our funders. The initial workshop was supported by the Swiss National Science Foundation (10CO15_136125), the Corti Foundation, and the IBME at the University of Zurich. Grants from the University Research Priority Program for Ethics (URPP for Ethics), also at the University of Zurich, and the Department of Global Health & Social Medicine, King's College London, allowed us to delegate the manuscript formatting and indexing. Carina's research has been financially supported for many years by the Swiss National Science Foundation (100012-120200 and 100017_146668). Funding from the People Programme (Marie Curie Actions) of the European Union's Seventh Framework Programme (FP7/2007-2013) under REA grant agreement No. 301816 gave Annette more time to focus on her writing.

Contributors

Sean Aas, MA, PhD, has been a postdoctoral fellow in the Department of Bioethics at the US National Institutes of Health since 2013. Previously, he was a fellow at the Center for Advanced Studies Justititia Amplificata in Frankfurt, Germany. He works at the intersection of bioethics and political philosophy, with particular focus on global justice and the ethics and politics of disability.

David V. Axelsen, PhD, is a postdoctoral fellow at the Department of Political Science, Aarhus University and the Department of Government, London School of Economics and Social Science. He works on global justice, national identity, political philosophical methodology, and, as in the case of the current contribution, distributive justice. He has recently published two articles in the *Journal of Political Philosophy* (one of which is coauthored with Lasse Nielsen). When not engaged in academia, he enjoys competing in the Danish sport, flaghelmet.

Pelham M. Barton, PhD, is a reader in Mathematical Modeling in the Health Economics Unit and director of the MSc program in Health Economics and Health Policy at the University of Birmingham, UK. He has more than 70 publications, of which approximately 50 are academic papers published in peer-reviewed journals, including *The BMJ, Health Economics, Health Technology Assessment,* and *Journal of Health Services Research & Policy.* He is an internationally recognized expert in modeling applied to health care provision, both preventative and curative. His methodological work includes adoption of ideas from outside health economics to resolve the tension between adequacy, efficiency, and transparency of models.

Joanna Coast, PhD, is Professor in the Economics of Health & Care in the School of Social and Community Medicine, University of Bristol, UK. Her research interests lie in the theory underlying economic evaluation (including capability), developing broader measures of outcome for use in economic evaluation (including measures of capability), health care decision-making, the economics of antimicrobial resistance, and the organization of care. She also has a methodological interest in the use of qualitative methods in health economics. She has published extensively in all of these areas. Work on capability has included methodological work in relation to health economics as well as empirical applications in health and end-of-life care. She has led the development of the ICECAP capability instruments. She has received major grants from the Medical Research Council and the European Research Council. She is Senior Editor (Health Economics) for *Social Science and Medicine*.

Leonard M. Fleck, PhD, is Professor of Philosophy and Medical Ethics in the Center for Ethics, College of Human Medicine, Michigan State University. He is author of *Just Caring: Health Care Rationing and Democratic Deliberation* (Oxford University Press, 2009) and is coeditor with Marion Danis, Samia Hurst, Reidun Forde, and Ann Slowther of *Fair Resource Allocation and Rationing at the Bedside* (Oxford University Press (OUP), 2014). His published essays address a wide range of topics related to health care justice, rational democratic deliberation, health care rationing, and ethical issues related to precision medicine and emerging genetic technologies.

Carina Fourie, PhD, is the Benjamin Rabinowitz Assistant Professor of Medical Ethics at the Department of Philosophy, University of Washington, and a member of the Department's Program on Values in Society. She works on a variety of topics in medical ethics and also in social and political philosophy, with particular interest in social justice and equality and their application to public health and health care policy. Her recent publications include "Moral Distress and Moral Conflict in Clinical Ethics" (*Bioethics*, 2015) and the collected volume *Social Equality: On What It Means to Be Equals* (coedited with Fabian Schuppert and Ivo Wallimann-Helmer; OUP, 2015).

Ewout van Ginneken, PhD, is Coordinator of the Berlin hub of the European Observatory on Health Systems and Policies, at the Berlin University of Technology. His topics of interest include international health systems, health insurance, health financing, cross-border health care, pharmaceutical policy, and the impact of European Union law. He is the author of "Implementing Insurance Exchanges—Lessons from Europe" (with Kathy Swartz; *New England Journal of Medicine*, 2013) and "Coverage for Undocumented Migrants Becomes More Urgent" (with Bradford Gray, *Annals of Internal Medicine*, 2013).

Axel Gosseries, PhD, is Senior Research Fellow at the Fonds de la Recherche Scientifique (FNRS, Brussels) and Professor at the University of Louvain (Hoover

Chair in Economic and Social Ethics, UCL, Belgium). As a political philosopher, his research focuses on theories of intergenerational justice and on democracy within organizations. He has authored more than 50 papers in philosophy, law, and economics, as well as one book on intergenerational justice (Flammarion, 2004). He has edited three books, including *Intergenerational Justice* (with L. Meyer; Oxford University Press, 2009) and *Intellectual Property and Theories of Justice* (with A. Marciano and A. Strowel; Palgrave, 2008).

Iwao Hirose, PhD, is Associate Professor at the Philosophy Department and the School of Environment, McGill University in Canada. He works on a wide range of topics in normative ethics, including projects on egalitarianism, justice in health and health care, and climate justice, as well as in the philosophy of economics. He is author of *Moral Aggregation* (OUP, 2015), *Egalitarianism* (Routledge, 2015), and *The Ethics of Health Care Rationing* (with Greg Bognar; Routledge, 2014), as well as the editor of *The Oxford Handbook of Value Theory* (with Jonas Olson; OUP, 2015) and *Weighing and Reasoning* (with Andrew Reisner; OUP, 2015).

Robert Huseby, PhD, is Professor of Political Science at the University of Oslo. His research interests include distributive justice and climate ethics. Among his recent publications are "Should the Beneficiaries Pay?" *Politics, Philosophy & Economics*, 2015, and "John Rawls and Climate Justice—An Amendment to The Law of Peoples," *Environmental Ethics*, 2013.

Paul T. Menzel, PhD, is Professor of Philosophy emeritus at Pacific Lutheran University. He has written widely on moral questions in health economics and health policy. Publications include "A Cultural Moral Right to a Basic Minimum of Accessible Health Care," *Kennedy Institute of Ethics Journal* (2011); *Prevention vs. Treatment: What's the Right Balance?* (coedited with H. S. Faust; OUP, 2012); and "Advance Directives, Dementia, and Withholding Food and Water by Mouth" (coauthored with M. C. Chandler-Cramer), *Hastings Center Report* (2014).

Paul Mark Mitchell, PhD, is Senior Research Associate at the School of Social and Community Medicine, University of Bristol. His research interests are in measuring capabilities and the theory and methods for conducting health economic evaluations. First author publications by Paul include "Assessing sufficient capability: a new approach to economic evaluation", *Social Science & Medicine* (2015); "The Relative Impacts of Disease on Health Status and Capability Wellbeing: A Multi-Country Study", *PLoS ONE* (2015).

Lasse Nielsen, PhD, is a postdoctoral fellow at the Department of Political Science and Government, Aarhus University in Denmark. He works on topics in political philosophy, such as the value of equality and sufficiency in distributive justice and the applicability of the capability approach to health and health care ethics. He is coauthor of the article, "Sufficiency as Freedom from Duress" in *Journal of Political Philosophy* (2015). He is author of the article, "Why Health Matters to Justice: A Capability Theory Perspective," in *Ethical Theory and Moral Practice* (2014). He is a keen participant in the Danish sport, flaghelmet.

Dimitra Panteli, MD, DrPH, is a research fellow at the Department of Health Care Management, Berlin University of Technology. Her research topics include evidence-based decision-making in health care with a focus on health technology assessment (HTA) and clinical guidelines, health systems research, pharmaceutical policy, and cross-border care. She coordinates the department's teaching on HTA and health systems and is a member of the editorial team of the European Observatory on Health Systems and Policies.

Govind Persad, JD, PhD, is Assistant Professor in the Berman Institute of Bioethics and Department of Health Policy and Management at Johns Hopkins University. His research bridges applied ethics, political philosophy, and health law. Recent projects focus on the normative implications of socioeconomic mobility as well as the ethical dimensions of health care financing and health insurance. His publications include "Priority-Setting, Cost-Effectiveness, and the Affordable Care Act" (*American Journal of Law and Medicine,* 2015) and "The Ethics of Expanding Access to Cheaper, Less-Effective Treatments" (with Ezekiel Emanuel; *Lancet,* 2016).

Efrat Ram-Tiktin, PhD, is a lecturer at the Department of Philosophy, Bar-Ilan University. Her research topics include political philosophy and various issues in medical ethics, such as triage of patients under extreme scarcity of resources. She has also developed a theory of sufficiency of basic human functional capabilities that she applies to questions surrounding justice in health and health care. Among her publications are "The Right to Healthcare as a Right to Basic Human Functional Capabilities" in *Ethical Theory and Moral Practice* (2012) and "Possible Effects of Moral Bioenhancement on Political Privileges and Fair Equality of Opportunity" (2014) in the *American Journal of Bioethics.*

Annette Rid, MD, is a Senior Lecturer in Bioethics and Society in at the Department of Global Health & Social Medicine at King's College London and an Elected Fellow of the Hastings Center. She works in a variety of areas in bioethics, including research ethics, clinical ethics, justice in health and health care, and ethics in transplantation medicine. Her publications on justice in health and health care include "Justice and Procedure: How Does 'Accountability for Reasonableness' Result in Fair Limit-Setting Decisions?" (*Journal of Medical Ethics*, 2009) and "The Importance of Being NICE" (with Peter Littlejohns, James Wilson, Benedict Rumbold, Katharina Kieslich, and Albert Weale; *Journal of the Royal Society of Medicine*, 2015).

Tracy E. Roberts, PhD, is Professor of Health Economics and head of the Health Economics Unit at the University of Birmingham, UK. She has specific research interests in the area of economic evaluation and in particular of testing and screening programs, especially in the areas of sexual health, obstetrics, and gynecology, and has published widely. She has also developed interest in pursuing outcome valuation for use in economic evaluation in these clinical specialties. She leads two applied research themes within the unit: women's health and infection. She also works within the two main methodological themes of modeling and capabilities.

Harald Schmidt, PhD, is Assistant Professor at the Department of Medical Ethics and Health Policy and Research Associate at the Center for Health Incentives and Behavioral Economics, both at the University of Pennsylvania's Perelman School of Medicine. His work centers around fairness in resource allocation, public health ethics, and personal responsibility for health. Publications include "Public Health, Universal Health Coverage, and Sustainable Development Goals: Can They Coexist?" (with Lawrence Gostin and Ezekiel Emanuel; *Lancet*, 2015) and "Equity and Non-communicable Disease Reduction Under the Sustainable Development Goals" (with Anne Barnhill; *PloS Medicine*, 2015).

Liam Shields, PhD, is a lecturer in political theory at the University of Manchester. He has previously held research positions at the McCoy Family Center for Ethics, Stanford University and the Institute of Advanced Study, University of Warwick. His main areas of research interest are distributive justice, especially sufficientarianism, equality of opportunity, justice in education, and justice in childrearing. He has published in journals such as *Utilitas, Canadian Journal of Philosophy* and *Politics, Philosophy and Economics* and has a monograph forthcoming titled *Just Enough: Sufficiency as a Demand of Justice* (Edinburgh University Press, 2016).

David Wasserman, JD, MA (psychology) has been a visiting scholar at the Department of Bioethics at the US National Institutes of Health since January 2013. Previously, he was Director of Research at the Center for Ethics, Yeshiva University. He has written extensively on ethical and policy issues in disability, reproduction, genetics, health care, biotechnology, and neuroscience. He has coauthored *Disability, Difference, Discrimination* (with Anita Silvers and Mary Mahowald, 1998) and *Debating Procreation* (with David Benatar, 2015). He has co-edited *Genetics and Criminal Behavior* (2001); *Quality of Life and Human Difference: Genetic Testing, Health-Care, and Disability* (2005); and *Harming Future Persons: Ethics, Genetics, and the Nonidentity Problem* (2009). He has also coedited special journal issues on bioethics and risk and on the ethics of enhancement. He is on the editorial boards of *Ethics* and the *Journal of Applied Ethics,* and he is a fellow of the Center.

What Is Enough?

Introduction

Carina Fourie and Annette Rid

WHAT DO WE owe future generations in terms of their health? How much should we invest today in technologies to eradicate diseases in the future? An intuitively appealing claim is that we should invest enough that future generations have sufficient health. What about our obligations here and now? What do we owe our fellow citizens today in terms of health care? It seems prima facie reasonable to claim that everyone should be provided with "enough" health care for maintaining a good quality of life. These answers seem to point to the idea that sufficiency of health or health care could be an important aim of social justice and public policy.

The notion of sufficient health or health care can be contrasted, for example, to conceptions of justice that promote equal health, provide the worst off with the best possible health, or maximize the total health of the population. Helping individuals to achieve sufficient life spans seems to be an intuitively more appealing aim of health policy than, for instance, helping them achieve equal life spans. Also, although giving priority to the worst off may be a fair strategy below certain thresholds of health, its appeal might wane if the worst off are actually quite healthy—or what might be called "sufficiently" healthy.

Yet despite the intuitive attraction of the sufficiency view, what sufficiency is, why we need it, and how it applies to practical challenges—such as the distribution of health care and the social determinants of health—still require much analysis. This is true of the broad philosophical discussion as well as debates within applied fields. With regard to the ethics of distribution, for example, the conflict between favoring equality or giving priority to the worst off is usually the central focus. A handful of authors explicitly defend a sufficientarian approach to health or health care justice, although—on closer examination—a number of scholars, who one might not initially associate with sufficientarianism, seem to be committed to a notion of sufficiency. However, these latter scholars typically focus on specifying other aspects of their approach to health justice, such as how health and capabilities are linked or to what extent individuals should be made responsible for their health-related behaviors.

The paucity of scholarship on sufficiency is surprising. This is especially true for the bioethical literature, given that a common-sense notion of sufficiency might be seen as already shaping health policy and practice. Countries with universal access to health care are delineating "basic" health care packages that all health insurance plans are obliged to cover, as opposed to services that individuals may access by purchasing voluntary, additional insurance plans or by paying out of pocket. These basic packages aim to provide an adequate amount of health care or, alternatively, a set of services that seeks to achieve adequate health within the population. Arguably, a notion of sufficiency underlies—or should underlie—the delineation of these basic health care packages. One might also argue that some of the most commonly discussed criteria for rationing health services, such as minimal effectiveness or age, reflect sufficientarian intuitions. This suggests that sufficiency already plays an important, albeit implicit and undertheorized, role in health care policy and practice.

A skeptic may argue that the paucity of literature on sufficientarianism indicates that the approach is flawed. For example, some critics claim that sufficientarian approaches tend to be ambiguous with regard to where the sufficiency threshold should be set or, when they are not ambiguous, where they draw the line between "enough" and "insufficient" is arbitrary. However, it would be premature to abandon interest in sufficientarianism on the basis of the existing criticisms. To understand its potential merits and flaws, we need to further specify and develop sufficiency views and assess how they might be defended from objections, if at all. In the field of health and health care, we need to investigate whether or not a sufficientarian approach to health justice is plausible and what aiming for sufficiency in health might look like—or already looks like—in practice. This book aims precisely to address these questions. It is divided into four main parts: Part I: Groundwork; Part II: The Sufficiency View; Part III: Sufficiency, Health, and Health Care Justice; and Part IV: Implementing Sufficiency in Health Care Policy and Economics.

Part I: Groundwork

The first two chapters of the volume introduce the reader to sufficientarianism as a component of a general theory of distributive justice and, specifically, as applied to health and health care. In Chapter 1, Carina Fourie distinguishes the sufficiency view from other distributive views such as distributive egalitarianism and identifies the most significant components that a sufficiency view would need to specify, such as its justification and the weight it accords sufficiency. A number of influential criticisms of the sufficiency view are also highlighted in this chapter. In Chapter 2, Annette Rid provides an overview of the existing sufficientarian approaches to health or health care justice, as well as concepts or policies that seem to be committed to the idea of ensuring "enough" health—notably, the moral right to an "adequate" level of health services and so-called "two-tiered" health systems that provide basic services to everyone but allow the private purchase of additional, faster or higher quality services.

Part II: The Sufficiency View

Why adopt a sufficientarian approach? To understand the sufficiency view's appeal, we need to identify and assess the most convincing versions of sufficientarianism, evaluating how well they can be defended from criticism. The four chapters that comprise this section flesh out compelling views of sufficiency and indicate how they can counter influential objections.

In Chapter 3, Iwao Hirose argues that according to a plausible sufficientarian ethos, we should minimize the disvalue of well-being below the sufficiency threshold rather than maximizing the amount of people at or above the threshold. Hirose specifies an axiological formula based on this ethos, claiming that sufficientarianism of this sort will avoid many of the counterintuitive consequences associated with, for example, Harry Frankfurt's influential account of sufficientarianism. Hirose does note, however, that even this improved version of sufficientarianism will be subject to "the very sadistic conclusion." This conclusion counterintuitively insists that having a small population with awful lives, well below the sufficiency threshold, can be preferable to having a larger population with much greater well-being, although they are still under the threshold. As Hirose argues, however, alternative axiological principles—for example, prioritarian or utilitarian principles—also have some counterintuitive consequences, and thus this particular problem with the sufficiency view should not be a reason to abandon it.

Like Hirose, Robert Huseby aims to present a convincing version of sufficiency that can escape certain common objections in Chapter 4. Huseby's sufficientarianism identifies two thresholds: a minimal threshold of basic needs and a maximal threshold at which an individual is content, or as well off as possible, without threatening general sufficiency over time. Using this theory as a basis, Huseby investigates two objections to sufficientarianism. One of these objections is that a sufficiency approach will reject aggregation even when aggregation seems to be morally required. Aggregation allows benefits to some individuals to outweigh losses to others. This objection, Huseby argues, is incorrect. In order to achieve general sufficiency over time, sufficientarianism will be able to support aggregation where it is indeed necessary and reject it in cases in which it seems morally unacceptable. In this way, he argues, sufficientarianism is superior to prioritarianism, which is unable to rule out many forms of morally problematic aggregation.

Whereas Hirose and Huseby each defend a specific version of sufficientarianism, in Chapter 5 Liam Shields considers how various forms of sufficientarianism could be defended from criticism. He indicates how what is known as "upper-limit sufficientarianism" could counter the criticism that it is implausible to be indifferent to benefitting those above the threshold. In addition, he argues that maximizing the number of people who have enough ("headcount sufficientarianism") is not necessarily as implausible as is often claimed, even when this occurs at the expense of the least advantaged. Although Shields argues that it is possible to formulate defenses of these two forms of sufficientarianism, he endorses neither, arguing instead that certain pluralist forms of sufficientarianism appear especially promising but require further analysis. He highlights two kinds of pluralist views that have particular appeal—a combination of a sufficiency view and responsibility–sensitivity and a combination of a sufficiency view and an emphasis on self-ownership rights.

In Chapter 6, the last contribution to this section, David V. Axelsen and Lasse Nielsen are also concerned with identifying forms of sufficientarianism that are able to avoid widespread criticisms. Sufficiency views are often criticized for ambiguity, and when they are made less ambiguous, they are then frequently accused of arbitrariness. Axelsen and Nielsen argue that the problem is not with sufficiency per se but, rather, with particular sufficientarian theories that lack "thick" notions of sufficiency thresholds. A thick notion of sufficiency will specify when sufficiency has been attained and why attaining sufficiency is so morally urgent. An example of a thick account of sufficiency is one that relies on a notion of autonomy and that can be understood according to what it means to live a flourishing life. Not only will such an account escape the accusations of ambiguity and arbitrariness, Axelsen and Nielsen argue, but also it avoids the criticism that a sufficiency view is underdemanding. In addition, unlike a number of other sufficientarian approaches, such a thick account of sufficiency is able to condemn many forms of discrimination and unfair burdens and thus cannot be accused of being "morally blind" to these significant injustices.

Part III: Sufficiency, Health, and Health Care Justice

The chapters in this section investigate how the sufficiency view might apply to health care policies, as well as how best to understand the concept of health in relation to sufficiency. Justice between generations is Axel Gosseries' focus in Chapter 7. He provides a sketch of the kinds of problems associated with *intra-generational* justice—that is, justice between age groups. His primary concern, however, is with *intergenerational* justice—for example, justice between those alive today and those who will be alive in the the future. Gosseries identifies the unique features of sufficientarianism in comparison to other views, such as egalitarianism, in the context of intergenerational justice. For example, he argues that sufficientarianism will allow generational dis-savings as long as these do not lead to insufficiency in the basic needs of future generations. After specifying the distinctiveness of intergenerational sufficientarianism and assessing defenses thereof, he applies a sufficiency principle to three specific concerns of intergenerational health and health care justice: patent length for drugs and medical devices, disease eradication versus control, and antibiotic resistance.

Whereas Gosseries focuses on intergenerational justice, in Chapter 8 Efrat Ram-Tiktin argues that in determining the just distribution of health care benefits for people alive today, we should aim for sufficiency in each of the nine key systems of basic human functional capabilities (BHFCs). Only individuals below the BHFC thresholds have legitimate claims of justice to health care resources. According to Ram-Tiktin, the BHFCs do not represent the only sufficiency thresholds; a lower personhood threshold represents the point at which we can say that someone has the capabilities required for the essential features of a human life. When we decide for whom to prioritize health care resources, both thresholds should be taken into account. In addition, the size of a health care benefit and the amount of people who will be benefitted should play a role in how we prioritize health care benefits below the sufficiency thresholds.

Ram-Tiktin claims that the distribution of health care should be determined not by its effects on health per se but, rather, on the BHFCs, which she describes as a state of "intactness" rather than a state of health. How to define health and related notions, such as intactness or the absence of disease, is a central challenge in the bioethics literature. If a sufficientarian approach claims that we require "enough" health, it faces the additional challenge of having to specify what makes someone healthy enough for the purposes of justice. In Chapter 9, Sean Aas and David Wasserman address this latter challenge by developing a narrow conception of health for the purposes of health justice, which makes the task of deciding how much health is "enough" a less daunting one precisely because it is so narrow. Using disability as a starting point, they claim that it is important to distinguish between disadvantages that are due primarily to social causes and those that are due to biological functioning. They argue that most conceptions of health in the bioethical literature, whether biostatistical or goal-oriented accounts, are unable to recognize this distinction. As an alternative account, the authors argue that being more or less healthy means being more or less free from "disease processes" that cause or threaten to cause certain harms, notably premature death, pain, or life-disrupting loss of function.

In Chapter 10, Carina Fourie, similar to Ram-Tiktin, presents a sufficientarian capabilities approach applied to health care justice. However, unlike Ram-Tiktin, who is focused on the capabilities usually directly associated with health care justice, Fourie examines how a general theory of justice—one that includes all the central capabilities—should be taken into account in determining health care policy. Fourie argues that a sufficiency of capabilities approach seems to justify certain forms of two-tiered health care systems—that is, systems in which some are able to buy health care services or benefits that others cannot. Such systems, she claims, are vulnerable to criticism from social–relational egalitarians. She shows, however, that specifying a capabilities approach and its sufficientarianism in certain ways can help to accommodate social egalitarianism. If, for example, we recognize that the distribution of health care resources should not violate the capability of affiliation, a capability not traditionally associated with health or health care, then we may be able to rule out socially inegalitarian forms of two-tiered health care systems.

While Fourie and Ram-Tiktin advocate a sufficientarian approach, Paul T. Menzel and Leonard M. Fleck take a more critical stance. In Chapter 11, Menzel discusses whether sufficientarian theories of the right to a decent minimum of health care are better able to specify this right than other theories. Menzel compares his own "patchwork" approach to specifying the right to a decent minimum of care—which is rooted, among others, in the principle of opportunity for welfare—with the sufficiency of well-being approach developed by Madison Powers and Ruth Faden. He uses age-related health care prioritization as a test case for evaluating the two approaches. He concludes that Powers and Faden's sufficientarian approach is no better at delineating the content of the right to a decent minimum of care than plausible non-sufficientarian alternatives such as his own approach, and indeed, his approach may be superior.

Fleck puts sufficientarian approaches to health or health care justice to a "practice test." In Chapter 12, he examines to what extent a range of potential and existing sufficientarian approaches help to address concrete problems in health care rationing. For example, Fleck explores whether patients with a serious life-threatening cardiac condition have a just claim to an artificial heart or other costly forms of cardiac surgery according to Powers and Faden's sufficiency of well-being approach, even when they have serious underlying conditions. He argues that their approach, as well as other sufficientarian approaches, is unable to yield clear and unambiguous moral guidance regarding similarly contentious problems of health care justice. Fleck grants, however, that other principled conceptions of health care justice—whether egalitarian, prioritarian, or something else—do not fare better. He concludes that processes of rational democratic deliberation are necessary to identify what citizens in a just and caring society judge to be a just enough policy.

Part IV: Implementing Sufficiency in Health Care Policy and Economics

Many aspects of current health policy and practice give the impression, at first glance, that they rest on sufficientarian foundations. For example, two-tiered health care systems could be viewed as embodying the idea that the key goal of health care justice is to ensure "enough" health or health care for everyone. However, as highlighted by Annette Rid in Chapter 2, no one to our knowledge has explicitly examined to what extent current practice is based on notions of sufficiency.

The first two chapters in this part of the book begin to close this gap in the literature by analyzing policies around essential health care benefit packages from a sufficientarian perspective. In Chapter 13, Dimitra Panteli and Ewout van Ginneken review how essential benefit baskets are defined in nine high-income countries. They examine the regulations that underpin coverage decisions in these countries and find that most of them invoke ordinary language notions of sufficiency, for example, by requiring the coverage of "adequate," "basic," or "essential" health services. The authors then develop a methodology for analyzing to what extent essential benefit baskets are consistent with a sufficientarian approach. They do so by examining the breadth, depth, and height of coverage—or who is covered, what is covered, and whether patients have to pay out of pocket for health services. In practice, they show that sufficiency of health or health care can be compromised in any or all of these three dimensions of coverage. For example, Panteli and van Ginneken find that some countries likely have a sufficient depth of coverage but risk falling short in breadth or height by excluding certain groups from access to care (e.g., undocumented migrants) or by requiring high copayments for certain services.

In Chapter 14, Govind Persad and Harald Schmidt investigate the relationship between depth and height of health care coverage in more detail using the recent health reforms in the United States as a case study. Persad and Schmidt examine what level of costs individuals can justifiably be asked to bear in order to access health care services. They argue that the costs of these services should not be so high as to threaten excluding individuals from participating in society—meaning that these costs should not undermine their ability to cover a decent minimum of food, clothing, housing, transportation, and so on. The authors show that the recent health care reforms in the United States allow citizens to control their health expenditures only by choosing different cost-sharing arrangements for a fixed basket of health services—for example, by choosing insurance that covers 60% or 90% of the benefit basket—but not by choosing baskets that include more or fewer services. This arrangement, Persad and Schmidt argue, encourages citizens to purchase health care insurance with cost-sharing arrangements that they cannot afford in case of illness, leading to insufficient access to otherwise sufficient care.

Chapter 15 offers a perspective on how notions of sufficiency might guide health policy and practice in the future. Paul Mark Mitchell, Tracy E. Roberts, Pelham M. Barton, and Joanna Coast discuss how the debate about the economic evaluation of health has evolved over time and how a new approach to health evaluation based on people's capabilities has emerged in recent years. This approach is based on the work of Amartya Sen and Martha Nussbaum and, inspired by their work, aims for sufficiency of capabilities rather than maximizing quality-adjusted life-years (QALYs), which is the traditional approach to health economic evaluation. Mitchell and colleagues show that measures for "years of sufficient capability" can make a real difference in how resources for health services are allocated compared to the traditional maximization of QALYs. Their chapter illustrates, among other things, how the philosophical discussion of the capability approach and health justice—which is further developed by Ram-Tiktin and Fourie in this volume—has significant potential to influence health policy and practice.

This volume covers much ground in terms of both the general philosophical debate about the significance of sufficiency and the application of sufficiency to health and health care. However, like any scholarly work, it has some gaps. For example, sufficiency as part of a theory of global justice or global health justice, although undoubtedly significant, is not a central theme in the volume. Similarly, how sufficiency might be able to address concerns about the social determinants of health is not specifically examined and requires further analysis. The book nonetheless offers a wide range of new, original, and in-depth investigations that advance our understanding of the sufficiency view, both philosophically and in terms of its bioethical implications. Sufficientarianism, we as editors came away thinking, has considerable potential as a principle of distributive justice in theory and in practice.

PART I

Groundwork

1

The Sufficiency View

A PRIMER

Carina Fourie

HOW SHOULD WE judge the justice of social, political, and economic institutions and their policies? One way to answer this question is to examine the implication of policies on the amount, or comparable amount, of the spread of benefits and burdens among individuals. Policies could be considered to be just, at least partially, if they result in the "correct amount" (known as the pattern of distribution) of the "correct form" of benefits and burdens (known as the currency of distribution).[1] Thus, a policy could be judged as just or pro tanto just if, for example, it leads to equality of income or a sufficient level of health. Theories of equality are fairly well represented in the political philosophy literature; sufficiency views, in contrast, are relatively underexplored.

As a preliminary description, we can say that according to a sufficiency view (or sufficientarianism) justice requires that individuals achieve a threshold level of primary social goods (or whatever the currency of justice should be).[2] The intuitive appeal of sufficientarianism rests, at least partially, on two common-sense claims.

---

1. Not everyone agrees that justice requires a specific distributive pattern. For example, you may believe that we require only a certain set of procedures to achieve justice. See, for example, Elizabeth Anderson's discussion of procedural rules and distributive patterns; "Justifying the Capabilities Approach to Justice," in *Measuring Justice Primary Goods and Capabilities*, ed. Harry Brighouse and Ingrid Robeyns (New York: Cambridge University Press, 2010), 81–82.

2. Alternatively, for example, a sufficiency view could be seen as an axiological view that does not claim that we require sufficiency for justice but, rather, because it is a better state of affairs (Shlomi Segall, "What Is the Point of Sufficiency?" *Journal of Applied Philosophy*, 2014, Early View). However, for the purposes of this primer, we refer to the sufficiency view as a requirement of justice, at least partially because this is how it is considered in most chapters

The first, inspired by the concern that so very many people lead lives of deprivation, ill-health, and stigma, is that we have obligations to ensure that everyone can
lead a decent life. The second is the claim that once people do live decent lives, our
moral obligations to provide them with further benefits are diminished. In order
to determine whether sufficientarianism can remain appealing beyond merely
these common-sense claims, it needs in-depth scrutiny.

This primer serves to provide background on sufficientarianism and estab-
lishes the context for the chapters of this volume. It presents an overview of
distinctions between sufficiency and other distributive views (Section 1), six significant aspects of a sufficiency theory (Section 2), and a selection of influential
criticisms of sufficiency views (Section 3).[3]

1. Distinguishing the Sufficiency View: The Basics

Among the many strands of debate that the publication of John Rawls' *A Theory of
Justice* motivated was an intense focus on the nature and value of equality. Rawls'
principles of justice demand equality in liberties and fair opportunities. They also
require that the worst off should be in the best possible position with regard to
the remaining distribution of the primary social goods, once the social bases for
liberties and opportunities have been distributed equally.[4] The theory thus encompasses an element that is not strictly egalitarian and, as will become clear from the
following discussion, includes a form of the priority view. Underlying the Rawlsian
principles, it has been argued, is a fundamental commitment to equal respect or
social–relational equality or both.[5] Central contemporary debates in social justice,
in no small measure spurred on by Rawls' theory, include assessments of what
the currency of justice should be—Rawls claims that this should be the primary
social goods—as well as whether equality per se has value and, if so, which kinds
of equality have value.

---

in this volume. A notable exception is Iwao Hirose's chapter in this volume (Chapter 3),
which deals explicitly with axiological sufficientarianism.

3. I do not provide a comprehensive summary of sufficientarian views and criticisms against
them. For an excellent list of sufficientarian literature, see Liam Shields' bibliography at his
website, http://liamshields.com/teaching-and-study-materials.

4. John Rawls, *A Theory of Justice*, rev. ed. (New York: Oxford University Press, 1999), IV–V,
171–292, especially V–47, p. 266.

5. R. M. Dworkin, "The Original Position," in *Reading Rawls: Critical Studies on Rawls'
A Theory of Justice*, ed. Norman Daniels (Stanford, CA: Stanford University Press, 1989), 16–
53; Elizabeth Anderson, "What Is the Point of Equality?" *Ethics* 109, no. 2 (1999): 287–337.

When we refer to a sufficiency view as a claim about the pattern of justice, it is usually understood as part of this debate on the value of equal distribution. A sufficiency view is most often seen to be an *alternative* to a distributive equality view. Harry Frankfurt is one of the first contemporary philosophers to have attempted to articulate a sufficiency principle explicitly as an alternative to distributive equality, and during the last two decades, a number of rival understandings of sufficiency have been further developed.[6] One of the best starting points for understanding sufficiency views is to examine how they can be distinguished from alternative views about the pattern of justice. In the remainder of this section, I provide a sketch of how four influential views—utility, equality, priority, and sufficiency views—might compare the justice of two policies.

Consider the graph shown in Figure 1.1, representing the outcomes of two health care policies on two population groups of the same size. The *y*-axis indicates the outcome of these policies on health, measured here numerically and ranging from 0 to 100, with 0 being "dead" and 100 being "in perfect health." If policy 1 is implemented, the individuals in group A will reach 80, thus health that is relatively high on the scale, whereas group B will have 20, thus health that is relatively low on the scale. The outcome of policy 2 is that the health in each group is equal—at the level of 50. Imagine that there are no (arguably) relevant differences between these population groups that might influence how we would view the justice of the outcome of each policy. For example, members of one group are no more reckless in terms of looking after their health than are members of the other group). What would views about the pattern of justice have to say about these distributions?[7]

According to a *utility view or utilitarianism*, which judges the justice of distribution according to whether the currency of justice is maximized (here it is health), there is no principled ethical difference between policies 1 and 2 because the total level of health in society remains the same, whichever policy is implemented—that is, it is 100.

---

6. Harry Frankfurt, "Equality as a Moral Ideal," *Ethics* 98, no. 1 (1987): 21–43; Harry Frankfurt, "Equality and Respect," *Social Research* 64, no. 1 (1997): 3–15; Roger Crisp, "Equality, Priority, and Compassion," *Ethics* 113, no. 4 (2003): 745–763; Yitzhak Benbaji, "The Doctrine of Sufficiency: A Defence," *Utilitas* 17, no. 3 (2005): 310–332; Paula Casal, "Why Sufficiency Is Not Enough," *Ethics* 117, no. 2 (2007): 296–326; Robert Huseby, "Sufficiency: Restated and Defended," *Journal of Political Philosophy* 18, no. 2 (June 1, 2010): 178–197; Liam Shields, "The Prospects for Sufficientarianism," *Utilitas* 24, no. 1 (2012): 101–117; David V. Axelsen and Lasse Nielsen, "Sufficiency as Freedom from Duress," *Journal of Political Philosophy* (2014): Early View.

7. Crisp's explanation, in "Equality, Priority, and Compassion," of the different patterns has been particularly beneficial for helping me to formulate the discussion here.

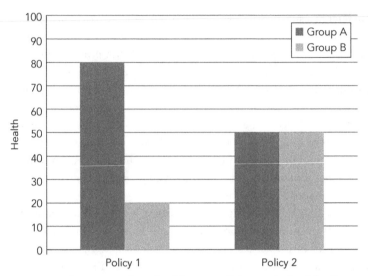

FIGURE I.I Outcomes of two health care policies on the health of two groups.

Many people claim that, intuitively at least, the utilitarian view does not seem correct. Policy 2 is in some way better than policy 1. Advocates of a *distributive equality view* would claim that the distribution following the implementation of policy 2 is indeed morally preferable to that of policy 1 because it is equal.[8] Even advocates of utilitarianism may claim to prefer policy 2 to policy 1, simply as a tie-breaker. However, distributive egalitarians will insist that we have reason to value an equal distribution even if the total level of health was less than we could achieve through an alternative policy, which would lead to greater total health but would be distributed unequally between groups. Advocates of the utilitarian view would reject the idea that there is value to such an equal distribution.

Those who advocate a *priority view* would agree that policy 2 is preferable; however, they would claim that egalitarians have not identified the fundamental reason for this. The fact that policy 2 is egalitarian is not in itself what makes it preferable. It is preferable, rather, because the worst off have the best possible health; their health is only at level 20 under policy 1, whereas it is at level 50 under policy 2. Imagine policy 2a. This policy actually leads to greater inequality than policy 1, but the worst off are still better off under policy 2a than they are under policy 1. Then policy 2a would be preferable despite the greater inequality it caused.

8. I refer to views that advocate an actual equal distribution as *distributive* egalitarianism. Egalitarianism without the qualifier refers to a broader category of views, which may include distributive egalitarianism but could also include other kinds, such as social-relational egalitarianism.

Under this understanding of the priority view, principles that are most often known as "prioritarian" are one *version* of the priority view but do not encapsulate this view. Indeed, certain versions of prioritarianism can be understood not simply as a kind of priority view but as a hybrid priority–utility view, which combines a concern with the position of the worst off with a concern for maximizing the currency of justice.[9,10]

What would a *sufficiency view* stipulate? On the basis of the current information, it would be unable to judge the justice of these distributions. This is because we cannot assess the justice of an outcome without knowing where the *threshold* for sufficiency lies. If, for example, it lay at 90, neither policy would be just. If it lay at 20, both distributions would be just, or at least minimally just. However, both 90 and 20 seem unlikely as indications of a sufficiency threshold: If 100 represents perfect health and 0 represents death, then thresholds of 90 and 20, which are close to these extremes, seem prima facie too high and too low, respectively.

Let us assume that 50 is the sufficient threshold for health. Then sufficientarians would argue that policy 2 is preferable but it is not because of the equality in outcome or because of the position of the worst off that it is so; rather, it is preferable because everyone has reached a sufficient threshold of health.

Having provided a rough guide to distinctions between these views, three more general remarks need to be made to help clarify them further; these concern comparativeness, non-instrumentality, and pluralism. The equality view is necessarily comparative—whether or not justice has been achieved is fundamentally concerned with whether some have more or less than others. For most versions of the utility, priority, and sufficiency views, justice has to do with absolute (meaning noncomparative) levels of the currency of justice. For example, for a sufficiency view, we do not determine the justice of a policy by considering how it will affect those below the sufficiency threshold in comparison to those above the threshold; we need merely understand how the policy will affect sufficiency in the currency of justice. Similarly, for a priority principle, we merely need to know

---

9. For example, Richard Arneson, "Distributive Justice and Basic Capability Equality," in *Capabilities Equality: Basic Issues and Problems*, ed. Alexander Kaufman (New York: Routledge, 2006), 27.

10. Sufficiency views are often directly contrasted to prioritarianism rather than the more general priority view described here as a single end committed to achieving the best position for the worst off. For the purposes of this discussion, it is useful to use this latter understanding of the priority view. First, it helps provide a clear distinction between the utilitarian and the priority views. Second, it will include under a priority view a number of views that have no commitment to the total maximization of distributive currency required by utilitarianism (e.g., maximin or leximin). Last, the priority view structurally resembles the other views described here.

which policy leads to the best possible position for the worst off no matter how well off the better off are.

Second, consider that in these descriptions, we are concerned with the *ultimate* pattern and currency of distribution. In the previous example, we considered health as the ultimate goal of distribution. The allocation of health care benefits or other determinants of health could be described as needing to be equal or sufficient, without this meaning that the view we hold is an equality view or a sufficiency view, respectively, if this pattern of allocation is not the ultimate aim of the allocation of goods. If, as a matter of justice, what we require is that individuals within society have *sufficient health*, then the way in which health-related goods are allocated is instrumental to achieving this ultimate, underlying pattern of distribution. The upshot of this is that one can recommend an egalitarian allocation of goods—for example, equal access to health care—without being committed to the equality view, as understood here, if the aim of such equal access is (merely) instrumental to achieving some form of sufficiency.

Assessments about instrumentality and non-instrumentality can quickly become complicated, so two qualifications are highlighted here. First, analyzing and assessing *instrumental* versions of sufficiency principles can still be significant, and although the rest of this chapter considers only non-instrumental versions, much of the discussion about how to specify sufficiency principles could apply to instrumental versions.[11] Second, it is not necessarily obvious whether a sufficiency principle is non-instrumental or not. I take it that a sufficiency principle is non-instrumental if it is *not a means to another distributive pattern principle*, although it may be constitutive of something else (e.g., justice or a life of dignity).

Last, for this section, as I have mainly described them here, the views are commitments to single ends, but they could be combined to form pluralist or hybrid views. I have already indicated that the view most commonly referred to as prioritarianism could be understood as a pluralist view. In Section 2.2, we examine pluralist sufficiency views in more detail.

2. Specifying a Sufficiency Principle

As a starting point, I described the sufficiency view as a theory that stipulates that individuals should achieve a threshold level of the currency of justice.[12] A more

---

11. See also Shields on non-instrumental reasons for sufficiency: "The Prospects for Sufficientarianism," 112–113.

12. That is, as much as this is socially possible to achieve. Some may not be able to reach the threshold. In Sections 2.4 and 3, I consider some concerns that this might raise.

comprehensive account of sufficiency would have to specify at least six significant elements, which I discuss in this section:

1. The currency of sufficiency
2. The positive and positioning claims
3. Justifications for sufficiency principles
4. Weighting rules
5. Setting sufficiency thresholds
6. The scope of sufficiency[13]

Factors such as currency and scope would be important for other distributive pattern views to specify and justify as well.[14] However, a sufficiency view will have some unique challenges, such as setting sufficiency thresholds.

2.1. The Currency of Sufficiency

A sufficiency principle must specify "sufficiency of what?," or in other words what is the currency of justice. Sufficiency of needs, welfare, or capabilities (or even a combination of these) are three popular currencies of sufficientarian theories.[15] A fuller theory of justice should specify and justify the currency and its pattern; however, in this primer, I focus almost exclusively on the *pattern* of sufficiency. It is worth raising the question, without the scope to explore an answer here, whether the pattern of sufficiency is more plausible when combined with certain currencies of justice rather than with others.[16]

---

13. The order in which I discuss these factors is useful for explanatory purposes but is not an indication of their primacy. Ultimately, the justification of the view would be one of its most significant features.

14. There are additional factors that are important for distributive views to specify, although I do not consider them in any detail here. For example, they should all address the issue of time—Are we concerned about inequality over a complete lifetime or within a particular slice of time (Dennis McKerlie, "Equality and Time," *Ethics* 99, no. 3 (1989): 475–491)?

15. For example, see Gillian Brock on needs, Crisp on welfare, and Anderson on capabilities (Gillian Brock, "Sufficiency and Needs-Based Approaches to Distributive Justice," in *Oxford Handbook of Distributive Justice*, ed. Serena Olsaretti (New York: Oxford University Press, forthcoming); Crisp, "Equality, Priority, and Compassion"; Anderson, "Justifying the Capabilities Approach to Justice").

16. Although this edited volume tends to focus on sufficiency, a number of chapters discuss aspects related to the currency of justice. Consider, for example, Huseby's discussion of subjective welfare, Axelsen and Nielsen on autonomy and capabilities, and Efrat Ram-Tiktin, Carina Fourie, and Paul Mark Mitchell et al. on capabilities (Chapters 4, 6, 8, 10 and 15, respectively).

2.2. The Positive and Positioning Claims

It has become common to describe sufficiency views as having two primary parts, a positive and a negative thesis.[17] Claiming that a sufficiency view requires a "negative thesis," as the name implies, means that in order to be sufficientarian, one must deny other distributive views. Because this fails to take into account that a sufficiency view may also affirm (certain) other views, I suggest instead that sufficiency views have a positive and a positioning claim.

The positive claim commits the sufficientarian to the moral significance of a non-instrumental sufficiency threshold, encapsulating the idea that it is a priority for individuals to reach or not to fall under such a threshold.[18] Summaries of positive claims, or aspects of positive claims, could be as follows: (1) We should maximize the number of people who are at the sufficiency threshold or (2) benefitting those below the threshold should have weighted priority in comparison to those above the threshold.

The positioning claim "positions" the sufficiency view in relation to other views. This includes a negative thesis that specifies which other kinds of views are rejected. However, it need not consist of a negative thesis alone. In positioning the view, it will indicate whether or not it *affirms* certain other views. A monist view, for example, will be committed to the claim that our *only* aim is to benefit those who fall under the sufficiency threshold, or those who are in danger of falling under the threshold,[19] and thus such a sufficiency view only has a negative thesis. In contrast, sufficiency views could be hybrid or pluralist instead, which means that they affirm certain other views.

There are two kinds of significant pluralist forms that the positioning claim could specify.[20] The first indicates pluralism in distributive views—in other words, a pluralism in distributive patterns. This is what I call pattern pluralism. It indicates that there is more than one kind of distributive pattern that has non-instrumental value; other distributive patterns are not merely instrumental to achieving sufficiency in this case but can have non-instrumental value themselves. Thus, for example, a sufficiency view may require maximizing the currency of justice above

---

17. Benbaji, "The Doctrine of Sufficiency," 311; Paula Casal, "Why Sufficiency Is Not Enough," 297–304.

18. I use the singular throughout for ease of description, although there may be more than one sufficiency threshold. See Sections 2.3 and 2.4.

19. Sufficiency views care about those below the threshold as well as those in danger of falling below it. In what follows, for short, I refer only to "those below the threshold" but take that to include considerations of those who are above it but in danger of falling below it.

20. See also Fourie's discussion of pluralism in Chapter 10.

the threshold, making it a sufficiency–utility hybrid.[21] How much weight to give to the sufficiency threshold in relation to maximizing goals above the threshold would need to be determined (weighting rules are discussed in Section 2.4).

Sufficiency views, whether they affirm or deny pattern pluralism, could also be pluralist in at least one other sense. These accept other values or goals of justice besides sufficiency (or other distributive patterns)—this is what I call external pluralism. External here merely indicates that this kind of view of justice requires something other than a particular distributive pattern. Frankfurt, for example, rejects the idea that we should care about patterns of distribution besides sufficientarian ones, and thus he rejects pattern pluralism. He insists, however, that we also need a principle of respect to evaluate the ethics of policies and not only a sufficientarian principle of distribution.[22] Thus, we could say that he is an external pluralist. A principle of respect need not, however, be external to a sufficientarian pattern; it is merely so in Frankfurt's description. Indeed, "sufficiency of respect" may well be an aim of a sufficiency view.[23]

One could be both a pattern pluralist and an external pluralist. The two are not mutually exclusive; however, one need not be both and could advocate pattern pluralism without external pluralism, and vice versa.[24]

The sufficiency view is often associated with a vehement denial of the moral significance of equality. Although this often depends on which kind of equality we are talking about—for example, it is most likely the significance of *distributive egalitarianism* that sufficientarians will deny—a number of prominent sufficientarians deny the plausibility of any form of (non-instrumentally valuable) egalitarianism.[25] There is no need to deny that equality has value if one is a sufficientarian

21. An example of such a view is Ram-Tiktin's, "The Right to Health Care as a Right to Basic Human Functional Capabilities," *Ethical Theory and Moral Practice* 15, no. 3 June 1, 2012): 337–351. See also Ram-Tiktin's chapter in this volume (Chapter 8).

22. Harry Frankfurt, "Equality and Respect."

23. Madison Powers and Ruth Faden, *Social Justice: The Moral Foundations of Public Health and Health Policy* (New York: Oxford University Press, 2006), 22–24.

24. A number of chapters in this volume assess pluralism and embrace or reject various forms of it. See, for example, Hirose, Huseby, and Axelsen and Nielsen's rejection of pattern pluralism (Chapters 3, 4 and 6). Huseby, however, affirms external pluralism, whereas Axelsen and Nielsen affirm a different kind of pluralism to the ones discussed here—pluralism in the currency of justice. A primary purpose of Shields' chapter (Chapter 5) is to indicate that there are a number of promising forms of pluralism that a hybrid sufficiency view could take and that need to be explored further.

25. For example, J. R. Lucas, "Against Equality," *Philosophy* 40, no. 154 (1965): 296–307, and Frankfurt, "Equality as a Moral Ideal"; Frankfurt, "Equality and Respect"; Benbaji, "The Doctrine of Sufficiency."

(or vice versa), however, and, as indicated in the next section, some sufficiency principles are rooted in notions of equality.[26]

It is popular to claim that sufficientarianism should be defined by both a positive thesis and a negative thesis.[27] However, in keeping with the emphasis placed on understanding these views as commitments to single ends, which could be combined with other principles into pluralist views, I consider the positive claim to be enough for claiming that a view is sufficientarian. This is also in keeping with how other distributive principles are often described; for example, all that need be true of distributive egalitarianism is that it is committed to seeing value in a pattern of distributive equality (not that it necessarily also denies other pattern views). In other words, what makes a view sufficientarian requires only a commitment to the non-instrumental moral significance of a sufficiency threshold, which is a priority for individuals to reach or under which they should not fall. A theory of justice could then be called a sufficiency view if it has such a positive claim. However, if it is not monist, we would need to add whichever further values it embraces to describe it accurately—for example, we could describe it as a sufficiency–equality view.

2.3. Justifications for Sufficiency Principles

Why would one adopt a sufficiency principle? The justifications that are often provided can be divided into two categories: negative reasons, which emphasize problems with other distributive views, and positive reasons, which specify why sufficiency itself is significant.

Negative reasons for supporting sufficiency often consist of pointing to implausible implications of other views. This will often justify the negative thesis of the positioning claim. The priority view, for example, has often been questioned for its commitment to the claim that we should care about benefitting the rich because they are not as well off as they could be (the existence of the super-rich shows us that the rich could be even better off).[28] In addition, a number of

---

26. In this volume, Fourie considers how sufficientarianism and social–relational egalitarianism may or may not be compatible. For more on the relationship between equality and sufficiency, see also Gillian Brock, "Sufficiency and Needs-Based Approaches to Distributive Justice"; Liam Shields, "Egalitarianism and Sufficientarianism: A Difficult Relationship," unpublished paper, n.d.

27. Casal, "Why Sufficiency Is Not Enough"; Axelsen and Nielsen, "Sufficiency as Freedom from Duress." Liam Shields, in contrast, argues that it is the combination of the positive thesis and a *shift* thesis that makes a sufficiency view distinctive (Shields, "The Prospects for Sufficientarianism," 108). See also Shields' chapter in this volume (Chapter 5).

28. Crisp, "Equality, Priority, and Compassion," 754–755.

sufficientarians endorse the leveling down objection (LDO) against distributive egalitarianism. The LDO denies what these egalitarians should affirm: that there is value to making the advantaged as badly off as the disadvantaged, without the disadvantaged being made better off.[29]

Negative reasons alone cannot provide support for a sufficiency principle. Indeed, a danger of focusing on the "implausible" implications of other views is that sufficiency views (indeed any distributive view) will also have some counterintuitive consequences. Furthermore, and more important, we cannot justify a sufficiency principle without justifying the moral significance of the sufficiency threshold itself. Positive reasons that have been offered for supporting the sufficiency view include the following:

- Sufficiency of basic needs or in basic social goods is required to ensure that no one suffers severe deprivation.[30]
- Sufficiency of welfare would be recommended by an impartial compassionate spectator.[31]
- Sufficiency of capabilities is required so that citizens are able to function as democratic equals.[32]
- Sufficiency of capabilities is required for living a life of human dignity.[33]

The sufficiency view seems least controversial, and often garners widespread agreement, when it claims that everyone should have their basic needs covered, or something similar, such that they should not suffer deprivation.[34] However, this tends to indicate a low sufficiency threshold, and it could seem particularly implausible to claim that this is all that justice requires. If this form of sufficiency is promoted, it is likely to be pluralist; what would then need to be determined

---

29. Crisp, "Equality, Priority, and Compassion"; Huseby, "Sufficiency," 186.

30. Casal, "Why Sufficiency Is Not Enough," 304–305; Shields, "The Prospects for Sufficientarianism," 115.

31. Crisp, "Equality, Priority, and Compassion."

32. Elizabeth Anderson, "What Is the Point of Equality?"; Anderson, "Justifying the Capabilities Approach to Justice."

33. Martha Nussbaum, *Women and Human Development: The Capabilities Approach* (New York: Cambridge University Press, 2000).

34. See Casal, "Why Sufficiency Is Not Enough" and Shlomi Segall, *Health, Luck, and Justice* (Princeton, NJ: Princeton University Press, 2010) for examples of views that are critical of high thresholds of sufficientarianism, and of monist sufficiency views, but accept that something like sufficiency of basic needs could be plausible or even required, as part of a pluralist view of distribution.

is what other values such a theory also encompasses and how to weigh those values against each other. This aspect of a sufficiency view—its significance and its weighting rules—is discussed in the next section.

An alternative, however, is that the sufficientarianism we should embrace, whether monist or pluralist, is actually of a different kind—sufficiency of capabilities or welfare—which is often likely to imply a higher threshold than sufficiency of basic needs. A further possibility is that there is more than one sufficiency threshold. It could be claimed, for example, that it is most morally urgent for a lower threshold to be achieved, such as a threshold of basic needs, whereas above this threshold there will be a second and higher threshold, for example, of welfare or capabilities.[35]

2.4. Weighting Rules

Sufficiency views must claim that achieving sufficiency is morally significant, but they need not claim that it is the most significant goal.[36] A complete sufficiency view would need to determine the moral significance of sufficiency (this would be true also, for example, of distributive egalitarian views, which would need to establish the significance of equality). Whether a view is monist or pluralist will set parameters for the significance of achieving sufficiency. For a monist view, for example, sufficiency is the only goal of moral significance, whereas pluralist views must establish the weight of achieving sufficiency in comparison to the other moral demands that it recognizes.

The significance of sufficiency will help to determine what can be called "weighting rules."[37] For an external pluralist view, the significance of achieving a pattern of sufficiency may need to be weighed against values other than distributive patterns, such as procedural justice or social–relational equality. For a pattern pluralist view, it would be particularly important to determine how much weight we should give to benefitting those below the threshold compared to those who are above the threshold. In this case, sufficientarian theories could be committed to *absolute* (or *lexical*) *weighting*, which means we should first help everyone to achieve sufficiency, or to get as close to it as possible, before we start benefitting

---

35. See Huseby's chapter (Chapter 4) for the view that there are two sufficiency thresholds—of basic needs and of welfare—and Ram-Tiktin's chapter (Chapter 8), in which she identifies a personhood threshold and a basic functionings threshold. For more on multiple thresholds, see also Benbaji, "The Doctrine of Sufficiency"; Huseby, "Sufficiency."

36. Also see, for example, Liam Shields, "The Prospects for Sufficientarianism," 105–106.

37. These are often called "priority" rules because they help to establish how much priority one moral value or principle has over another. Priority rules have nothing directly to do with the priority view, and in order not to cause confusion, I refer rather to weighting rules.

those above it. In contrast, they could be committed to *qualified weighting*. These sufficientarians claim that although ensuring that people are at a sufficient level of advantage is morally more urgent than providing benefits to those above that threshold, at times, benefitting those above the threshold could outweigh benefitting those below it (e.g., depending on how large the benefits are and how many people will be benefitted).

Rules also need to be established to determine how we weigh benefits for those below the threshold. A sufficiency view is likely to be suspect if it insisted only on the moral significance of individuals *reaching* the threshold. If it did so, this would imply that benefits for those who are below the threshold and cannot reach it should be sacrificed to provide for those who are actually better off and able to reach the threshold.[38] Rules under the threshold could include taking into account how many people would benefit, how far below the threshold they are, as well as how much they would gain from being benefitted.[39]

Another kind of weighting rule that a sufficiency view might need to specify is how to weigh different sufficiency thresholds. Multiple sufficiency thresholds can be described as vertical or horizontal.[40] Vertical thresholds indicate higher and lower points on a continuum. For example, Benbaji claims that there could be a number of thresholds, or priority lines (e.g. luxury, pain, and personhood), that help to indicate who requires preference when we have benefits to distribute.[41] Thresholds could also be horizontal, meaning that there are distinct and independent sufficiency thresholds; Powers and Faden, for example, claim that there are six dimensions of well-being, and sufficiency in each of these dimensions has moral significance.[42] In cases of multiple thresholds, we are likely to need weighting rules to help establish, for example, if a policy that promotes sufficiency of health but that threatens sufficiency of respect could justifiably be adopted.

---

38. For more on this, consider, for example, the "excessive upward transfers objection" (Shields, "The Prospects for Sufficientarianism," 103). See also Shields' chapter in this volume (Chapter 5): Sometimes we do indeed think that benefitting the better off is morally required, for example, as part of triage after a natural disaster.

39. Consider, for example, Benbaji's description and criticism of this as part of what he refers to as absolute sufficientarianism; "Sufficiency or Priority?" *European Journal of Philosophy* 14, no. 3 (2006): 327–344, at 331–344. For a view that combines sufficiency with the priority view below and above the threshold, see Campbell Brown, "Priority or Sufficiency ... or Both?" *Economics and Philosophy* 21, no. 2 (2005): 199–220.

40. David V. Axelsen and Lasse Nielsen, "Sufficiency as Freedom from Duress," 8–9.

41. Benbaji, "Sufficiency or Priority?" 338–344. See also Benbaji, "The Doctrine of Sufficiency," 320–321.

42. Powers and Faden, *Social Justice*.

2.5. Setting Sufficiency Thresholds

Imagine we agree that health care policies should be prioritized for those under a certain threshold of life-years. Furthermore, we agree with Crisp that sufficiency is justified according to the compassion of a neutral spectator—where that spectator's compassion is likely to run out is where the threshold should be. Should we then agree with Crisp that "eighty years of high-quality life on this planet is enough"?[43] This latter claim, and more generally, where sufficiency thresholds should be set, may cause substantial disagreement.

Where to set sufficiency thresholds poses the methodological question of how thresholds should be set. A number of sufficientarians are wary of the idea that philosophers, in isolation, should be setting thresholds.[44] They claim that we require deliberative consultation with policymakers, scientists, and the public, among others, to interpret what it means to live a life of dignity or a minimally decent life. This consultation is also necessary to highlight relevant facts against which thresholds should be set, such as how technologically advanced a society might be.

If indeed particular facts about a society help to establish where a threshold should lie, this means that thresholds are relative to context rather than being rigid. Taking the example of life-years again, although sufficiency of life might be an important universal ideal, where the threshold for a sufficient life can be drawn (if indeed it can and should be drawn) could be seen to be relative to what is possible within a society (or across societies). If, for example, the better off tend to live on average to 80 years, whereas those who are worse off tend to live to 60 years, sufficientarians can point to the longer lives of the better off as an indication that under the right circumstances the worse off could live longer and that this would need to be taken into account in setting a context-sensitive threshold. If we accept this, we will, at times, need to compare the positions of the worst off and the better off to establish thresholds, and thus we accept that sufficientarianism has a comparative element. However, note that there is still a difference between this and the claim that the *inequality* or the relationship between the better off and the worse off is itself morally significant. Hence, the recognition of the relevance of comparisons between these two groups does not commit a sufficientarian to the recognition of the relevance of non-instrumental equality.

---

43. Crisp, "Equality, Priority, and Compassion," 762.

44. Powers and Faden, *Social Justice*, 57–64; Martha Nussbaum, "Constitutions and Capabilities: 'Perception' Against Lofty Formalism," *Harvard Law Review* 121 (2007): 15–16.

2.6 The Scope of Sufficiency

A sufficiency view need not promote sufficiency for all people globally and for all generations. There are two central questions about the way in which the scope of a sufficiency view could be set. The first is whether sufficientarianism is a claim about what we owe those within a society, and thus a claim about domestic justice, or whether it is rather (or also) a claim about what we owe people throughout the world—in other words, a claim about global justice.[45] For some theorists, what we owe globally should be less demanding than what we owe domestically. Because monist sufficiency views that set low sufficiency thresholds tend to be less demanding than other pattern views, they can be appealing to a number of theorists as an understanding of global justice, even though these theorists may believe we have more stringent obligations when it comes to distributive justice within our own societies.

A second significant aspect of scope would be to determine whether sufficiency applies on an intragenerational or intergenerational level. We may reject the idea that sufficiency is what is owed individuals within our society or globally, but we may still be tempted to be sufficientarians in our understanding of what we owe future generations. A number of philosophers have argued that the sufficiency view provides a cogent basis for determining intergenerational justice—for example, we owe future generations, at least, sufficiency, and what we owe future generations should not jeopardize our own sufficiency.[46]

3. Criticisms of Sufficiency Views

Each distributive pattern view—utility, equality, priority, and sufficiency—attracts a variety of criticisms. A sufficiency view is, in certain ways, more challenging to specify than, for example, a distributive equality view: "Calculating the size of an equal share is plainly much easier than determining how much a person needs in order to have enough."[47] This is not a criticism of sufficiency views; it is merely how they are per definition. Sufficiency views encompass a *qualitative* aspect in

---

45. See, for example, David Miller for a sufficientarian view of global justice: *National Responsibility and Global Justice* (Oxford: Oxford University Press, 2007).

46. In Chapter 7, Axel Gosseries identifies the distinctiveness of a sufficientarian view of intergenerational justice and indicates how this might apply to three aspects of health policy. For further discussions of sufficiency and intergenerational justice, see, for example, Edward A. Page, *Climate Change, Justice and Future Generations* (Cheltenham, UK: Elgar, 2007); Lukas H. Meyer and Dominic Roser, "Enough for the Future," in *Intergenerational Justice*, ed. Axel Gosseries and Lukas H. Meyer (Oxford: Oxford University Press, 2009).

47. Frankfurt, "Equality as a Moral Ideal," 23–24.

determining whether justice has been achieved—that is, the morally significant sufficiency threshold: "The sufficientarians must accomplish an additional task, namely, proving that the well-being space contains a qualitative morally privileged distinction between good and bad lives."[48] In contrast with distributive equality views, as long as we can agree on what we are measuring, we usually require no specific qualitative information about people's actual levels of advantage to be able to judge if justice has been achieved—all we need to know is whether or not they are equal in the requisite sense.[49]

In the final section of this primer, I consider four particularly influential criticisms of sufficiency views. These are not necessarily only applicable to the sufficiency view—for example, the "bottomless pit" problem, in its most well-known form, has been applied to the priority view.[50] Furthermore, each of these criticisms may apply to certain kinds of sufficiency views but not to others. I provide a brief indication of some of the views that would be particularly susceptible to these criticisms and those that are less likely to be. Primarily, I do not provide a defense of sufficiency views from these criticisms; particular theories of sufficiency would need to counter these objections based on how their theories have been specified.[51]

3.1. The Arbitrariness of the Sufficiency Threshold

Sufficiency views are often criticized for being morally arbitrary. The claim is that along a continuum of well-being, wherever we draw a threshold, it will lack the moral significance ascribed to it by sufficientarians. Arneson, for example, claims that well-being is a matter of degree; we can have more or we can have less. What does not make sense, he claims, is to try to justify a level of well-being that is of the utmost moral importance for individuals to reach, but once they have reached it, their well-being is no longer morally relevant.[52] How susceptible a sufficiency

---

48. Benbaji, "The Doctrine of Sufficiency," 332.

49. Although, when it comes to interegenerational justice, who the future parties will be is not clear, and, interestingly, in this case, equality might be harder to judge than sufficiency because 'equality between whom?' cannot be specified. I thank Fabian Schuppert for emphasizing this point.

50. For example, Kenneth J. Arrow, "Some Ordinalist–Utilitarian Notes on Rawls's Theory of Justice," *Journal of Philosophy* 70, no. 9 (1973): 245–263, at 251–252.

51. For a detailed understanding of particular sufficiency views and how they can be defended from criticisms, consider Chapters 3–6 by Iwao Hirose, Robert Huseby, Liam Shields, and David V. Axelsen and Lasse Nielsen, respectively.

52. Richard J. Arneson, "Why Justice Requires Transfers to Offset Income and Wealth Inequalities," *Social Philosophy and Policy* 19, no. 1 (2002): 187–191; Arneson, "Distributive Justice and Basic Capability Equality," 28–29.

view is to this specific criticism is partially related to how much weight it places on reaching sufficiency; a monist view is more likely to be particularly susceptible because it emphasizes the threshold at the expense of all else.

3.2. The Indifference Objection

Imagine that we have resources to distribute to one of two groups, both of which have an above-threshold level of well-being. One group's well-being is at sufficiency; the other is far above sufficiency. Another central objection that has been directed against certain forms of sufficientarianism is that they will claim that justice is indifferent to which group should be benfitted because it is indifferent to the plight of those above the threshold.[53] Intuitively, however, many would claim that we should benefit the worse off, and it is a failure of a sufficiency view that it cannot direct us to this conclusion.

The lower the threshold of sufficiency, the more susceptible a monist theory is likely to be to this criticism. Views with higher thresholds seem more plausible in terms of the claim that sufficiency is all we should care about.[54] Pluralist sufficiency views can avoid the criticism all together because they do not necessarily claim that we should be indifferent to benefiting those above the threshold. These latter theories will then, however, require an explanation as to why there is a shift in our reasons for benefitting individuals once they reach a certain threshold.[55]

3.3. The Problem of Prioritizing the Better Off

Imagine a group of people with an illness that made them suffer excruciating pain—this group is far below the sufficiency threshold of health or well-being. Another group is suffering from a far less severe illness but one that pushes them slightly below the sufficiency threshold. We can distribute a treatment to members of the worse off group, which will greatly improve their health and alleviate their pain, although they will still be slightly below the threshold. Alternatively, we can provide members of the better off group with a treatment that will increase their health slightly so that they reach the threshold. Some sufficiency views will indicate, counterintuitively according to many, that we should benefit those who

---

53. Arneson, "Why Justice Requires Transfers to Offset Income and Wealth Inequalities."

54. See also, for example, Shields and Casal for discussions of the susceptibility to particular criticisms for views committed to low or high thresholds (Shields, "The Prospects for Sufficientarianism," 104–105; Casal, "Why Sufficiency Is Not Enough," 315–316).

55. Shields, "The Prospects for Sufficientarianism."

are able to reach the threshold through treatment.[56] This seems counterintuitive because we will be benefitting those who are better off at the expense of those who are worse off. Sufficiency views that aim, for example, to maximize the number of individuals at the sufficiency threshold are especially susceptible to this criticism.[57] In order to avoid this objection, a sufficiency view could adopt a weighting rule that will give some weight to those who are further away from the threshold in comparison to those who are still beneath it but who are better off.

3.4. The Bottomless Pit Problem

If a sufficiency view gives weight to benefitting those who are furthest from the threshold and avoids the problem of prioritizing the better off, it could be susceptible to the bottomless pit problem.[58] It can be accused of potentially exhausting all of society's resources to help those who are particularly badly off without helping them to achieve sufficiency and still leaving many who are better off, but below the threshold, without any benefits. A way of avoiding this is for weighting rules below the threshold to take into account not only how badly off someone is but also how great the benefit is (and how closely it will thus bring her to sufficiency), as well as how many individuals can be benefitted.

Distributive equality and priority views are also subject to a host of objections, and as mentioned previously, even some of the criticisms of sufficiency views described here are also applicable to some of the other distributive views. This list of criticisms does not imply that sufficientarianism is necessarily particularly difficult to defend in relation to other views. To choose between these distributive views, or pluralist versions of them, we need to find the positive justifications for adopting the view convincing. Then, in terms of the criticisms against the view, we could assess whether it is able to defend itself from the most worrying of objections.

In this primer, I aimed to provide readers with an introduction to the topic of sufficientarianism by focusing on distinguishing the most influential distributive views, identifying six significant elements that a sufficiency view would need to specify, and highlighting a number of influential criticisms of sufficientarianism. This can help readers to place particular sufficientarian principles, and the chapters in this volume, in the context of the debate.

---

56. Richard J. Arneson, "Egalitarianism and Responsibility," *Journal of Ethics* 3, no. 3 (January 1, 1999): 225–247; Arneson, "Why Justice Requires Transfers to Offset Income and Wealth Inequalities."

57. See, for example, Shields in this volume (Chapter 5).

58. Arrow, "Some Ordinalist–Utilitarian Notes on Rawls's Theory of Justice"; Powers and Faden, *Social Justice*, 176–177.

Acknowledgments

I thank Annette Rid for the joint planning of the introductory chapters and for her helpful questions and comments. I also very much appreciate Sebastian Muders, Fabian Schuppert, Philipp Schwind, Diego Silva and an anonymous reviewer's comments that helped me to revise this chapter. Last, I am grateful for the financial support that the Swiss National Science Foundation has provided.

2

Sufficiency, Health, and Health Care Justice

THE STATE OF THE DEBATE

Annette Rid

HEALTH IS NOW widely recognized to be relevant for distributive justice, given that it has important value for individuals as well as societies. Being healthy—and, in particular, being free from pain and suffering—is a good in itself and a precondition for many valuable activities, such as engaging in meaningful relationships or work and learning. Furthermore, ample empirical literature shows that health is, at least in part, determined by the conditions in which people are born, grow, live, work, and age.[1] The fact that health is both critical to people's quality of life and so strongly influenced by social, economic, and other factors makes it an appropriate focal point of justice.

A burgeoning literature is exploring questions about health and health care justice. This literature discusses what is the right concern or "currency" of justice—for example, resources, welfare, or capabilities—and how health or health care are linked to these currencies, including whether they should be considered a currency of justice. The questions of what is health, and how should it be measured in practice are central topics for debate in this context.[2] Discussion also revolves

---

1. For two classic texts, see Michael Marmot and Richard Wilkinson, eds., *Social Determinants of Health* (New York: Oxford University Press, 2005, 2nd edition); Lisa F. Berkman, Ichiro Kawachi, and M. Maria Glymour, eds., *Social Epidemiology* (New York: Oxford University Press, 2014, 2nd edition).

2. In Chapter 9, Sean Aas and David Wasserman develop a novel conception of health for the purposes of health justice. Paul Mitchell and colleagues discuss recent

around whether health or health care should be distributed according to a particular principle or pattern—for example, whether policies should promote equal health or the health of the worst off—and, if so, which principle or combination of principles the distribution should follow.[3]

Whereas some authors are skeptical that a unified set of distributive principles can be developed,[4] others have linked health to different currencies and principles of distributive justice with the goal of developing systematic, although not necessarily all-encompassing, accounts of health or health care justice.[5] Among these authors, relatively few focus specifically on the sufficiency principle—that is, the principle according to which everyone should have "enough" health or health care. Of course, in the broadest sense, all approaches to health justice aim to justify how much health or health care is enough as dictated by the tenets of their preferred theory. For example, Norman Daniels argues that a health insurance package is providing enough services when it helps to preserve normal functioning and hence fair equality of opportunity.[6] However, this does not make Daniels a sufficientarian in the narrower, more specialized sense of sufficiency that implies a commitment to *achieving a threshold level of whichever currency of justice is deemed appropriate.* The remainder of this chapter uses the terms "sufficiency" and "sufficientarian" in this narrower sense. Understood as such, it

---

developments in the economic evaluation of health in Chapter 15, focusing in particular on new health measures that are based on Amartya Sen's and Martha Nussbaum's capability approach.

3. For an overview of different distributive principles of justice, see Carina Fourie's primer on the sufficiency view in this volume (Chapter 1).

4. For example, Allen Buchanan, *Justice and Health Care: Selected Essays* (New York: Oxford University Press, 2009); Leonard Fleck, *Just Caring: Health Care Rationing and Democratic Deliberation* (New York: Oxford University Press, 2009); Tom L. Beauchamp and James F. Childress, *Principles of Biomedical Ethics* (New York: Oxford University Press, 2013).

5. In particular, Madison Powers and Ruth Faden, *Social Justice: The Moral Foundations of Public Health and Health Policy* (New York: Oxford University Press, 2006); Yukiko Asada, *Health Inequality: Morality and Measurement* (Toronto: University of Toronto Press, 2007); Norman Daniels, *Just Health: Meeting Health Needs fairly* (New York: Oxford University Press, 2008); Shlomi Segall, *Health, Luck and Justice* (Princeton, NJ: Princeton University Press, 2010); Jennifer Prah Ruger, *Health and Social Justice* (New York: Oxford University Press, 2010); Sridhar Venkatapuram, *Health Justice* (Cambridge, UK: Polity, 2011); Rosamund Rhodes, Margaret P. Battin, and Anita Silvers, eds., *Medicine and Social Justice: Essays on the Distribution of Health Care* (New York: Oxford University Press, 2012, 2nd edition); Nir Eyal, Samia A. Hurst, Ole F. Norheim, and Dan Wikler, eds., *Inequalities in Health: Concepts, Measures, and Ethics* (New York: Oxford University Press, 2013).

6. Daniels, *Just Health.*

is noteworthy that very few scholars have begun specifying the significant elements of a sufficiency view in relation to health and health care.[7,8]

This is not to say that sufficientarian ideas play no role in the work of other authors. Indeed, a significant number of scholars embrace sufficiency as a distributive principle, although they may not develop the sufficientarian element of their theory in detail or self-identify as sufficientarians. For example, Sridhar Venkatapuram largely focuses his work on capabilities as a currency of health justice, but—like Martha Nussbaum's capabilities approach on which his view is partially based—he also argues that achieving threshold levels of certain capabilities is a minimal requirement of justice.[9] However, Venkatapuram does not further develop where a sufficiency threshold (or thresholds) should be set, how resources should be prioritized below and above the threshold(s), how sufficiency is positioned in relation to other distributive principles of justice, and so on. It nevertheless seems appropriate to classify these approaches as "sufficientarian" because they are fundamentally committed to the idea that achieving a critical threshold of welfare, capabilities, or some other currency of justice is morally significant.

Finally, in addition to this theoretically oriented literature, there is a body of conceptual and normative work on concepts or practices in health policy that resonate with sufficientarian ideas. This applies in particular to the moral right to an "adequate" level of health services and to so-called "two-tiered" health systems that provide basic services to everyone but allow the private purchase of additional, faster or higher quality services.

This chapter provides an overview of the existing sufficientarian approaches to health or health care justice, as well as concepts or policies that seem to be

---

7. The key authors are Powers and Faden, *Social Justice*; Allen Andrew A. Alvarez, "Threshold Considerations in Fair Allocation of Health Resources: Justice Beyond Scarcity," *Bioethics* 21 (2007): 426–438; Efrat Ram-Tiktin, *Distributive Justice in Health Care* (PhD diss., Bar-Ilan University, 2009); Efrat Ram-Tiktin, "A Decent Minimum for Everyone as a Sufficiency of Basic Human Functional Capabilities," *American Journal of Bioethics* 11 (2011): 24–25; Efrat Ram-Tiktin, "The Right to Health Care as a Right to Basic Human Functional Capabilities," *Ethical Theory and Moral Practice* 15 (2012): 337–51. See also Ram-Tiktin's contribution in this volume (Chapter 8), which is not included in the present overview of the literature.

8. In Chapter 1, Fourie discusses six significant elements of the sufficiency view: (1) the currency of sufficiency; (2) the positive and positioning claims that commit sufficientarians to the independent moral significance of achieving sufficiency and "position" sufficiency in relation to other values or distributive principles of justice; (3) justification(s) for sufficiency principles; (4) weighting rules that specify the moral importance of achieving sufficiency in relation to other distributive principles of justice or values other than justice (if any); (5) guidance on where and how sufficiency thresholds should be set; and (6) the scope of sufficiency—for example, whether it applies to all people globally or to all generations.

9. Venkatapuram, *Health Justice*, 65 and 117–119.

committed to the idea of ensuring "enough" health. The key goal is to orient readers about the most prominent lines of argument and positions; hence, several caveats apply. The chapter does not provide a comprehensive literature review, and it does not engage critically with the specific views or claims under consideration. Moreover, the focus is on literature that takes a distinctly normative approach to the issues at hand, meaning that the authors aim to specify when the distribution of health or health care *should* be considered just. This implies, in particular, that important health policy literature without this normative orientation is not considered.

1. Sufficientarian Approaches to Health or Health Care Justice

The following sections use Fourie's six significant elements of a sufficiency view in order to summarize the existing sufficientarian approaches to health or health care justice.[10] Currently, three sufficientarian approaches are specified in significant detail: Powers and Faden's sufficiency of well-being approach;[11] Efrat Ram-Tiktin's sufficiency of basic human functional capabilities approach;[12] and Allen Andrew Alvarez's sufficiency of vital capacities approach.[13] All three approaches primarily focus on health or health care justice within national boundaries—two in the context of high-income countries (Powers and Faden and Ram-Tiktin) and one in the context of low-income countries (Alvarez). Moreover, all three approaches regard sufficiency in health or health care as a morally urgent requirement of justice that matters in and of itself, meaning that it does not matter for the sake of some other requirement of justice.

1.1. Sufficiency of Well-Being

The sufficiency of well-being approach (SWA) was developed by Powers and Faden with the goal of positioning health justice within the wider context of social justice. Its outlook is decidedly non-ideal; in the authors' words, SWA is "intended to offer practical guidance on questions of which inequalities matter most when just background conditions are not in place."[14]

---

10. For a summary of the significant elements, see footnote 8.

11. Powers and Faden, *Social Justice*.

12. Ram-Tiktin, *Distributive Justice*; Ram-Tiktin, "A Decent Minimum"; Ram-Tiktin, "The Right to Health Care."

13. Alvarez, "Threshold Considerations."

14. Powers and Faden, *Social Justice*, 30.

The currency of sufficiency is well-being, and this is composed of six essential elements: health, personal security, reasoning, respect, attachment, and self-determination.[15] According to SWA, the job of social justice is to secure and maintain "the social conditions necessary for a sufficient level of well-being in all of its essential dimensions for everyone."[16] The underlying justification is that threshold levels of each of the identified dimensions of well-being are typical of a "decent life." As Powers and Faden state, "A life substantially lacking in any one of these [dimensions] is a life seriously deficient in what it is reasonable for anyone to want, whatever else they want."[17]

Powers and Faden do not systematically position SWA in relation to other theories of health justice. They seem to reject the non-instrumental relevance of other distributive principles above the sufficiency threshold, which suggests that concerns about justice no longer obtain once individuals and populations have achieved sufficiency of well-being. Below the sufficiency threshold, SWA refers to the notion of giving priority to the worst off. However, it does not seem to endorse a priority principle in its own right, given that the worst off are defined with respect to the sufficiency threshold—namely with respect to how far away an individual is from the threshold or how many elements of his or her well-being are insufficient. SWA thus appears to endorse the notion of prioritizing the worst off on sufficientarian grounds.

Equally, SWA endorses egalitarian distributive principles only when they serve to promote sufficiency of well-being.[18] For example, Powers and Faden argue that inequalities in wealth and income matter only insofar as they "contribute to . . . deprivations in any of the dimensions of well-being below the level of sufficiency"; this implies that equality is of "derivative importance."[19] Egalitarian principles are especially important for the dimensions of respect and attachment because sufficiency of these dimensions cannot be achieved in the presence of substantial or systematic inequalities. The authors write, "Respect . . . has its value for any

---

15. Powers and Faden, *Social Justice*, 16. The six dimensions of well-being resonate with Martha Nussbaum's list of 10 central human functional capabilities, although Powers and Faden emphasize actual well-being rather than capabilities. Martha C. Nussbaum, *Women and Human Development: The Capabilities Approach* (New York: Cambridge University Press, 2000).

16. Powers and Faden, *Social Justice*, 50.

17. Powers and Faden, *Social Justice*, 29. The authors are quick to note that a life deficient in some of the essential dimensions of well-being can still be valuable, and those leading it are entitled to the same moral concern as others. However, in their view, the positive aim of justice is to strive for sufficiency in each of the six dimensions of well-being.

18. Powers and Faden, *Social Justice*, 176–177.

19. Ibid., 57–58.

individual or group of individuals only when the social conditions that promote and sustain it are equal for all persons."[20]

SWA adopts an ordinary-language conception of health as the dimension of well-being that is mediated through the biological functioning of the body.[21] It seems to require, at a minimum, that everyone have "enough health over a long enough life span to live a decent life."[22] Powers and Faden "do not think it plausible to attempt to specify in the abstract precisely what constitutes a sufficiency of health,"[23] and hence they are hesitant to provide more detail on where and how a health sufficiency threshold should be set. Although the threshold is influenced both by particular social contexts and by what is technologically feasible, they argue that "in the world we inhabit, there are many clear instances in which populations or population subgroups fall below a level of sufficiency in health."[24]

In a similar vein, Powers and Faden believe that there is no "generally right answer" regarding how resources should be prioritized to assist those below the sufficiency threshold or to prevent those just above it from falling below the threshold.[25] SWA does require, however, that priority be given to the worst off below the sufficiency threshold.[26] This requirement is viewed as stringent but not absolute. Individuals in very poor health thus should be given priority, and their claims may be discounted only when little can be done to improve their health or when what can be done would exhaust most of the resources available.

Finally, given that health is only one of six essential dimensions of well-being, SWA requires that any distribution of health care or public health resources be judged according to the effect it has on sufficiency in the other dimensions of well-being. One implication is that cases of multiple disadvantage, in which individuals or populations suffer insufficiency in a number of dimensions of well-being, are particularly morally urgent to address.[27] Similarly, the needs of children equally deserve priority, both because they cannot achieve sufficient well-being on their own and because some dimensions of well-being have to be promoted in early life in order to achieve sufficient well-being over the life course.[28]

---

20. Ibid., 63.

21. Ibid., 16–18.

22. Ibid., 61. See pages 60–64 for their discussion of health sufficiency.

23. Ibid., 61.

24. Ibid., 61.

25. Ibid., 176.

26. Ibid., 176–177.

27. Ibid., 64–79.

28. Ibid., 158–167.

1.2. Sufficiency of Basic Human Functional Capabilities

Another approach that specifies a sufficiency view in significant detail is Ram-Tiktin's sufficiency of basic human functional capabilities approach, or for short sufficiency of capabilities approach (SCA).[29] Unlike Powers and Faden's SWA that positions health justice within the wider context of social justice, SCA focuses more narrowly on justice in the distribution of resources for medical care—notably interventions aimed at treating or preventing illness. SCA also differs from SWA in that it takes an ideal approach. This implies that SCA aims to delineate distributive principles that should govern just institutions rather than offering guidance on how to make institutions and their policies more just in the face of background injustices.

Capabilities—the things that a person can do or be—are the currency of sufficiency and, specifically, the basic physiological and psychological capabilities that advance the goals of an individual in his or her social environment. According to the SCA, justice demands that health institutions guarantee individuals sufficiency of these basic human functional capabilities because such sufficiency enables individuals "to live dignified lives and implement their life plans."[30]

SCA holds that basic human functional capabilities cluster in nine key systems—for example, "digestion and metabolism," "movement and balance," and "thinking and emotions."[31] Sufficiency thresholds within these systems are set by first determining the relevant norm values for a given physical or psychological capability and then evaluating to what extent deviations from the norm prevent affected individuals from executing their life plans within the given society. For example, one sufficiency threshold in the system of digestion and metabolism is a blood glucose level of 70–100 mg/dl. This reflects the normal range for blood glucose, outside of which it is difficult or impossible to pursue one's life goals. Furthermore, in the case of blood glucose, this latter statement is probably true independent of social context. SCA requires that sufficient functioning in all nine capability systems be achieved in order to attain sufficiency of basic human capabilities.

SCA rejects the relevance of other distributive principles for achieving just health outcomes once sufficiency has been achieved. Individuals or populations have no claims of *justice* to medical care resources above the sufficiency threshold,

29. Ram-Tiktin, *Distributive Justice*; Ram-Tiktin, "A Decent Minimum"; Ram-Tiktin, "The Right to Health Care."

30. Ram-Tiktin, "The Right to Health Care," 342.

31. Ibid., 341.

unless they are in concrete jeopardy of falling below it.[32] However, where the claims of justice have been met, *beneficence* seems to require satisfying individual preferences above the threshold, and any remaining resources should be directed toward the greatest benefit to as many people as possible.[33] Moreover, providing certain services to those above the sufficiency threshold—notably health education, preventive services, and follow-up care—can be justified on grounds of justice when they are necessary to prevent individuals from falling below a sufficient level of basic human capabilities.

In addition, SCA endorses other distributive principles for distributing resources below the sufficiency threshold, although it is not entirely clear whether these principles matter because they promote sufficiency or because they are important in and of themselves. Below the threshold, SCA holds, "benefiting people matters more the worse off those people are, the greater the size of the benefit in question, and the more of those people there are."[34] Furthermore, the size of the benefit has more importance than the number of beneficiaries, and cross-personal aggregated benefit is generally irrelevant.[35] SCA also stipulates that special priority be given to those who may die or lose capabilities that are fundamental for human life, such as patients at risk of falling into coma.[36] Only in the rarest of circumstances is it justified not to give priority to those below the threshold—for example, when tremendous benefits accrue to a great number of people above the threshold.

1.3. Sufficient Capacity to Perform Vital Tasks

The sufficiency of vital capacities approach (SVCA) was developed by Alvarez to address situations of extreme scarcity in low- and middle-income countries.[37] SVCA's currency is the basic physical and mental capacity to perform vital tasks, such as earning a living for adults or growing up to be a productive member of society for children.[38] The approach rests on the idea that achieving a threshold

---

32. Ram-Tiktin, "A Decent Minimum," 347; Ram-Tiktin, "The Right to Health Care," 347–349.

33. Ram-Tiktin, "The Right to Health Care," 349.

34. Ibid., 343.

35. Ibid., 343–344.

36. Ibid., 343.

37. Alvarez, "Threshold Considerations."

38. Ibid., 436.

level of capacity to perform vital tasks is the primary goal of justice when resources are extremely limited. SVCA defines health as the "physical/mental capacity for basic living" and posits that thresholds of sufficient health should be set using an "absolute, universal, and more objective measure of threshold health" in order to avoid unwarranted variation between different social contexts.[39]

SVCA justifies its commitment to sufficiency based on the principle's intuitive appeal and its apparent endorsement in international instruments, such as the World Health Organization's *Declaration of Alma-Ata*.[40] Moreover, according to SVCA, alternative distributive principles of justice jeopardize health and vital functioning under conditions of extreme scarcity. Specifically, few will reach or maintain a sufficient level of health when extremely limited resources are distributed with the goal of promoting equal health or prioritizing the worst off.[41]

SVCA is explicitly pluralist in that it embraces several distributive principles of justice and, in particular, directly acknowledges the relevance of equality and priority above the sufficiency threshold. SVCA maintains that sufficiency should be given "lexical [or absolute] priority" under conditions of extreme scarcity while using the available resources so as to minimize the gap between current health status and the sufficiency threshold.[42] However, once sufficiency has been attained, justice seems to require that resources be distributed according to prioritarian or egalitarian principles.[43]

1.4. Sufficientarian Approaches That Primarily Focus on the Currency of Justice

In addition to the previously mentioned approaches that specify sufficiency views in significant detail, several authors include a sufficientarian element in their theories of health or health care justice, although typically without developing it in depth or self-identifying as "sufficientarians." Broadly, these latter approaches can be grouped according to whether they primarily focus on justifying or specifying the currency of

---

39. Ibid., 436.

40. Ibid., 426–427.

41. Ibid., 427–428.

42. Ibid., 430, 432.

43. I take the above to reflect Alvarez's position, although he is not always clear about his views. For example, Alvarez claims that efficiency considerations should play a role only after sufficiency has been attained. However, he also seems to suggest that equality, priority, and efficiency can help to make decisions about "extraordinary medical care"—for example, dialysis—even when sufficiency has not been achieved. Alvarez, "Threshold Considerations," 437–438.

justice or whether they primarily focus on justifying or specifying distributive principles other than sufficiency or values other than justice.

One group of approaches seems to endorse sufficiency but focuses mostly
on specifying the currency of justice. For example, Venkatapuram developed a
capabilities-based approach to health justice that, like that of Nussbaum, is committed to achieving threshold levels of the capabilities as a minimal requirement
of justice. Venkatapuram argues, for example, that "ensuring each member [of
society] achieves a threshold level of these ten central capabilities becomes a primary political goal."[44] Moreover, he emphasizes that different societies will determine threshold levels of each capability depending on their history and resources,
even though thresholds should not be wholly determined by local circumstances.
He also acknowledges that a meaningful application of the capabilities approach
needs to specify priority rules for distributing resources above and below the
threshold and, for example, tackle questions about aggregation and trade-offs between improving the capabilities of those below and above the threshold "head
on."[45] However, Venkatapuram does not explore these questions in depth, partly
because he seems to be wary of "thought experiments" that, in his view, tend to
force us to make moral errors by considering only some of many morally significant dimensions of priority-setting problems.[46] Instead, he focuses mainly on
defending the capability to be healthy as the right currency of health justice.

Similarly, Jennifer Prah Ruger is a capabilities theorist who endorses the sufficiency principle but primarily defends (central) health capabilities as the currency
of health care justice.[47] Prah Ruger states that her approach, "while eschewing
a call for complete equality, is a hybrid of sufficiency and priority principles."[48]
She sketches several of the significant elements of a sufficiency view.[49] In particular, Prah Ruger argues that achieving a threshold level of central health capabilities has priority over achieving a threshold level of noncentral capabilities,[50] and
that the threshold for central health capabilities should be set at an "optimal or

---

44. Venkatapuram, *Health Justice*, 65.

45. Ibid., 117–119.

46. Ibid., 119.

47. Ruger, *Health and Social Justice*. In addition to a theoretical defense of her health capabilities paradigm, Ruger devotes significant time to discussing its implications for health policy.

48. Ibid., 88.

49. See Carina Fourie's primer on the sufficiency view in Chapter 1.

50. Central health capabilities are prerequisites for other health capabilities and other capabilities more broadly, such as the capacity of our organs and systems to function. Ruger,
Health and Social Justice, 76–77.

maximal absolute average level"—amounting to the highest population average for the given capability worldwide. Moreover, the health of individuals below the threshold should be promoted efficiently, and no individual should be required to sacrifice his or her central health capabilities for the sake of another.[51] However, Prah Ruger does not develop these sufficientarian elements further and, similar to Venkatapuram, she focuses mainly on defending the health capabilities as the right currency of health justice.

1.5. Sufficientarian Approaches That Primarily Focus on Principles Other Than Sufficiency

Another group of approaches with a sufficientarian element endorses the idea that everyone should have enough health or health care—either to promote justice or to promote values other than justice, such as equal respect. However, with regard to justice, these approaches focus on specifying distributive principles other than sufficiency.

One example is Shlomi Segall's luck prioritarian approach to health care justice, which aims to incorporate considerations of personal responsibility into health care.[52] A common objection to responsibility-sensitive approaches is that they are too harsh on individuals who suffer ill health as a result of not having acted responsibly with respect to their health. For example, a responsibility-sensitive approach might recommend not covering the care for injuries that individuals sustain while engaging in risky sports, such as skiing. However, not caring for such injuries seems hard-hearted, especially when an injury, such as a bone fracture, is both serious and treatable.

To avoid what is known as the "harshness objection" to responsibility-sensitive approaches, Segall develops a version of luck prioritarianism that supports the moral significance of personal responsibility as a matter of justice while constraining it based on values other than justice. Specifically, he argues that meeting the basic needs of all members of society is an independent moral requirement and that individuals' basic health needs should therefore be met whether or not they have acted responsibly with respect to their health. For care that goes beyond meeting basic needs, however, justice requires giving priority to those who have taken responsibility for their health. In addition, when there are several people, all of whom have invested equal amounts of effort into looking after their health, those in worse health should be given priority.[53]

---

51. Ibid., 115–116.

52. Segall, *Health, Luck and Justice*.

53. Ibid., 118–120.

Segall grants that this line of argument adds a "layer of sufficientarian distribution" to his luck egalitarian approach, and he suggests that sufficiency of capabilities is one way of understanding what it means to meet basic needs.[54] Thus, although he focuses primarily on specifying the luck prioritarian element of his approach, Segall arguably is a sufficientarian as well—even though he endorses sufficiency not as a matter of justice but, rather, as a matter of meeting basic needs.[55]

2. Sympathizers with a Sufficientarian Approach

Finally, there are authors who do not include a sufficientarian element in their own approach to health or health care justice but argue that their approach fulfills the requirements of sufficiency. A key example is Norman Daniels, who extends John Rawls' approach to justice to the realm of health and health care.[56] Rawls famously argued that a social contract among free and equal members of a society would include three general principles of justice: a principle protecting equal basic liberties, a principle guaranteeing fair equality of opportunity, and a principle limiting inequalities to those that benefit the least advantaged.[57] Daniels adds that health—defined as species-typical functioning—contributes to the range of exercisable opportunities open to us. Justice, he then argues, requires promoting and restoring health in order to ensure that everyone has a fair opportunity range within the given society.

Daniels' approach to health justice does not include a sufficientarian element. However, he argues that preserving species-typical functioning under reasonable resource constraints—and generally abiding by Rawls' distributive principles—will result in a sufficient level of capabilities on both the individual and the population level. In other words, Daniels argues that his approach to health justice converges with a sufficiency of capabilities approach.[58] Thus, although he does not

---

54. Ibid., 69. On p. 76, Segall explicitly writes that "I am happy here to rely on the list of capabilities provided by Amartya Sen and Martha Nussbaum as summing up those basic needs."

55. Readers should note, however, that Segall is critical of sufficientarianism when it is an axiological principle—that is, when it claims that a sufficientarian state of affairs is better in itself without grounding it in justice or the requirement to meet basic needs, for example. Shlomi Segall, "What Is the Point of Sufficiency?" *Journal of Applied Philosophy* 33, no. 1 (2016): 36–52.

56. Daniels, *Just Health*.

57. Rawls, John, *A Theory of Justice* (Cambridge, MA: Harvard University Press, 1971).

58. Daniels, *Just Health*, 66–71. According to Daniels, Martha Nussbaum—a proponent of the sufficiency of capabilities approach—similarly notes that "the conditions for assuring

embrace sufficiency as a distributive principle of justice, he is eager to show that his approach satisfies the requirements of sufficiency.

3. Debates Related to Sufficiency

In addition to the theoretically oriented literature, a considerable body of work explores concepts in health policy and practice that resonate with sufficientarian ideas—most notably, the moral right to an adequate level of health services and two-tiered health systems.

3.1. The Moral Right to an Adequate Level of Health Services

A recent literature survey shows that the moral right to health is typically understood as a right to a certain set of health-related programs, not as a right to be healthy.[59] Few argue that the moral right to health entitles its holders to receive— and places an obligation on society to provide—all technologically possible goods and services that they might need to be in perfect health. Such an extensive right would both put an intolerable burden on society and fail to respect the demands of other rights or socially valuable goals on the available collective resources, such as providing education and security. The moral right to health is therefore typically viewed as entitling individuals to an adequate level of health services, or—depending on what is considered adequate or required by the demands of justice—a reasonable or basic or decent minimum of services.[60]

It might seem that most authors rely on notions of sufficiency to ground the moral right to health; after all, terms such as a "basic minimum" and "decent minimum" seem to evoke sufficientarian ideas. A closer look at the literature, however, reveals that this is not the case. Consistent with the broad sense of "enough"

such development [of a sufficient set of capabilities] may well converge with some of Rawls' principles of justice" (p. 70).

59. Benedict E. Rumbold, "Review Article: The Moral Right to Health: A Survey of Available Conceptions," *Critical Review of International Social and Political Philosophy* (2015): in press. DOI: 10.1080/13698230.2014.995505. See also Jonathan Wolff, *The Human Right to Health* (New York: Norton, 2012). The conception of the right to health as a right to be *healthy* is widely rejected because it fails even the most basic feasibility requirement, given that some people will remain ill regardless of how many resources are spent on their health.

60. Historically, the discussion has largely focused on the right to a decent minimum of health care, not health *services* that include, for example, public health interventions. Presumably this is because the literature on the social determinants of health (see footnote 1) was still in its beginnings.

health or health care discussed at the beginning of this chapter, one group of authors draw on their theory of health or health care justice to justify that individuals are entitled to basic health services.[61] Insofar as their approach endorses the sufficiency principle, their justification is—at least in part—a sufficientarian one. For instance, Ram-Tiktin argues that the moral right to health care entitles individuals to those goods and services that ensure sufficiency of basic human functional capabilities.[62] Yet several authors defend the moral right to an adequate level of health services based on accounts of health justice that do not endorse sufficiency. For example, Daniels argues for a basic level of services that preserves normal functioning and hence fair equality of opportunity,[63] and Julian Savulescu defends the right to a decent minimum of health care from a consequentialist viewpoint.[64]

Other authors eschew a systematic approach to the moral right to adequate health services and instead offer a patchwork defense.[65] Allen Buchanan, for example, finds that principles or theories of justice either do not provide a firm basis for the right to a decent minimum of health care or encounter serious difficulties in specifying the right's content.[66] Instead, he argues, it is preferable to ground this right in a plurality of considerations, including arguments from special (as opposed to universal) rights to health care, harm prevention, and prudential arguments. Similarly, Paul Menzel maintains that a moral right to accessible basic health care can be generated in the US context by combining the legal requirement of access to emergency care with widely held moral and prudential principles.[67]

---

61. Among others, this includes Daniels, *Just Health*, 313–332; Ram-Tiktin, "The Right to Health Care"; Julian Savulescu, "Justice and Healthcare: The Right to a Decent Minimum, Not Equality of Opportunity," *American Journal of Bioethics* 1 (2001): 1a–3a; Venkatapuram, *Health Justice*, 181–184. For a discussion of basic health care and its relationship to basic needs, see, for example, David T. Ozar, "What Should Count as Basic Health Care?" *Theoretical Medicine* 4 (1983): 129–141.

62. Ram-Tiktin, "The Right to Health Care."

63. Daniels, *Just Health*.

64. Savulescu, "A Decent Minimum."

65. President's Commission for the Study of Ethical Problems in Medicine and Biomedical and Behavioral Research, *Securing Access to Health Care: The Ethical Implications of Differences in the Availability of Health Services, Volume One* (Washington, DC: U.S. Government Printing Office, 1983), 20; Allen Buchanan, "The Right to a Decent Minimum of Health Care," *Philosophy and Public Affairs* 13 (1984): 55–78 (reprinted in Buchanan, *Justice and Health Care*, 17–36); Paul T. Menzel, "A Cultural Moral Right to a Basic Minimum of Accessible Health Care," *Kennedy Institute of Ethics Journal* 21 (2011): 79–120.

66. Buchanan, "The Right to a Decent Minimum."

67. Menzel, "A Cultural Moral Right." See also Paul Menzel's chapter in this volume (Chapter 11), in which he compares his "patchwork defense" of the right to a basic minimum of health services to a sufficientarian approach.

With regard to specifying an adequate level of health services and deciding which services to include and exclude, many authors end up endorsing a deliberative process that may or may not be constrained by their prior normative commitments. Some hold that their particular justification for the moral right to an adequate level of health services offers some general or mid-level guidance on which services a basic benefit package should include. For example, Menzel claims that his justification for basic health care supports the coverage of emergency, primary, and preventive care as well as post-emergency acute services, but a deliberative process is needed to specify further details.[68] Other authors, by contrast, have little faith in the practical utility of applying a particular set of distributive principles of justice. For instance, Leonard Fleck argues that basic health benefits should be defined through rational democratic deliberation that is loosely constrained by a plurality of principles.[69]

3.2. Two-Tiered Health Systems

If justice requires providing an adequate level of health services but not everything that is technologically possible, the question arises whether health systems should allow individuals to purchase additional health services. This question has received considerable attention in the literature, both in relation to the right to an adequate level of health services and in relation to other topics, notably specific health policies.[70]

---

68. Menzel, "A Cultural Moral Right."

69. Leonard Fleck, "Just Caring: Defining a Basic Benefit Package," *Journal of Medicine and Philosophy* 36 (2011): 589–611; Fleck, *Just Caring*. See also Leonard Fleck's contribution in this volume (Chapter 12).

70. Some representative papers are Allen Buchanan, "Public and Private Responsibilities in the U.S. Health Care System," in Allen Buchanan, *Justice and Health Care: Selected Essays* (New York: Oxford University Press, 2009), 77–88 [originally published in 1992]; H. Tristram Engelhardt Jr., *Foundations of Bioethics* (New York: Oxford University Press, 1996, 2nd edition), 398–402; Benjamin J. Krohmal and Ezekiel J. Emanuel, "Access and Ability to Pay: The Ethics of a Tiered Health Care System," *Archives of Internal Medicine* 167 (2007): 433–437; Allen S. Brett, "Two-Tiered Health Care: A Problematic Double Standard," *Archives of Internal Medicine* 167 (2007): 430–432; Benjamin J. Krohmal and Ezekiel J. Emanuel, "Tiers Without Tears: The Ethics of a Two-Tier Health Care System," in *The Oxford Handbook of Bioethics*, ed. Bonnie Steinbock (New York: Oxford University Press, 2007), 175–189; Daniels, *Just Health*, 258–259; Benjamin Sachs, "Extortion and the Ethics of 'Topping Up'," *Cambridge Quarterly of Healthcare Ethics* 18 (2009): 443–445; Ruger, *Health and Social Justice*, 150–153; Ruud ter Meulen, "How 'Decent' Is a Decent Minimum of Health Care?" *Journal of Medicine and Philosophy* 36 (2011): 612–623; Elizabeth Fenton, "Mind the Gap: Ethical Issues of Private Treatment in the Public Health System," *New Zealand Medical Journal* 124 (2011): 89–96; Norman Daniels, "Justice and Access to Health Care," in *The Stanford Encyclopedia of Philosophy*, ed. Edward N. Zalta (Spring 2013 edition),

Many authors argue that the purchase of additional, faster or higher quality services in a "second tier" should be allowed—provided that services in the "first tier" are set at an adequate level, and the second tier does not undermine the quality or sustainability of services in the first tier.[71] Broadly, the argument for this view is that allowing the purchase of second-tier services leads to a pareto improvement under these conditions. Healthwise, those acquiring additional services are made better off without making anyone else worse off. Furthermore, disallowing the purchase of these services restricts the liberty of individuals who otherwise have discretion to spend their (after-tax) income as they see fit. Following this line of argument, it would seem difficult to justify this restriction, especially when services in the first tier are adequate and not compromised by those provided in the second tier.

At the same time, tiered health systems raise concerns that go beyond their impact on health or individual liberty. For example, it has been argued that tiering can undermine equal respect for all members of society, especially when access to basic services requires means testing,[72] or that it can undermine solidarity—understood as mutual respect, personal support, and the commitment to a common cause.[73] Due to the pressures they can create on basic services, tiered health systems might also exacerbate inequities within or between patient groups.[74] Importantly, the potential links between two-tiered health care systems and sufficientarianism have not yet been adequately highlighted and assessed.[75]

4. Sufficiency in Practice?

At first sight, it might appear as if current health policy and practice rest on sufficientarian foundations. The majority of health systems in high-income countries operate two-tiered services, and the content of "essential benefit baskets" in these

---

available at http://plato.stanford.edu/archives/spr2013/entries/justice-healthcareaccess (accessed December 20, 2015); Beauchamp and Childress, *Principles*, 272–274.

71. For a good exposition of the following line of argument, see Buchanan, "Public and Private Responsibilities." Krohmal and Emanuel, "Tiers Without Tears," provide a helpful discussion of the various ways in which second-tier services might undermine the first or basic tier.

72. Krohmal and Emanuel, "Access and Ability to Pay"; Krohmal and Emanuel, "Tiers Without Tears."

73. Ter Meulen, "How 'Decent'."

74. Fenton, "Mind the Gap."

75. Carina Fourie's chapter in this volume is one of the first attempts to link two-tiered health care and a sufficientarian approach (see Chapter 10).

systems is much debated.[76] Key international instruments and guidance might also be regarded as invoking sufficientarian ideas. For example, *The Universal Declaration of Human Rights* states that "everyone has the right to a standard of living *adequate* [emphasis added] for the health and well-being of himself and of his family, including food, clothing, housing and medical care and necessary social services."[77] Moreover, the World Health Organization's initiative to promote universal health coverage in low- and middle-income countries requires, among other things, that the "quality of health services is *good enough* [emphasis added] to improve the health of those receiving services."[78] All of this—tiering in existing health systems, debates about essential services, and so on—might seem to embody the idea that everyone should have enough health or health care.

However, as discussed in the previous sections, these practices need not necessarily rest on a principle of sufficiency. Most, if not all, approaches to health or health care justice are committed to ensuring access to a certain level of but not maximum health services, and tiering of services seems to be broadly endorsed when the above mentioned conditions are met. Accordingly, the existing policies and practices may not be guided by sufficientarian ideas. At the same time, it is difficult to determine whether or to what extent current policy and practice aim for sufficiency. Despite my best efforts, I was unable to identify scholarship that explicitly addresses this question from the bottom up, by analyzing current practice in light of the philosophical or bioethical debate about sufficientarian approaches to health justice. There is an extensive empirical and bioethical literature on how priorities for health and health care are set in various countries;[79] however, so far no one seems to have examined explicitly whether current practice is consistent with, or driven by, notions of sufficiency in health or health care.[80]

---

76. For an overview of selected countries, see Dimitra Panteli and Ewout van Ginneken's Chapter in this volume (Chapter 13).

77. *The Universal Declaration of Human Rights*, Article 25. Available at http://www.un.org/en/ documents/udhr (accessed December 20, 2015).

78. World Health Organization, "What Is Universal Coverage?" Available at http://who. int/health_financing/universal_coverage_definition/en (accessed December 20, 2015). However, another requirement is "equity in access to health services—those who need the services should get them, not only those who can pay for them," which may exclude tiered services.

79. For a selected discussion of priority-setting in several high-income countries, see Dimitra Panteli and Ewout van Ginneken's contribution in this volume (Chapter 13).

80. For two innovative papers on this topic, see the contributions by Dimitra Panteli and Ewout van Ginneken (Chapter 13), and by Govind Persad and Harald Schmidt (Chapter 14).

Acknowledgments

I thank Carina Fourie for planning the two introductory chapters to this volume and for her very helpful comments and suggestions on this chapter. I also thank Benedict Rumbold, Benjamin Sachs, Diego Silva and Sridhar Venkatapuram for their valuable discussion or input on earlier versions of this chapter, and I thank Rose Mortimer for help with formatting. This work was supported by funding from the People Programme (Marie Curie Actions) of the European Union's Seventh Framework Programme (FP7/2007-2013) under REA grant agreement No. 301816.

PART II

The Sufficiency View

3

Axiological Sufficientarianism

Iwao Hirose

1. Introduction

There are different ways to approach what has become known as *sufficientarianism* in the recent literature of distributive justice. One way is to conceive it as an axiological principle—that is, a criterion for ranking the states of affairs in terms of goodness. In this chapter, I focus on this particular way of understanding sufficientarianism and attempt to elucidate the formal structure and theoretical scope. Specifically, I (1) elucidate the basic aspiration of sufficientarianism, (2) present an axiological formula, and (3) consider what sufficientarianism implies in cases in which the number of individuals in a population is variable.

Unfortunately, there is a difficulty in attempting to pin down the axiological formula of sufficientarianism. This is because different philosophers make different claims concerning what sufficientarianism implies. Furthermore, whereas many philosophers have implicated *some* axiological features that are distinctive to sufficientarianism, to my knowledge, few have presented an axiological formula.[1] The axiological formula I present in this chapter will, I hope, serve to better understand the nature of sufficientarianism.

For the sake of simplicity, I make four assumptions throughout this chapter. First, I confine my analysis to the *welfarist* framework. In other words, I consider only people's well-being and ignore other non-welfarist features, such as desert, responsibility, and freedom. Thus, I take *well-being* to be the currency of distributive

1. See Campbell Brown, "Priority or Sufficiency . . . or Both?" *Economics and Philosophy* 21, no. 2 (2005): 199–220; Roger Crisp, "Equality, Priority, and Compassion," *Ethics* 113, no. 4 (2003): 745–763; Robert Huseby, "Sufficiency: Restated and Defended," *Journal of Political Philosophy* 18, no. 2 (2010): 178–197.

judgment. Second, I use the notion of well-being in its broadest sense. There are different accounts of well-being: the subjective account, the objective list account, and so on. For the sake of structural analysis of sufficientarianism, I set aside the issue concerning the appropriate account of well-being. Third, I focus on a single sufficiency level. The results of my analysis in this chapter can easily be generalized to the multiple sufficiency-level cases. Fourth, I set aside the issues concerning whether the sufficiency level can be determined in a non-arbitrary way and how the sufficiency level is determined. I assume a well-defined sufficiency level.

The chapter is structured in the following way. In Section 2, I first formulate Harry Frankfurt's doctrine of sufficiency in the axiological form and show that his doctrine is untenable as an axiological principle. I then elucidate the basic aspiration of sufficientarianism, which I call the sufficientarian ethos. In Section 3, I consider how the disvalue of sub-sufficiency well-being should be measured. In Section 4, I first consider how the value of well-being above the sufficiency level should be taken into consideration and then offer a definite formula of axiological sufficientarianism. In Section 5, I examine what axiological sufficientarianism implies in cases in which the number of individuals in a population is variable (the variable-population size cases). Sufficientarianism avoids a much discussed problem in population ethics—Derek Parfit's repugnant conclusion. However, it implies another highly counterintuitive conclusion.

By axiological principle, I mean a principle that identifies a betterness ordering of states of affairs. Let X be a finite set of states of affairs and T be the sufficiency level. Let $N(x) = \{1, 2, \ldots, n\}$ be a set of individuals in $x \in X$, and let $S(x) \subset N(x)$ be a set of individuals below T in x. w_i denotes the well-being of person $i \in N(x)$. Define a weak betterness relation on X such that, for any pair $x,y \in X$, x is at least as good as y. For the present purpose, I assume that the betterness relation constitutes a complete weak ordering—that is, that it is reflexive, transitive, and complete.[2]

2. Frankfurt's Doctrine of Sufficiency and the Sufficientarian Ethos

The idea of sufficientarianism is commonly traced back to Harry Frankfurt's *doctrine of sufficiency*. His doctrine inspired and motivated a number of versions of sufficientarianism in the recent literature. Therefore, it is fitting to use Frankfurt's doctrine as a starting point of my axiological analysis.

---

2. A betterness relation on a set X is reflexive if and only if, for all $x \in X$, x is at least as good as x. It is transitive if and only if, for all $x,y,z \in X$, (1) x is at least as good as y and (2) y is at least as good as z together imply that x is at least as good as z. It is complete if and only if, for all $x,y \in X$, either x is at least as good as y or y is at least as good as x.

Frankfurt states the rough idea of the doctrine as follows:

> What is important from the point of view of morality is not that everyone should have the same, but that each should have enough. If everyone had enough, it would be of no moral consequence whether one had more than others.[3]

The main goal of Frankfurt's paper is to argue for the moral irrelevance of economic equality. It is not his main goal to put forward the doctrine of sufficiency as an axiological principle of well-being distribution. However, in passing, Frankfurt hints what the axiological claim of the doctrine would look like: "Another response to scarcity is to distribute the available resources in such a way that as many people as possible have enough or, in other words, to maximise the incidence of sufficiency."[4] In this passage, Frankfurt claims that the doctrine of sufficiency aims to maximize the number of individuals at or above sufficiency. It is not clear how seriously Frankfurt is committed to this claim because he does not elaborate it any further. However, in order to motivate the need for a precise axiological formula, I start by examining what this claim implies when it is understood as a general criterion for determining the relative goodness of states of affairs. The following is the direct translation of Frankfurt's claim into axiological language:

> **Frankfurt sufficientarianism (FS)**: A state of affairs x is at least as good as another y if and only if the number of individuals at or above T in x is at least as large as that in y.

According to FS, the relative goodness of states of affairs is determined solely by the number of individuals at or above T. Five remarks on FS are in order:

1. When the population size is fixed, FS is equivalent to the principle of *minimizing* the number of individuals below T: A state of affairs x is at least as good as another y if and only if the number of individuals below T in x is at least as small as that in y.
2. In cases in which the population size varies, FS is not equivalent to the minimization of the number of individuals below T. In these cases, FS judges the relative goodness of states of affairs, regardless of the number of individuals below T. Let us assume that $T = 10$ (in the rest of this chapter, I assume that $T = 10$). Compare a distribution of well-being for two persons, (0,10), with a distribution of well-being for four persons, (0,0,10,10). FS implies that (0,0,10,10)

---

3. Harry Frankfurt, "Equality as a Moral Ideal," *Ethics* 98, no. 1 (1987): 21.

4. Ibid., 31.

is strictly better than (0,10). Thus, according to FS, the number of individuals below *T* is an irrelevant consideration in the variable-population size cases.

3. The well-being level of individuals above *T* does not affect the relative goodness of states of affairs. Compare (0,10,10) and (0,20,20). FS implies that (0,10,10) is just as good as (0,20,20) because the number of individuals above *T* is two in both states.

4. The total size of shortfall from *T* does not affect the relative goodness of states of affairs. Compare (1,1,10) and (9,9,10). FS implies that (1,1,10) is just as good as (9,9,10).

5. The distribution of well-being among individuals below *T* does not affect the relative goodness of states of affairs. Compare (1,9,10) and (5,5,10). FS implies that (1,9,10) is just as good as (5,5,10). Furthermore, FS is insensitive to the absolute level of the worse-off individuals below *T*. Compare (0,10) and (4,6). FS implies that (0,10) is strictly better than (4,6).

Remarks 2–5 may each appear counterintuitive. Not surprisingly, the conjunction of these remarks shows that FS is even more counterintuitive. Compare (1,1,1,10) and (9,9,50). From remarks 2–4, FS implies that (1,1,1,10) is just as good as (9,9,50). This implication, however, is counterintuitive. FS seems to fail to capture what Frankfurt really wanted to say or what advocates of contemporary sufficientarianism aspire.

In order for the doctrine of sufficiency to serve as a reasonable axiological principle, we need to offer a different axiological formula without losing its basic aspiration. I speculate what Frankfurt and other advocates of sufficientarianism aspire to is to minimize the *disvalue* associated with the well-being of individuals below *T*, regardless of the aggregate value of well-being above *T*. I stated it as the *sufficientarian ethos*:

> **Sufficientarian ethos (SE):** The disvalue associated with well-being below *T* is to be minimized, regardless of the aggregate value of well-being at and above *T*.

According to SE, the primary concern for sufficientarianism is the disvalue associated with well-being below *T*, not the number of people above *T*. The value of well-being above *T* may or may not be a relevant consideration. However, the concern for the disvalue associated with well-being below *T* dominates the concern for the value of well-being above *T*. What I have to do now is to identify (1) how the disvalue associated with well-being below *T* should be measured and (2) how the value of well-being above *T* should be taken into account in determining the relative goodness of states of affairs. In Sections 3 and 4, I attempt to provide answers to both these issues and propose a precise formula that best represents SE in the fixed-population-size cases. I then examine the implications of this formula in the variable-population-size cases in Section 5.

3. The Disvalue of Sub-sufficiency Well-Being

In this section, I argue that the disvalue associated with well-being below T should be measured in such a way that a greater weight is given to benefits to the worse-off than the better-off below T.

Before starting my analysis, two qualifications are needed. First, it is incorrect to formulate sufficientarianism as the principle that aims to maximize the sum of well-being below T. This is because, if this formulation is correct, the outcome is made strictly better by taking some benefits from a person above T and lowering his or her well-being to the level below T. For example, compare (5,9) and (5,12). If sufficientarianism is understood as aiming to maximize the sum of well-being below T, it implies that (5,9) is strictly better than (5,12). However, such an implication is absurd. Thus, axiological sufficientarianism is not as simple as the maximization of the sum of well-being below T.

Second, it is also incorrect to formulate sufficientarianism as the principle that aims to minimize the sum of well-being below T. This is because, if this formulation is correct, the outcome is made strictly better by taking some benefits from any person below T and lowering the absolute level of his or her well-being. For example, compare (1,1,12) and (5,5,12). If sufficientarianism is formulated as the principle aiming to minimize the sum of well-being below T, (1,1,12) is strictly better than (5,5,12). However, such a judgment is absurd. The measurement of the value or disvalue of sub-sufficiency well-being is more complicated than the simple maximization or minimization of the sum of well-being below T.

The goal of SE is the minimization of the disvalue associated with the well-being below the sufficiency level. In what follows, by the disvalue of sub-sufficiency well-being, I mean the disvalue associated with the well-being below T. However, I do not mean that well-being below the sufficiency threshold is something sufficientarianism should aim to minimize.

Let me start with the simplest measure: the *head count method*.[5] According to the head count method, the disvalue is measured by the number of individuals below T. That is, the smaller the number of individuals below T, the better the state of affairs. As noted in remark 1 about FS, in the fixed population-size cases,

---

5. For the analysis of the head count method and total shortfall method (and the implausibility of these methods as the measure of poverty), see James E. Foster, "On Economic Poverty: A Survey of Aggregate measures," in *Advances in Economietrics*, ed. Robert Basmann and George Rhodes (Greenwich, CT: JAI Press, 1984), vol. 3, 215–251; Amartya Sen, "Poverty: An Ordinal Approach to Measurement," *Econometrica* 44, no. 2 (1976): 219–231.

the head count method is equivalent to FS. However, it is quite different from FS in the variable population-size cases. The head count method avoids the counterintuitive implication in remark 2. In remark 2, I noted that, according to FS, (0,0,10,10) is strictly better than (0,10). In contrast, the head count method judges that (0,10) is strictly better than (0,0,10,10).

However, the head count method is susceptible to the counterintuitive implications in remarks 4 and 5. Consider the example in remark 4—that is, the comparison between (1,1,10) and (9,9,10). The head count method implies that (1,1,10) is just as good as (9,9,10). However, (9,9,10) seems strictly better than (1,1,10). Why? Because (9,9,10) is strictly better than (1,1,10) for every person below T. Thus, the head count method and FS share the implausible implication in remark 4.

Next, consider the second example in remark 5–that is, the comparison between (0,10) and (4,6). The head count method implies that (0,10) is strictly better than (4,6). However, this implication seems counterintuitive: Many people would judge that (4,6) is indeed strictly better than (0,10). Why counterintuitive? That is because the well-being of the better-off person is brought up to T by lowering the well-being of the worse-off person. The head count method can justify the claim that we should take some benefits from people far below T and give them to people just below T because this reduces the total number of people below T. Many proponents of sufficientarianism would disagree. They would claim that the measure of the disvalue of sub-sufficiency well-being should be sensitive to the deterioration of the state of the worse-off below T. Thus, it is not plausible to measure the disvalue of sub-sufficiency well-being solely on the basis of the head count method.

Next, we consider a different method: the *total shortfall method*. The total shortfall method simply adds up the shortfall from T across people below T and takes the unweighted sum to be the measure of the disvalue of sub-sufficiency well-being. According to this method, (9,9,10) is strictly better than (1,1,10), although, as discussed previously, the head count method supports the contrary. In this respect, the total shortfall method is more plausible than the head count method.

However, the total shortfall method does not avoid the other problem that the head count method encounters. Compare again (0,10) and (4,6). In both states, the total shortfall is 10. Therefore, the total shortfall method judges that these two states are equally good. This means that, according to the total shortfall method, the outcome is insensitive to the distribution of well-being among individuals below T. This feature has the following implication: It is not better or worse even if we take some benefits from a person who is far below T and transfer them to a person who is just below T insofar as the total short fall remains unchanged. Like the head count method, the total shortfall method is insensitive to the deterioration of the state of the worse-off below T. Again, that is not, I suspect, what SE aims at.

Neither the head count method nor the total shortfall method is sensitive to the state of the worse-off individuals below T or the distribution of well-being below *T*. A plausible measure of the disvalue of sub-sufficiency well-being should take the distribution of well-being among people below *T* so that (4,6) is judged to be better than (0,10). How? The standard way is to impose the *Pigou–Dalton condition*.[6] The Pigou–Dalton condition holds that a transfer from a better-off person to a worse-off person decreases the disvalue of sub-sufficiency well-being when both persons are below *T* and the relative position of the two persons is not altered. When the Pigou–Dalton condition is imposed, given the total shortfall being constant, the disvalue of sub-sufficiency well-being is minimized when people's well-being is equally distributed below *T*. Thus, the Pigou–Dalton condition adds the egalitarian bias to the measurement of the disvalue of sub-sufficiency well-being.

The most general way to incorporate the Pigou–Dalton condition is to assign a greater weight to benefits to the worse-off than the better-off below *T* in the interpersonal aggregation of sufficiency shortfall. That is, the disvalue of sub-sufficiency well-being is measured by a weighted sum of different people's shortfall with the greater weights to the worse-off.

There are two ways to determine the weights of well-being below *T*. One is the *nonrelational approach*. According to the nonrelational approach, the weight is determined by the absolute shortfall of a person below *T*. Specifically, a greater weight is given to a greater absolute shortfall than a smaller absolute shortfall. When the nonrelational approach is adopted, the disvalue of the sub-sufficiency well-being in *x*, $V^{NR}(x)$, is given by the following general formula:

$$V^{NR}(x) = \sum_{i \in S(x)} f(T - w_i), \tag{3.1}$$

where $f()$ is some strictly increasing, strictly convex function.

"Strict convex" function is a function with an upward-curving graph. An example of this general formula is the sum of squares of different people's shortfall:[7]

$$V^{NR}(x) = \sum_{i \in S(x)} (T - w_i)^2. \tag{3.2}$$

In order to verify that this formula provides the desired result, consider (0,10) and (4,6) again. The disvalue of sub-sufficiency well-being in (0,10) is $(10 - 0)^2 +$

---

6. See Foster, "On Economic Poverty"; Sen, "Poverty."

7. This formula is somewhat similar to what economists call the *Foster–Greer–Thorbecke poverty measure* (FGT). See James E. Foster, Joel Greer, and Erik Thorbecke, "A Class of Decomposable Poverty Measures," *Econometrica* 52, no. 3 (1984): 761–766. The FGT measure normalizes each person's shortfall by the sufficiency level *T* and the weighted sum of shortfall by the total number of people for the purposes of inter-state comparison.

$(10 - 10)^2 = 100$, whereas that in $(4,6)$ is $(10 - 4)^2 + (10 - 6)^2 = 52$. Hence, the disvalue in $(0,10)$ is greater than the disvalue in $(4,6)$, as required.

According to the nonrelational approach, the weights are determined by the absolute size of each person's shortfall from T. According to this approach, the weight of a person's shortfall increases as the absolute distance from T becomes greater. In other words, the weight of a person's shortfall increases as the absolute level of his or her well-being becomes lower below T.

It is obvious that the nonrelational approach is *prioritarian* below T. According to the standard understanding of prioritarianism, the relative overall goodness of states of affairs is judged on the basis of a weighted sum of different people's well-being, where the weights are determined by an increasing, strictly concave function. That is, the marginal moral value of a person's well-being diminishes as the absolute level of his or her well-being gets higher. Prioritarianism is nonrelational in the sense that the weights are determined by the absolute level, not the relative position to other people's well-being.[8] The nonrelational approach to the measurement of the devalue of sub-sufficiency well-being uses a similar idea. The marginal moral disvalue of a person's shortfall from T increases as the absolute level of his or her well-being gets lower. This means that benefits to the worse-off matter more than benefits to the better-off insofar as their well-being is below T. Thus, the nonrelational approach is prioritarian below T.

The weights do not need to be determined by the absolute size of the shortfall. The weights may be determined in the relational manner. The *relational approach* determines the weights on the basis of the relative position of people below T.[9] Specifically, the disvalue is measured by a weighted sum of different people's sufficiency gap with the weights being determined by the rank-order position of the person in the ranking by well-being level below T. In other words, the relational approach assigns greater weights to benefits to the worse-off than the better-off below T, and it adds up the weighted shortfall. According to the relational approach, giving some benefit to the relatively worse-off person reduces a greater amount of disvalue than giving it to the relatively better-off person because the weight for the worse-off is greater than that for the better-off. Thus, the relational approach gives priority to benefits to the relatively worse-off people below T.

The following is an example of relational axiological sufficientarianism. Let $S'(x) = \{i, j, \ldots, m\}$ be a permutation of $S(x)$ such that $w_i \geq w_j \geq \cdots \geq w_m$. Let $s =$

8. See Iwao Hirose, *Egalitarianism* (London: Routledge, 2015); Derek Parfit, "Equality or Priority?" in *The Ideal of Equality*, ed. Matthew Clayton and Andrew Williams (Basingstoke, UK: Palgrave Macmillan, 2000), 81–125.

9. The relational approach is similar to what economists call the *ordinalist approach* to poverty measurement. See Sen, "Poverty."

#*S'*(*x*) be the number of individuals below *T* in *x*. Then, one type of relational sufficientarianism estimates the disvalue of sub-sufficiency well-being in *x*, $V^R(x)$, as follows:

$$V^R(x) = \frac{1}{s^2}[(T - w_i) + 3(T - w_j) + \cdots + (2s - 1)(T - w_m)]. \tag{3.3}$$

Both nonrelational and relational approaches assign greater weight to benefits to the worse-off below *T*. However, the two approaches assign weight in different ways. The nonrelational approach determines weight with reference to the absolute distance from *T*, whereas the relational approach determines weight with reference to the rank-order position. This difference is not merely a technical one. It implies two important theoretical differences, which are worth discussing briefly.

The first is that the nonrelational approach requires only *ordinal* level comparability, whereas the relational approach requires interpersonal comparable *cardinal* measure. Interpersonal comparable cardinal measure is more demanding than ordinal level comparability. If sufficientarianism is concerned with income poverty, this difference may not be so important. However, in many cases, sufficientarianism is concerned with the interpersonal distribution of well-being, and the measure for well-being is quite different from that for income. When one believes that one has access to a cardinal interpersonally comparable measure of well-being, one can adopt the nonrelational approach. Otherwise, one should adopt the relational approach.[10]

The second difference is that the nonrelational approach satisfies the *subgroup consistency property*, whereas the relational approach does not.[11] The subgroup consistency property holds that the disvalue of sub-sufficiency well-being decreases if a subgroup of the population experiences a reduction in the disvalue of subsufficiency well-being, while the disvalue of sub-sufficiency well-being in the rest of the population remains unchanged. The nonrelational approach satisfies the subgroup consistency property, whereas the relational approach does not.

In the economic literature on poverty measurement, many people take the subgroup consistency property to be a desirable property. Therefore, they prefer the nonrelational approach to the relational approach. Their preference is reasonable because they are concerned with income poverty, and it is easy to measure income cardinally. However, it is highly debatable whether the absolute level of well-being can be measured cardinally. If it is thought that the absolute level

---

10. Sen, "Poverty."

11. See James E. Foster and Anthony F. Shorrocks, "Subgroup Consistent Poverty Indices," *Econometrica* 59, no. 3 (1991): 688.

of well-being cannot be measured cardinally, then the relational approach to the disvalue of sub-sufficiency well-being is more attractive than the nonrelational one. The issue about the relative plausibility of the nonrelational and relational approaches comes down to the measurability of distributive currency. Although this issue is important, I do not discuss it any further here.

4. The Value of Well-Being Above Sufficiency

Having established how we measure the disvalue of sub-sufficiency well-being, I now consider how the value of well-being above T should be taken into account. This is not an easy task because advocates of sufficientarianism are ambiguous about this. For example, it is not clear how Roger Crisp's version of sufficientarianism takes the value of well-being above T into account.[12] He considers the Beverley Hills Case, in which a fine bottle of wine is made available to give to either the Super-Rich or the Rich in Beverley Hills. According to Crisp, prioritarianism implies that we should give the bottle to the Rich because the Rich's well-being is at a lower absolute level than the Super-Rich's well-being. However, Crisp finds it counterintuitive, and this allegedly counterintuitive implication of prioritarianism motivates him to propose his version of sufficientarianism. Nonetheless, he does not discuss what his version of sufficientarianism must say in the Beverley Hills Case.

There are three possible states in the Beverley Hills Case:

S1 Neither the Rich nor the Super-Rich receives the bottle (e.g., the bottle is destroyed).
S2 The Super-Rich receives the bottle.
S3 The Rich receives the bottle.

Crisp thinks it implausible to choose to bring about S3 outright. This is all Crisp says. Presumably, Crisp implies that S3 is not strictly better than S1 or S2. I see no reason for judging that S1 or S2 is the best. As far as I can see, there are two possibilities. The first possibility is that we judge S1, S2, and S3 are equally good. This means that benefits to the person above T do not matter at all. The second possibility is that S2 and S3 are equally good but strictly better than S1. This means that benefits to the person above T do matter but that the distribution of their well-being does not matter.

These two possibilities are represented by two different views about the value of well-being above T. The first possibility is represented by what I call the *pure*

12. Crisp, "Equality, Priority, and Compassion," 755.

view. The second possibility is represented by the *lexical view*. Both views are consistent with SE.

Let me start with the pure view. According to the pure view, the well-being above T carries no moral weight whatsoever and hence should not affect our judgment about the relative goodness of states of affairs. The pure view implies that the increase or decrease in the well-being above T does not make the outcome morally better or worse. Frankfurt seems to support this view, and I formulated FS as a version of the pure view.

However, the pure view is nonsensical as far as axiological analysis is concerned. According to the pure view, well-being has moral value below T but no moral value above T. The pure view has the following implication. Imagine that the well-being of a person above T is lowered to the level below T. According to the pure view, other things being equal, adding well-being below T is a good thing, whereas reducing the well-being level above T is not a good or a bad thing. Thus, the pure view implies that the outcome is made strictly better if the well-being of people above T is lowered to the level below T. But this is absurd. Regardless of whether a person's well-being is above or below T, everyone's well-being must have some moral weight insofar as it is above the level worth living.

It is a mistake to conceive of SE as the view that holds that well-being above T has no moral value. What sufficientarianism should state is that there is some degree of *moral disvalue* attached to well-being below T, whereas there is no moral disvalue attached to well-being above T. As discussed in the previous section, the disvalue is the weighted shortfall from T. Well-being below T always has some degree of this disvalue. Well-being above T does not have this disvalue because there is no shortfall from T. This is why I formulated SE as the view that aims to minimize the disvalue of sub-sufficiency well-being.

The reinterpretation of sufficientarianism in terms of the disvalue of sub-sufficiency well-being does not commit advocates of sufficientarianism to the claim that well-being above T has no moral value. Nor does it commit them to the claim that the value of well-being above T can outweigh the disvalue of sub-sufficiency well-being. The reinterpretation can lead them to what I call the lexical view.

According to the lexical view, sufficientarianism first aims to minimize the disvalue of sub-sufficiency well-being, regardless of the value of well-being above T. This is perfectly consistent with SE. The lexical view then claims that sufficientarianism is allowed to consider the aggregate value of well-being above T, provided that the disvalue of sub-sufficiency well-being is the same. The lexical view thus gives a complete priority to the minimization of the disvalue of sub-sufficiency well-being over the maximization of well-being above T. The aggregate value of well-being above T merely plays the role of tiebreaker. Nonetheless, the lexical view implies that every person's well-being has moral value, regardless of whether it is below or above T. However, the distribution of well-being above T is not taken into account. Thus, the value of well-being above T is measured by a sum of people's well-being above T.

I can finally present the definitive axiological formula of sufficientarianism. Although I referred to two approaches to the measurement of the disvalue of sub-sufficiency well-being, I present the general formula in the nonrelational approach:

> *Axiological sufficientarianism (AS)*: A state of affairs x is strictly better than another state y if and only if either

$$\sum_{i \in S(x)} f(T - w_i) < \sum_{i \in S(y)} f(T - w_i) \quad \text{or}$$

$$\sum_{i \in S(x)} f(T - w_i) = \sum_{i \in S(y)} f(T - w_i) \quad \text{and} \quad \sum_{j \in N(x) \backslash S(x)} w_j > \sum_{j \in N(y) \backslash S(y)} w_j,$$

where $f()$ is an increasing, strictly convex function.

In plain words, a state x is strictly better than y if and only if either (1) the weighted sum of sufficiency gap in x is strictly smaller than that in y or (2) the weighted sum of sufficiency gap in x is the same as that in y and the unweighted sum of well-being above T in x is strictly greater than that in y.

Two remarks are in order. First, AS implies that when there is no person below T, sufficientarianism is equivalent to classical utilitarianism. Few sufficientarians are explicit about this implication. To my knowledge, only John Skorupski explicitly claims it.[13]

Second, consider the following example to understand another implication of AS. Imagine a situation in which we can transfer some benefits from a person above T to a person below T. There are two options: (1) taking the benefits from a person just above T and (2) taking the same size of benefits from another person far above T. AS is neutral between options 1 and 2, provided that neither person falls below T as a result of the transfer. Some advocates of sufficientarianism may find such an implication to be counterintuitive. They may be tempted to claim that we should take the benefits from the person far above T rather than the person just above T. In other words, they may be tempted to give greater weights to benefits to the worse-off both below and above T. Advocates of sufficientarianism, however, must suppress this temptation. The reason is as follows: If

---

13. John Skorupski, "Threshold Justice," in *Ethical Explorations* (Oxford: Oxford University Press, 1999), 90.

sufficientarianism gives greater weights to benefits to the worse-off both below and above *T*, there will be little difference between sufficientarianism and prioritarianism. Prioritarianism is a nonrelational axiological principle that assigns greater weights to benefits to the worse-off. Although prioritarianism is not committed to the morally privileged level of well-being such as the sufficiency level, it is perfectly consistent with the notion of sufficiency insofar as the level of sufficiency is determined absolutely. Thus, sufficientarianism may well be viewed as a version of prioritarianism—that is, prioritarianism with a kink at *T*.[14] If advocates of sufficientarianism do not want to lose its edge, then they must be indifferent between options 1 and 2.

5. Variable Population-Size Cases

My analysis so far has been confined to the fixed population-size cases. However, sufficientarianism cannot be viewed as a general axiological principle unless we examine how it works in the variable population-size cases. In this section, I examine three implications in the variable population-size cases.

First, consider the *empty world case*.[15] Imagine a state of affairs that contains no human well-being. Call it A. Imagine another state, in which one or more persons are below *T*. Call this state B. For the present purpose, it does not matter whether there are people above *T* in B. According to AS, A is strictly better than B because there is no disvalue of sub-sufficiency well-being in A, whereas there is some in B. Is it plausible to judge that A is strictly better than B?

Some people think that it is implausible to judge that A is strictly better than B. Paula Casal, for example, thinks that it is implausible to rank A above B. She further claims that sufficientarianism implies this allegedly implausible conclusion insofar as it is formulated as a minimizing principle of the disvalue of sub-sufficiency well-being. According to Casal, sufficientarianism must be formulated as a maximizing principle to avoid the allegedly implausible conclusion in the empty world case. In what follows, I show that Casal's claim is false. It does not matter whether sufficientarianism is formulated as a maximizing principle or a minimizing principle. We can rewrite AS as a maximizing principle:

---

14. I showed elsewhere that AS satisfies (1) the Pareto principle, (2) strong separability, and (3) the Pigou–Dalton condition, and that all three of these conditions are necessary and jointly sufficient conditions of prioritarianism. Thus, AS is a special case of prioritarianism. See Iwao Hirose, *Equality, Priority, and Aggregation* (St. Andrews, UK: University of St. Andrews, 2004).

15. See Paula Casal, "Why Sufficiency Is Not Enough," *Ethics* 117, no. 2 (2007): 298; Robert Huseby, "Sufficiency and Population Ethics," *Ethical Perspectives* 19, no. 2 (2012): 197.

Maximizing sufficientarianism (MS): A state of affairs x is strictly better than another state y if and only if either

$$\sum_{i \in S(x)} [g(w_i) - g(T)] > \sum_{i \in S(y)} [g(w_i) - g(T)] \quad \text{or}$$

$$\sum_{i \in S(x)} [g(w_i) - g(T)] > \sum_{i \in S(y)} [g(w_i) - g(T)] \quad \text{and} \quad \sum_{j \in N(x) \setminus S(x)} w_j > \sum_{j \in N(y) \setminus (S(y)} w_j,$$

where $g()$ is an increasing, strictly concave function.

Although MS has a maximizing principle, it still implies that A is strictly better than B. This means that sufficientarianism, be it in the maximizing or the minimizing form, makes the same judgment about the relative goodness of A and B. Thus, the empty world case is not the issue about the minimizing structure of sufficientarianism. It is about something else.

Here is my analysis about the empty world case: The original question (i.e., "Is it plausible to judge that A is better than B?") is misleading. If we attempt to answer this question directly, we will miss the real issue behind the empty world case. The real issue is about the *discontinuity* between the value of well-being above T and the disvalue of well-being below T. Specifically, it is about the lexical dominance of sub-sufficiency improvement over *any* above-sufficiency improvement. SE tells us to minimize the disvalue associated with well-being below T, no matter how large the aggregate value of well-being above T would be. Any reduction in the disvalue of sub-sufficiency well-being, no matter how small, outweighs any loss in the aggregate value of above-sufficiency well-being, no matter how large. This is a radical claim, but it is the claim to which advocates of SE are committed. Thus, advocates of SE do not find it implausible to judge that A is strictly better than B in the empty world case.

To illustrate my point, add a third state, A*, to the comparison of A and B. A* contains only one person's well-being at T. For the sake of argument, let me be more specific about B. Let us suppose that, in B, one person's well-being is just below T and 1 billion people have well-being far above T. Any intelligible axiological formulation of SE ranks these three states in the following descending order:

A*: One person's well-being is just above T.
A: No well-being.
B: One person's well-being is just below T and 1 billion people's well-being is far above T.

Any axiological formulation of SE implies that A* is strictly better than A and that A is strictly better than B. By transitivity, it follows that A* is strictly better than B. Some people would find it counterintuitive to judge that A* is strictly better than

B. In the same sense, they would find it counterintuitive to judge that A is better than B. They are opposed to discontinuity between the value of well-being above T and the disvalue of well-being below T.

In contrast, advocates of sufficientarianism find it perfectly plausible to judge that A is better than B in the same sense that A^* is better than B. For them, it is perfectly plausible to state that any gain for a person below T, no matter how small, outweighs any loss for people above T, no matter how large, because they are already committed to SE, which entails the discontinuity of value. The empty world case does not pose any distinctive problem to those who have already committed themselves to SE. It merely shows that sufficientarianism is radical. Needless to say, there is the issue concerning whether the discontinuity of value is acceptable. However, this issue is separate and more general.

Second, consider what Derek Parfit calls the *repugnant conclusion*. The repugnant conclusion states that

> for any possible population of at least ten billion people, all with a very high quality of life, there must be some much larger imaginable population whose existence, if other things are equal, would be better even though its members have lives that are barely worth living.[16]

Many people agree with Parfit that this conclusion is repugnant. However, many axiological principles, such as classical utilitarianism and prioritarianism, imply the repugnant conclusion.

Does sufficientarianism imply the repugnant conclusion? No, it does not.[17] To explain why, I need to introduce the notion of the level worth living. If a person's well-being is lower than the level worth living, then his or her well-being contributes to the goodness of a state of affairs negatively. If it is higher than the level worth living, then his or her well-being contributes positively. I believe it uncontroversial to assume that the level worth living is lower than T.

What does sufficientarianism say about the comparison between the population with a very high quality of life and the much larger population with well-being barely worth living? The population with a very high quality of life does not have the disvalue of sub-sufficiency well-being. In contrast, the "much larger population" has the disvalue of sub-sufficiency well-being. Therefore, according to sufficientarianism, the population with a very high quality of life is better than the much larger population with well-being barely worth living. Sufficientarianism does not imply the repugnant conclusion.

---

16. Derek Parfit, *Reasons and Persons* (Oxford: Oxford University Press, 1984), 388.

17. Huseby, "Sufficiency and Population Ethics," 193.

If sufficientarianism implies a variant of the repugnant conclusion, it must be in terms of cases in which there is no well-being below T or the disvalue of sub-sufficiency is constant. In those cases, we can consider the following variant of the repugnant conclusion: For any possible population of at least 10 billion people, all with a very high quality of life, there must be some much larger imaginable population whose existence, other things being equal, would be better even though its members have lives that are barely above T. It is clear that sufficientarianism implies this conclusion. However, the conclusion is not repugnant. Given that everyone in the "much larger population" has well-being above T, there is nothing repugnant in that conclusion. Thus, advocates of sufficientarianism happily endorse such a conclusion.

The third implication is that sufficientarianism implies what Gustaf Arrhenius calls the *very sadistic conclusion*: For any population with negative well-being (e.g., tormented lives), there is a population with positive well-being that is worse, other things being equal.[18] Imagine a state that contains a small number of individuals who endure severe suffering everyday during their entire lives. Their well-being is far below not only T but also the level worth living. Call this state C, and assume there are no other people. Imagine another state, which contains a large number of individuals who have well-being just below T but well above the level worth living. Call this state D. According to AS, C is strictly better than D if the disvalue of sub-sufficiency well-being in C is smaller than that in D. That is, AS may well judge that the population with well-being far below the level worth living is strictly better than the population with well-being just below T and well above the level worth living.

To visualize the very sadistic conclusion, consider an example. Suppose that the level worth living is 0, and that we use Eq. (3.2) as the measure of the disvalue of sub-sufficiency well-being. Compare two distributions: $(-2,-2)$ and $(4,4,\ldots,4)$. In $(-2,-2)$, there are two people, whose well-being is below the level worth living. In $(4,4,\ldots,4)$, there are many people, whose well-being is just below T but well above the level worth living. According to Eq. (3.2), if the number of people in $(4,4,\ldots,4)$ is eight, $(-2,-2)$ is as good as $(4,4,\ldots,4)$. If it is greater than eight, $(-2,-2)$ is strictly better, although there is no person whose life is worth living. Thus, AS implies the very sadistic conclusion.

Can the state, in which no person's well-being is worth living, really be better than the state in which all people's well-being is well worth living but below T? I do not think it can. Imagine that you are the only person who exists. Suppose that your well-being is above T. If you are asked to comapre (1) adding two people whose well-being is at -2 and hence below the level worth living and (2) adding

18. See Gustaf Arrhenius, "An Impossibility Theorem for Welfarist Axiologies," *Economics and Philosophy* 16, no. 2 (2000): 251.

nine people whose well-being is at 4 and hence above the level worth living (but below *T*), how would you rank these two alternatives? Few people would judge that (1) is better than (2). However, AS implies that (1) is better than (2) .

It may be argued that sufficientarianism can be saved from the very sadistic conclusion by introducing multiple sufficiency levels. One level is the sufficiency level, and the other level is the level worth living. According to this multilevel view, the disvalue of well-being below the level worth living dominates the disvalue of well-being below the sufficiency level. This view makes perfect sense. However, it does not avoid the very sadistic conclusion. The view implies the possibility that a small population with hellish life is strictly better than a larger population with well-being just below the level worth living. Thus, the multilevel sufficientarianism does not save sufficientarianism from the very sadistic conclusion.

Axiological sufficientarianism thus implies the very sadistic conclusion. This is bad news for sufficientarianism. However, there is consolation. To date, there is no alternative axiological principle that is perfectly plausible in the variable population-size cases.[19]

6. Conclusion

The main results I reported in this chapter are as follows:

- Frankfurt's original presentation of the doctrine of sufficiency is not tenable as an axiological principle.
- The sufficientarian ethos is to minimize the disvalue associated with well-being below sufficiency, regardless of the aggregate value of well-being above sufficiency.
- The measure of the disvalue associated with well-being below sufficiency should satisfy the Pigou–Dalton condition and assign greater weights, relational or nonrelational, to benefits to the worse-off below *T*.
- The pure view, which assigns no moral value to benefits to people above *T*, is nonsensical. The aggregate value of well-being above sufficiency should be measured by the sum of well-being above *T*.
- Axiological sufficientarianism holds that a state *x* is strictly better than *y* if and only if either (1) the weighted sum of the sufficiency gap in *x* is strictly smaller than that in *y* or (2) the weighted sum of the sufficiency gap in *x* is the same as that in *y* and the unweighted sum of well-being above sufficiency in *x* is strictly greater than that in *y*.

---

19. Gustaf Arrhenius, *Population Ethics* (Oxford: Oxford University Press, forthcoming).

• In the variable population-size cases, axiological sufficientarianism avoids the repugnant conclusion, but it implies the very sadistic conclusion.

Acknowledgments

I am grateful to Ralf Bader and the editors of this volume, Carina Fourie and Annette Rid, for helpful comments on an earlier version of this chapter.

4

Sufficiency, Priority, and Aggregation

Robert Huseby

1. Introduction

Few people would say, with a straight face, that we live in a just world. But even if many agree that injustice is rampant, there is less agreement on what justice in fact requires. In the current debate about distributive justice, at least the strand of it concerned with telic principles, four theories are extensively discussed and analyzed: egalitarianism, prioritarianism, sufficientarianism, and utilitarianism.[1] These theories come in different forms and shapes, and none of them are immune to criticism.[2] My own view is that, all things considered, a particular version of sufficiency is the most plausible account of what distributive justice demands.[3] This

---

1. Although most of the examples used in this chapter concern domestic settings, I take it that most telic principles are global in scope. Telic principles are principles in light of which we can judge some state of affairs as good or bad in itself, regardless of how it came about. For instance, a telic egalitarian would judge as bad a state of affairs in which people are unequally well off. A deontic egalitarian would have to know how that state of affairs came about in order to make a judgment. See Kasper Lippert-Rasmussen, "The Insignificance of the Distinction Between Telic and Deontic Egalitarianism," in *Egalitarianism: New Essays on the Meaning and Value of Equality*, ed. Nils Holtug and Kasper Lippert-Rasmussen (Oxford: Oxford University Press, 2007), 102.

2. I assume throughout that some form of welfare is the relevant currency of justice. I specify this in relation to sufficiency, but I make no attempt to argue that welfare is the superior currency of distributive justice.

3. The classic contemporary formulation of sufficiency is due to Harry Frankfurt, "Equality as a Moral Ideal," *Ethics* 98, no. 1 (1987): 21–43. For further defenses, see Elizabeth Anderson, "What Is the Point of Equality?" *Ethics* 109, no. 2 (1999): 287–337; Yitzhak Benbaji, "The Doctrine of Sufficiency: A Defence," *Utilitas* 17, no. 3 (2005): 310–332; Roger Crisp, "Equality, Priority, and Compassion," *Ethics* 113, no. 4 (2003): 745–763; and Liam Shields, "The

view has as its central concern that individuals should be sufficiently well off, and it requires, roughly, that insufficiency should be minimized, to the extent that this is compatible with sufficiency attainment over time. Sufficiency, both in this and other renderings, has implications that many find troubling. In this chapter, I single out two such implications and argue that they can be avoided, at least on a suitable formulation of the view. Moreover, this result, I claim, amounts to a comparative advantage over prioritarianism (and utilitarianism).[4]

In my discussion, I focus on prioritarianism—the view that benefits matter more the worse off the recipient is, the larger the benefit is, and the more recipients there are—as the most viable alternative to sufficiency.[5] The reason is mainly that prioritarianism incorporates, to a certain extent, some of the most intuitively appealing aspects of both egalitarianism and utilitarianism, without (it is generally assumed) taking on board the most problematic aspects of these two theories. Importantly, prioritarianism tends, in many cases, toward equality because it prioritizes the worse-off. At the same time, it sacrifices, in many cases, relatively little utility because the number of recipients and the size of the benefits matter too.

After presenting sufficiency and, briefly, prioritarianism, I introduce and rebut an objection pressed by Nils Holtug, Carl Knight, and Karl Widerquist. They argue that sufficientarianism, due to its aversion to some forms of aggregation, implies that we cannot, for instance, build a new road that will benefit thousands if the construction work is likely to bring a few (injured road workers, perhaps) below the sufficiency threshold.[6] This suggests that sufficientarianism is incompatible with social life as we know it. If the objection can be sustained, sufficientarians

---

Prospects for Sufficientarianism," *Utilitas* 24, no. 1 (2012): 101–117. The version of sufficiency that I defend here was first outlined in Robert Huseby, "Sufficiency: Restated and Defended," *Journal of Political Philosophy* 18, no. 2 (2010): 178–197. Note that Section 2 of the current chapter draws on and revises this account. For an influential criticism of sufficientarian theories, see Paula Casal, "Why Sufficiency Is Not Enough," *Ethics* 117, no. 2 (2007): 296–326.

4. There are several other objections to sufficiency, many of which have been discussed elsewhere. See Paula Casal, "Sufficiency Is Not Enough"; Larry Temkin, "Egalitarianism Defended," *Ethics* 113, no. 4 (2003): 764–782; Carl Knight, "Enough Is Too Much," unpublished manuscript; Benbaji, "The Doctrine of Sufficiency,"; Huseby, "Sufficiency: Restated"; Robert Huseby, "Sufficiency and Population Ethics," *Ethical Perspectives* 19, no. 2 (2012): 187–206; Shields, "Prospects for Sufficientarianism."

5. Nils Holtug, *Persons, Interests, and Justice* (Oxford: Oxford University Press, 2010); Richard J. Arneson, "Equality of Opportunity for Welfare Defended and Recanted," *Journal of Political Philosophy* 7, no. 4 (1999): 488–497; Carl Knight, *Luck Egalitarianism: Equality, Responsibility, and Justice* (Edinburgh, UK: Edinburgh University Press, 2009); Knight, "Enough Is Too Much." For a critical assessment, see Michael Otsuka and Alex Voorhoeve, "Why It Matters That Some Are Worse Off Than Others," *Philosophy and Public Affairs* 37, no. 2 (2009): 171–199.

6. Holtug, *Persons, Interests, Justice*, 236–237; Knight, "Enough Is Too Much," 29–30; Karl Widerquist, "How the Sufficiency Minimum Becomes a Social Maximum," *Utilitas* 22, no. 4 (2010): 474–480.

have compelling reason to abandon their theory. I argue, however, that sufficiency avoids this objection, largely because sufficientarianism entails that we have to balance immediate insufficiency against future insufficiency. Thus, sufficientarians need not oppose road-building on a principled basis.

I then consider the further objection, posed by Karl Widerquist, that sufficientarianism implies that all of society's surplus resources must be channeled toward persons who have difficulties reaching the sufficiency level. I argue that on my formulation of the view, this objection also fails.

2. Sufficiency

In my opinion, the following version of sufficientarianism seems plausible:

> *Sufficiency:* It is, in itself, bad if a person is not sufficiently well off. It is worse the farther below a sufficient level a person is, it is especially bad if a person's basic needs are unmet, and worse the more people that are not sufficiently well off.[7]

This formulation needs some specification, particularly with regards to (1) what counts as being sufficiently well off and (2) how we should prioritize between different insufficiently well-off individuals.

2.1. Minimal and Maximal Thresholds

The means to subsistence can reasonably be viewed as a necessary and morally fundamental part of sufficiency. It would be absurd to claim that a person lacking such means is sufficiently well off. In light of this, it makes sense to place the minimal threshold at the point where basic needs are met. Insufficiency below this level is especially problematic from a moral standpoint.[8] Access to the means of subsistence, however, is not a sufficient condition for sufficiency. Merely being able to maintain one's existence does not preclude further moral claims for distribution.

What about the maximal threshold, then? The basic, although imprecise, intuition driving my support of sufficientarianism is that people should have good lives, and that it is morally bad whenever they do not. In brief, I hold that people are in typical cases sufficiently well off if they are content[9] and in non-typical cases

---

7. Huseby, "Sufficiency: Restated," 180. For a related statement, see Crisp, "Equality, Priority, Compassion," 758. My interpretation of the principle, however, differs from that of Crisp in several respects.

8. See Huseby, "Sufficiency: Restated," 180.

9. Frankfurt, too, appeals to subjective contentment. Contentment, on his account, concerns money rather than welfare. See Frankfurt, "Equality as a Moral Ideal."

if they are as well off as possible without jeopardizing general sufficiency attainment over time.

In my view, individuals' subjective standpoints should be taken into account, but not exclusively. "Subjective" here refers to an individual's *overall* self-assessment of her welfare level. Intuitively, the extent to which individuals consider themselves sufficiently well off should influence the location of the maximal sufficiency threshold. As a first approximation, then, we could consider equating the maximal threshold with the welfare level at which an individual would herself be content.[10] Being content does not mean that one could not have wished for even more or that one has no interest in doing even better. I mean by content the sort of satisfaction one can have with one's life even though it is in some respects imperfect, and even though some others are better off than oneself.[11]

It might, for familiar reasons, be difficult to rely solely on subjective assessments because some people need huge resources in order to be content. Some might have preferences for costly goods, whereas others may require expensive support because of physical or mental impairments. Yet others would not be content even at a level of preference satisfaction with which most others would have been content (regardless of the price of their preferences), for instance, due to a gloomy or pessimistic character. Lifting these individuals to the maximum threshold of sufficiency may be prohibitively expensive. Thus, the subjective account must be curtailed to some extent.

One might ask why. If it is bad that some are insufficiently well off, and worse, the farther below the threshold they are, it seems that we really should prioritize the worst-off, come what may. However, this would mean that too many resources would be spent on a relatively small number of individuals, some of whom it might even be impossible to make sufficiently well off. This would jeopardize sufficiency for all over time. Because the aim is to minimize insufficiency, we have to balance shortfalls here and now against future shortfalls.

But how should we respond to the claims of those who have difficulties reaching a sufficient level of welfare? Here is one suggestion. Assume that every person has a number of preferences. These preferences can be more or less costly and also more or less difficult to satisfy (although not necessarily for reasons of cost). Assume further that these preferences can be ranked, from a first-person perspective, in terms of importance. For each individual, there are several combinations or sets of preferences (all of them including some of the more important ones) that are such that their simultaneous satisfaction would result in subjective

---

10. Huseby, "Sufficiency: Restated," 181.

11. Huseby, "Sufficiency: Restated," 181.

contentment. In addition, we can assume that for some individuals, it is the case that *all* sets of preferences the simultaneous satisfaction of which would result in subjective contentment include some preferences that, for different reasons, are either very costly or very difficult to satisfy.

Individuals who require the satisfaction of unduly expensive preferences, or of preferences that are very difficult to satisfy (and therefore sometimes expensive), will need large shares of resources in order to be content. The same is true for individuals who have difficulties achieving contentment because the sets of preferences the simultaneous satisfaction of which would make them subjectively content are few and large. Such people need not have expensive preferences, or preferences that are very difficult to satisfy, but they require unusually many of their preferences to be satisfied in order to experience subjective contentment.

I suggest that these three groups should split a share of resources that is as large as could be without undermining general sufficiency attainment either in the short or the long term. The assumption is that there is some portion of the available resources that is adequate for securing sufficiency for the majority over time and that the remainder is to be distributed among the minority, which consists of individuals who require more resources than others in order to be sufficiently well off.

On this account, then, the demands of sufficiency can be met even though some people are not in fact content, if the reason for their not being content is one of the following: (1) They require an unusually high level of preference satisfaction, (2) one or more of their preferences are very expensive, (3) one or more of their preferences are very difficult to satisfy, or (4) some combination of reasons 1–3.

2.2. Prioritization Between Insufficiently Well-Off Individuals

A further question is how we should distribute resources among those who have difficulties becoming sufficiently well off. The same question arises, of course, in situations of scarcity in which no one, or only a few, are sufficiently well off. These situations should be dealt with in the same way.

Sufficiency can be interpreted as a form of inverse and (doubly) constrained prioritarianism.[12] According to prioritarianism, benefiting a person matters more the worse off the person is. Much the same can be said about sufficientarianism. The difference is that whereas prioritarianism values morally weighted welfare, in the sense that benefits matter more the lower the welfare level of the recipient, sufficientarianism (on the account presented here) *disvalues* morally weighted

---

12. Huseby, "Sufficiency: Restated," 184–185. I say more about prioritarianism later.

shortfalls from the maximal threshold (and does not value welfare above that threshold).[13]

There are two constraints, both of which follow readily from the way the principle is formulated. First, welfare shortfalls are morally relevant only below the maximal threshold. Second, the badness of welfare shortfalls increases gradually only between the two thresholds. At the lower threshold, the badness of shortfalls increases nongradually because basic needs are especially urgent. On most versions of prioritarianism, in contrast, the moral weighting of welfare is gradual all the way down.

This specification is open to some interpretation, not least with respect to the exact significance of the lower threshold. Nevertheless, it should be sufficient to suggest the manner in which prioritization among insufficiently well-off individuals should be carried out. Note, however, that further concerns could also be relevant. To take one prominent example, many would think that those who are themselves responsible for their expensive preferences have weaker claims than those who are not thus responsible. I leave these questions aside here.

2.3. Relative (Maximal) Threshold and Deontological Constraints

The principle of sufficiency supposes that it is possible for individuals to be content even though not all of their preferences are satisfied and even if others have more. Both these assumptions strike me as plausible. However, it is arguably difficult to be subjectively content if one is *much* worse off than *many* others.[14] Given the subjective aspect of sufficiency, the maximal threshold will vary with societal welfare levels and distributive profiles.[15] This feature helps explain why even many non-egalitarians are hostile to certain inequalities.[16]

Sufficiency is also compatible with versions of deontic egalitarianism. Sufficiency is a telic principle according to which a state of affairs in which some people are not sufficiently well off is, for that reason, morally bad. This does not rule out the possibility that it may be bad, in a deontic sense, if A is

---

13. Huseby, "Sufficiency: Restated," 184–185.

14. Huseby, "Sufficiency: Restated," 184–185. See also Edward Page, *Climate Change, Justice and Future Generations* (Cheltenham, UK: Elgar, 2007), 94.

15. The same is not true of the minimal threshold. Basic needs are (more) objective. The extent to which my basic needs are met does not seem to depend on the extent to which your basic needs are met.

16. Note that there are of course further, instrumental, reasons to avoid large inequalities, for instance that large inequalities may lead to societal conflict.

rendered worse off than she used to be because of B's (morally unjustifiable) acts or omissions. This holds true even if A is still sufficiently well off. The unjustifiable acts or omissions may well be those denied by deontic theories (egalitarian or not).[17]

3. Prioritarianism

Prioritarianism is a forceful view of distributive justice, and it has been subject to substantial theoretical scrutiny and refinement by Derek Parfit, Nils Holtug, Richard Arneson, and others.[18] Egalitarians would agree with prioritarians in many cases because prioritarians will often prefer more equal outcomes.[19] However, because prioritarians do not believe that equality is intrinsically valuable, there is a real and interesting difference between the two principles.[20] The similarities between priority and sufficiency are also striking. Many sufficientarians agree with prioritarians in situations in which the worst-off are insufficiently well off. Prioritarians, however, reject any sufficiency line as a cutoff point for moral concern.

On Holtug's account, prioritarianism holds that "an outcome in which a benefit falls at a lower level is *intrinsically* better than an outcome in which an equal benefit falls at a higher level."[21] This means that the moral value of a benefit of a given size diminishes with the increasing welfare level of the person who receives it. As a principle for ranking outcomes, Holtug proposes the following:

> *Overall outcome welfare prioritarianism*: An outcome is intrinsically better, the larger a sum of weighted benefits it contains, where benefits are weighted such that they gain greater value, the worse off the individual to whom they accrue.[22]

While prioritizing the worst-off, this form of prioritarianism still allows larger gains at a higher level of welfare to outweigh smaller gains at a lower level. It is commonly assumed that sufficientarianism (and absolute prioritarianism) does not.[23]

---

17. Huseby, "Sufficiency: Restated," 185.

18. Arneson, "Equality of Opportunity"; Holtug, *Persons, Interests, Justice*; Derek Parfit, "Equality and Priority," *Ratio* 10, no. 3 (1997): 202–221.

19. Derek Parfit, "Another Defense of the Priority View," *Utilitas* 24, no. 3 (2012): 401.

20. Parfit, "Another Defense," 401.

21. Holtug, *Persons, Interests, Justice*, 132.

22. Holtug, *Persons, Interests, Justice*, 133.

23. I discuss this further later.

4. The Problem of Aggregation

In the context of distributive justice and moral theory, aggregation implies that benefits to some individuals can outweigh or justify losses to others, if the sum of the (morally weighted) benefits outweighs the sum of the (morally weighted) losses.[24] For instance, a large benefit to a badly off individual might outweigh small losses to 10 (or 1000) well-off individuals. However, by the same token, and depending on one's favored principle, a (very) large benefit to a well-off person might outweigh small losses to 10 (or 1000) badly off individuals.

Prioritarians and utilitarians have often been criticized because their theories allow intuitively problematic aggregation, or what I refer to as "negative" aggregation.[25] One famous illustration is provided by T. M. Scanlon:

> Jones has suffered an accident in the transmitter room of a television station. Electrical equipment has fallen on his arm, and we cannot rescue him without turning off the transmitter for fifteen minutes. A World Cup match is in progress, watched by many people, and it will not be over for an hour. Jones' injury will not get any worse if we wait, but his hand has been smashed and he is receiving extremely painful electrical shocks. Should we rescue him now or wait until the match is over? . . . It seems to me that we should not wait, no matter how many viewers there are.[26]

Prioritarians cannot accommodate this judgment, at least not if the benefits of uninterrupted World Cup action to millions outweigh Jones' injury and pain, which—at some point—we can assume to be the case. Recall, however, that even if prioritarianism allows aggregation in many cases, the values of the losses and gains are always morally weighted so that benefits and losses count for more (positively and negatively) the worse off an individual is. Whereas a utilitarian would simply sum up the benefits to the spectators and compare them with the loss (or harm) to Jones, a prioritarian would give more weight to Jones' harm and less weight to the benefits of the spectators (on the reasonable assumption that they are better off than Jones because he is currently in severe pain).[27] Sufficientarians,

---

24. Aggregation can be both interpersonal and intrapersonal. Here, I discuss only the former.

25. Casal, "Sufficiency Is Not Enough," 320–321; Crisp, "Equality, Priority, Compassion," 754; Knight, "Enough Is Too Much," 28–29.

26. T. M. Scanlon, *What We Owe to Each Other* (Cambridge, MA: Harvard University Press, 1998), 235.

27. Jones might still be better off than some or all viewers over the course of their lives. I leave aside here the question of whether one should adopt a whole-life or time-slice view of prioritarianism. For further discussion, see Parfit, "Another Defense."

on the other hand, gladly agree with Scanlon in the transmitter room case because to them, Jones' welfare matters more than the fans' welfare because he is insufficiently well off, to say the least.

As indicated previously, however, sufficientarians have trouble with aggregation too, perhaps equally severe. They can be charged with rejecting aggregation even in cases in which it really does make intuitive sense to let many small benefits outweigh substantial losses to a few. I refer to these cases as cases of "positive" aggregation.[28] For example, most of us accept some risk of injury and death on our roads in order to facilitate rapid and easy transport and communication.[29] Injury and death are severe losses to those individuals who suffer them, whereas the gains delivered by efficient transport are arguably quite small in most cases, at least when divided by the number of beneficiaries.

Thus, although aggregation has been used as ammunition against prioritarianism (and utilitarianism), it could readily backfire. The challenge for sufficientarians is to examine whether or not it is possible to distinguish between cases of intuitively "positive" and "negative" aggregation in a way that gives plausible reasons to accept the former and reject the latter.

In summary, then, prioritarianism runs the risk of accepting the negative kind of aggregation, whereas sufficientarianism runs the risk of rejecting the positive form of aggregation. Ideally, a theory of distributive justice should make neither error. In the following sections, I argue, first, that it is unlikely that prioritarianism can escape the implausibility of the negative form of aggregation and, second, that sufficientarianism can largely avoid the implausibility of denying the positive form.

4.1. Why Adjusted Prioritarianism Cannot Escape Cases of Negative Aggregation

Carl Knight has suggested that prioritarianism could be adjusted such that small benefits, below some threshold, do not count in the welfare calculations. If so, (sufficiently) minor benefits for the many can never outweigh substantial losses to a few. Can prioritarians get off the hook in this way? This does not seem likely. To be sure, such an adjustment might *reduce* the number of cases in which prioritarianism leads to negative aggregation, but there will be

---

28. I use these labels to signal what a sufficientarian would want to accomplish: Accept the positive and reject the negative. I also think the labels are intuitively acceptable to many people, even though some prioritarians and utilitarians would of course accept most forms of aggregation and would object to the proposed labels.

29. Widerquist, "Minimum Becomes a Maximum."

plenty of cases left, unless some form of absolute priority for the worse-off is accepted. Such absolutism, however, is shunned by most contemporary prioritarians,[30] and the problem of resource drainage associated with such views is, moreover, one of the most important objections prioritarians have against sufficientarianism.[31]

Knight's suggestion, of course, does not amount to absolutism. However, depending (to some extent) on where the threshold for non-minor benefits is set, there would still be many implausible cases. If a severe loss to a badly off person (e.g., the loss of his home) can be outweighed by many non-minor benefits to thousands of very well-off individuals (e.g., a free dinner at a top-notch restaurant, which at least counts as non-minor in my book), I would still think that aggregation would be wrong and suspect that others would think so as well. On the other hand, if the bar for non-minor benefits is raised very high, we would be approaching some form of semi-absolutism, and the resource drainage problem would surface again.

A different version of adjusted prioritarianism might hold that "the number of beneficiaries matters less the better off they are."[32] On this view, aggregation is again constrained in a way that makes it less likely that small benefits to the well-off outweigh substantial losses to the worse-off. This will also reduce the number of implausible cases, but not sufficiently so. There could still be instances in which minor benefits to a large number of moderately well-offs (to whom benefits still count for something) will outweigh the substantial losses to one or a few who are even worse off. The transmitter room case might be an example, assuming the viewers have an average level of welfare. Although this version of prioritarianism will be superior to ordinary prioritarianism, it will still have implausible implications in many cases.

This conclusion need not pose too much of a problem for prioritarians. The reason is that to the extent which they succeed in blocking some cases of negative aggregation, they also, it seems, rule out many cases of positive aggregation. For instance, one might ask if a shortened commute due to a new bridge is a minor or non-minor benefit. If it is minor, prioritarians of the adjusted type would not accept the bridge project. If it is a non-minor benefit, benefits of a similar size could add up to outweigh the imposition of lasting, severe pain, as the transmitter room case illustrates. In effect, adjusted forms of prioritarianism would not allow all the negative cases of aggregation that standard prioritarianism would allow,

30. Richard Arneson, "Equality of Opportunity"; Holtug, *Persons, Interests, Justice*; Knight, "Enough Is Too Much," 24.

31. Knight, "Enough Is Too Much."

32. Crisp, "Equality, Priority, Compassion," 754. See also Knight, "Enough Is Too Much," 29.

but for each such case they avoid, it is likely that they would deny a positive case of aggregation.

4.2. Sufficientarianism and Aggregation in Cases of Socially Useful Projects

As indicated previously, most of us seem willing to accept positive aggregation. We do not object to the building of large bridges, even if "some will predictably suffer death or serious injury, all for the sake of a shortened commute for many more."[33] Must sufficientarians ban the building of bridges, roads, and other socially useful projects because, predictably, such projects will harm a few? In my view, this is not the case.

First, many of the projects that apparently go against the grain of sufficientarianism are such that it is natural to view them as forms of societal *maintenance*. Roads, bridges, hospitals, airports, and railroad tracks, just like privately owned houses and cars, will deteriorate if not properly maintained. This does not mean that maintenance is exclusively tied to the refurbishing of already existing buildings, bridges, and so on. Much the same can be said of many new building projects as well. If a new bridge is not built, the old one will deteriorate due to ever increasing use. Given urbanization and other related developments, the public value of an old (narrow) bridge will lessen with increased population, even apart from the actual wear. Thus, in the absence of the maintenance of old bridges or the building of new bridges (or buildings or railroad tracks and so on), deterioration will set in. In cases of aggregation akin to Scanlon's transmitter room case, this aspect is absent. No societal values are protected from deterioration. Of course, more welfare stands to be realized, but this is not sufficient to render it morally permissible, or so many would argue.

This maintenance aspect is highly relevant from a sufficientarian perspective. Allowing important parts of society's infrastructure to deteriorate will inevitably lead to less welfare. If deterioration is allowed to progress unchecked, this will eventually push increasingly more people below the sufficiency threshold. This is part of the reason why it would seem absurd, also from the viewpoint of sufficientarianism, to allow society's infrastructure to severely deteriorate by banning new projects and large maintenance operations in the name of justice. Thus, although sufficientarianism certainly provides no reason for open-ended maximization of

---

33. Knight, "Enough Is Too Much," 29–30. Knight refers here to Holtug, *Persons, Interests, Justice*, 236–237, and Widerquist, "Minimum Becomes a Maximum," 474–480, who both make this argument. One might hold that these claims are false, and that people generally reject aggregation in these instances. My impression, for what it is worth, is that Knight et al. are correct on this score.

(weighted) welfare, it provides clear reasons against welfare reductions, if this pushes (or threatens to push) people below the threshold.[34]

This shows, I think, that it is too rash to simply conclude that sufficientarianism must ban all large building projects, as well as the use of cars, planes, and buses.[35] To the contrary, sufficientarianism implies that society should be maintained and developed in a way that secures (preferably with a good margin) a state of affairs in which citizens are sufficiently well off. Thus, a sufficientarian social planner would not simply weigh the loss to a few against the benefits of the many. Rather, she would (and should) weigh the insufficiency of the few against the (future) insufficiency of the many.

Note that this does not show that sufficientarianism allows *all* those cases of apparently socially useful projects that we would intuitively accept. Whether or not such projects are compatible with sufficientarianism depends crucially on whether or not the project's nonrealization will in fact threaten sufficiency attainment over time.

It is difficult to determine in advance which projects would fall into this category. Perhaps sufficientarians would sometimes opt for less risky and less welfare-inducing projects, but that would not be implausible. Suppose, for instance, that there is a choice to be made between building two different bridges. Functionally, they are equivalent; they will both reduce the time spent commuting to an equal extent, for the same number of people. One of the projects, however, envisages a very grand bridge of great aesthetic value. This will give many commuters a small surge of joy driving across it. Perhaps the bridge will also become an architectural landmark and boost tourism to a certain extent. The problem is that the construction work will be more risky on this bridge than on the more ordinary bridge. There is a significantly higher probability that a construction worker will be injured or killed than if the other, less grand bridge is realized. In such a case, it is likely that sufficientarians would choose the drab bridge, even if the net weighted welfare gain would be larger if the other, grander bridge were built.[36]

---

34. In this chapter, I follow the recent literature on this issue (Holtug, *Persons, Interests, Justice*; Knight, "Enough Is Too Much"; Widerquist, "Minimum Becomes a Maximum") in discussing cases involving bridges, airports, and so on. It is important to keep in mind, however, that (depending on a host of empirical questions) it could well be the case that many such projects might not, all in all, maintain (or increase) the aggregate welfare level over time, for instance, because of climate change. If this was to be the case, sufficientarianism, as well as prioritarianism and utilitarianism, would of course oppose projects that threaten less sufficiency-attainment or (weighted) welfare maximization over time.

35. Widerquist, "Minimum Becomes a Maximum."

36. Fortunately, there is no reason to assume that projects of great aesthetic value are generally more risky than other projects.

Furthermore, suppose a large project is completed and that Ms. Fortune, a construction worker, is injured in the process. A large number of people, then, have had their welfare slightly increased, whereas Ms. Fortune's welfare is substantially decreased and she is now below the sufficiency threshold. That surely sounds bad, from a sufficientarian standpoint. However, it also follows that in such a case, Ms. Fortune should be adequately *compensated*. Being insufficiently well off, she can claim resources in order to improve her welfare level. This is not to say that accidents and injuries are insignificant just because we compensate those who experience them. However, it does mean that the welfare loss to the few will to a large extent be recovered, which again makes aggregation more morally plausible. In practice, such compensation should be guaranteed through some universal public or private (state-sponsored if necessary) insurance scheme.

One could perhaps object that sufficientarianism cannot allow aggregation even in cases in which compensation is included. Before it materializes, Ms. Fortune has been harmed, and rendered insufficiently well off, for however short a period, and for that reason sufficientarians must oppose such proceedings. I do not think this objection holds. Consider a parallel objection to prioritarianism. Assume that everyone is equally badly off, and we have to choose between (1) maintaining the status quo and (2) allowing a few of the badly off to become even worse off for a short period of time, only to predictably move on to a situation in which everyone is very well off and equally so. It seems to me that prioritarians could reasonably argue that choice 2 should be allowed. Both sufficientarians and prioritarians can allow temporary affronts to distributive justice in order to subsequently secure (morally) superior states of affairs.

Notice that prioritarianism could perhaps also appeal to compensation in order to reduce the impact of negative aggregation in cases such as the transistor room case. Prioritarians could say that after the millions of spectators have enjoyed the game, they should compensate Jones. It is even likely that such compensation would increase the moral value of the outcome for prioritarians because Jones is badly off, the spectators are (we still assume) better off, and increased welfare to Jones matters more. However, this will always, implausibly in my view, be entirely contingent on the specifics of the welfare calculations.

A further relevant consideration is that sometimes people die in the course of building bridges. Will this again mean that sufficientarianism would lead to a society without roads and hospitals and other public goods people cannot do without? Again, the cumulative welfare loss of banning all the things that involve some risk of death ensures that at least some, arguably the most important, projects will be pursued. It would, however, be important to spread the risk and to invest heavily in safety for employees.

Last, it is worth repeating that sufficientarianism is not a monistic theory. Other values, apart from the disvalue of welfare shortfalls, are also important. It seems that to the extent that we allow individuals to take on personal risk in order to prevent future insufficiency for all, we should make sure that this happens voluntarily. This requires a labor market that gives people a reasonable measure of freedom in their choice of occupation. This, to be sure, is not a reason derived from sufficientarianism (unless it is true that the lack of such freedom endangers sufficiency), and it is also not a reason that is unavailable to (non-monistic) prioritarianism.

4.3. Sufficientarianism and Aggregation in Cases of Less Socially Useful Projects

However, the objection could be pressed further. Clearly, there are cases that are not plausibly viewed as necessary for societal maintenance. As Widerquist has argued, sufficientarianism seems to imply that chocolate factories and other potentially risky ventures that produce trivial goods (as opposed to vital infrastructure) should immediately be shut down.[37] (Some might be tempted to rebut that chocolate is not all that trivial, especially to the exporters of cocoa beans, but other examples could be devised to make the point.)

There is, admittedly, some risk involved in virtually all occupations. Should sufficientarians support closing down all coffee shops because a barista might burn herself on the milk steamer? I do not think this is necessary. There are some similarities between socially useful and (many) less obviously useful projects. Even projects and occupations that are not important from the viewpoint of societal maintenance may be important to maintain sufficiency over time. Shutting down all coffee bars, chocolate factories, and all other similar enterprises would lead to mass unemployment. This is surely not an insignificant consequence from a sufficientarian viewpoint because it would predictably push many below the sufficiency threshold. Here, too, however, sufficiency would require both compensation to those who are unfortunate enough to be harmed and reasonable freedom of occupation.

5. Sufficiency and Hard Cases

A different objection has been put forth by Widerquist. He argues that as sufficientarians, we must

> devote nearly the whole of our economic activity to the attainment of sufficiency for harder and harder cases, but because we will not attain it

---

37. Widerquist, "Minimum Becomes a Maximum," 478.

for everyone, we will have no resources left to consume above the sufficiency level.[38]

I do not think this criticism affects the version of sufficiency that I affirm. First, as I argued previously, there is a limit to the transfers that we are required to make to the hard cases. Second, this limitation is based on the fear that open-ended transfers to these hard cases undermine sufficiency, or the prospects of maintaining sufficiency, for most individuals in society. Third, contrary to Widerquist, I do not believe that sufficiency is best secured, or can at all be secured, by taxing all people's income that is not strictly necessary for keeping them above the threshold. Complete equality (for the majority) at the sufficiency level would probably lead to less economic activity due a loss of incentives and endanger sufficiency in the long term. In my view, the cutoff point for transfers to the hard cases, the point at which more transfers endanger sufficiency over time, is reached well before all surplus resources are spent.

Widerquist suggests that compared to Rawlsians, sufficientarians would have more trouble accepting incentives to the better-off in order to increase their economic activity.[39] To the contrary, I think that sufficientarians should have no trouble whatsoever with incentives. After all, welfare inequalities, within limits, are perfectly acceptable. It does not matter in and by itself that some are worse off than others. What is important is that people are sufficiently well off, as long as making them sufficiently well off does not threaten more extensive insufficiency later on.

It is worth noticing, however, that even if the stipulation that inequalities above the threshold are necessary for long-term sufficiency attainment turns out to be false, this should not bother sufficientarians. If all are sufficiently well off, and all are at the sufficiency threshold and hence equally well off, and there is no risk that less sufficiency is to be expected in the future, there would be little to complain about. By hypothesis, such a society could not have a higher rate of sufficiently well-off people. I do not think this sounds implausible, even if the total welfare level of course could have been higher, and perhaps much higher.

6. Conclusion

The upshot of this discussion, I think, is that sufficientarianism is compatible with most cases of intuitively acceptable aggregation and that sufficientarians can safely allow bridges, roads, and railroads to be built. Denying this would risk

---

38. Widerquist, "Minimum Becomes a Maximum," 478.

39. Widerquist, "Minimum Becomes a Maximum," 478.

undermining the chances to become or remain sufficiently well off for many, if not most, citizens. As I have noted, however, this does not license all risky large-scale projects. Sometimes sufficientarians would opt for a less risky (even if less welfare-inducing) project. Furthermore, sufficientarians have reasons to accept risk to a few even in connection with less socially necessary enterprises, to the extent that banning them would have detrimental economic consequences, which seems likely. Lastly, sufficiency, suitably formulated, does not imply that we must spend all available resources on hard cases. In summary, it seems that sufficiency deals more adequately with the challenges posed by aggregation than does prioritarianism.

Acknowledgments

This chapter was presented at the Gothenburg–Oslo Workshop in Political Theory at the University of Gothenburg in June 2014. I am grateful to Bengt Brülde, Jakob Elster, Fredrik Dybfest Hjorthen, and Göran Duus-Otterström for helpful comments. I am also grateful for the many useful comments and suggestions provided by the editors of this volume, Carina Fourie and Annette Rid.

5

Some Questions (and Answers) for Sufficientarians

Liam Shields

1. Introduction

Different laws and public policies alter the size and proportion of individual shares of wealth and well-being, as well as access to health care and education. For example, a decision to build a factory in one area of the country opens up job opportunities and economic prosperity for some at the expense of others. A decision to lower tax rates at the top rather than the bottom of the income distribution directly affects how much income individuals will have to promote their welfare. These decisions affect the distribution of benefits and burdens in ways that can be evaluated as just or unjust.

Distributive justice is concerned with general principles capable of identifying what distributions fall into these categories. In conjunction with a good deal of empirical work, the principles can then be used as a guide by those making decisions about laws and public policies. Debates about distributive justice have primarily focused on clarifying both the currency of justice (e.g., welfare, resources, and capabilities)—that is, the currency for which we should care about the distribution—and the pattern or way that currency should be distributed or shared out (e.g., equal, sufficient, or as large as possible).[1]

Now, consider the following approach to problems of distributive justice. If someone were to say to you that it is important that you secure enough of some

---

1. For some discussions of the "equality of what" debate, see G. A. Cohen, "On the Currency of Egalitarian Justice," *Ethics* 99 (1989): 906–944; Ronald Dworkin, *Sovereign Virtue* (Cambridge, MA: Harvard University Press, 2000), 285–306; Amartya Sen, "Equality of What?" in *The Tanner Lectures on Human Values*, ed. Sterling M. McMurrin (Salt Lake City, UT: University of Utah Press, 1980), vol. 1, 195–220.

goods, such as health, wealth, and well-being, you would probably think that it is so obviously true as to not really be worth saying. If someone were to say to you that the *only* thing that matters is that you secure enough of those goods, you would probably think that this is so obviously false as to not really be worth saying. At the very least, you would think much more needs to be said about what it means to say that people have *enough* of those goods before you would be convinced.

With regard to distributive justice, sufficientarians make claims about the importance of securing enough that are not dissimilar from those mentioned previously. Some claims they make seem true, perhaps trivially so. Other claims seem false or at least raise very tricky questions that have not been answered satisfactorily. If sufficientarians are correct that the idea of sufficiency should play a very important role in our thinking about the distribution of benefits and burdens, such as wealth and well-being, then they must avoid making statements that are either trivially true or obviously false. Throughout the years, sufficientarianism has been thought by many critics to invite difficult questions.[2] For sufficientarianism to prove acceptable, proponents of the view must show that these questions can be answered in at least plausible ways.

This chapter defends some answers to these questions. First, I set out a capacious definition of sufficientarianism that allows a wide variety of distinctive views to count as distinctively sufficientarian. Second, I raise some questions that can be derived from some common objections. I then suggest some ways of answering these questions. Third, I specify several less familiar sufficientarian views and show how these views may answer questions to which they give rise. Overall, I have two aims: (1) to show that sufficientarians have at least adequate responses to many of the questions that have been asked of them and (2) to describe some relatively underexplored pluralist sufficientarian views and identify their strengths. Achieving each of these aims would provide general support for sufficientarianism as well as indicate some promising ways forward.

2. What Is Sufficientarianism?

Sufficientarians endorse the moral relevance of securing enough. They hold that whether people have *enough* has a significant effect on how we should regard them

---

2. Richard Arneson, "Distributive Justice and Basic Capability Equality," in *Capabilities Equality: Basic Issues and Problems*, ed. Alexander Kaufman (New York: Routledge, 2006); Paula Casal, "Why Sufficiency Is Not Enough," *Ethics* 117, no. 2 (2007): 296–326; Robert Goodin, "Egalitarianism, Fetishistic and Otherwise," *Ethics* 98, no. 1 (1987): 44–49; Shlomi Segall, "What Is the Point of Sufficiency?" *Journal of Applied Philosophy* 33, no. 1 (2016): 36–52; Karl Widerquist, "How the Sufficiency Minimum Becomes a Social Maximum," *Utilitas* 22, no. 4 (2010): 474–480.

as possible beneficiaries or burden-bearers in the allocation of whatever goods are deemed to matter. For instance, most sufficientarians hold that it is more important to benefit someone who lacks enough than to benefit someone who has enough, at least when we can benefit those who lack enough by at least as much as those who have enough.

More precisely, sufficientarians make two claims. The first claim is the *positive thesis*, which states that it is important that some individuals secure enough of some goods. Note that this does not commit sufficientarians to the claim that it is always better to be above rather than below the threshold. Nor does it commit them to claiming that we always have more reason to move a person above rather than below the threshold. Although they make many additional claims, sufficientarians need only insist, as a matter of definition, that it is valuable or important to secure enough. The second claim is the *shift thesis*, which states that once individuals have secured enough, our reasons to benefit them further change or shift.[3] There is a shift in our moral reasons to benefit or burden some people once they have enough. As such, the nature of the claim that they can press on distributive decisions is different depending on whether they are above or below the sufficiency threshold. The shift is what makes a view sufficientarian. The different kinds of shifts that are possible specify different versions of sufficientarianism. Next, I briefly survey some possible shifts for purely illustrative purposes.

A shift could specify that our reasons to benefit a person diminish more quickly or slowly once the person has enough or that there is some sudden decrease in the importance of benefitting a person once he or she has enough. A shift could specify that once a person has enough, we should ensure that the person has an equal share or that benefits should be distributed in accordance with merit or desert. A shift could specify that once a person has secured enough, we have much stronger reasons to distribute in a way that is responsibility sensitive. A shift could specify that once a person has enough, we should be solely or primarily concerned with equality, whereas prior to the achievement of universal sufficiency we should not be concerned with equality. The type of shift is only one area of variation and difference among sufficiency views, but it can be seen that there are a wide variety of possible shifts, some of which will raise different sorts of theoretical questions than others and will issue different guidance.

Having discussed the basic idea of sufficientarianism, I next discuss the most common versions of that view and consider the questions that have been raised and answers that may be given to them. I then discuss pluralist sufficientarian views and explore the questions that can be raised to these views and set

---

3. This characterization was originally set out and defended in Liam Shields, "The Prospects for Sufficientarianism," *Utilitas* 24, no. 1 (2012): 101–117.

out some possible answers. I conclude with some remarks about the future of sufficientarianism.

3. Upper-Limit Sufficientarianism

One of the most widely discussed versions of sufficientarianism views securing enough as a kind of upper limit, above which claims for further benefits lack normative force. There are many different advocates of this view, most notably Roger Crisp and Harry Frankfurt.[4] The common idea is that as long as people have enough, it is not important to give them more or to prioritize the worse-off or to equalize individual shares of benefits.

Crisp motivates this position by asking us to consider a hypothetical example called the Beverly Hills case, in which everyone is very well off. In such cases, it seems we do not have particularly strong moral reasons to be concerned with the inequality, vast though it is. However, in response, Paula Casal notes that if everyone has enough but we can distribute some further benefits, it seems that it is apt to have some concern for equality. Casal's case is as follows:

> Suppose that having provided every patient with enough medicine, food, comfort, and so forth, a hospital receives a fantastic donation, which includes spare rooms for visitors, delicious meals, and the best in world cinema. If its administrators then arbitrarily decide to devote all those luxuries to just a few fortunate beneficiaries, their decision would be unfair.[5]

Although this is a forceful counterexample to upper-limit sufficientarianism, it does not settle the matter decisively against the view. Rather, it raises a question that proponents may find difficult to answer. That is,

> Q1: Why should we be indifferent once people have enough?

In light of this, sufficientarians need to explain why it is that indifference is the appropriate response to securing enough. I believe that at least two decent answers that can be given.

3.1. Noncomparative Ambitions

The first answer that I consider takes inspiration from work by Harry Frankfurt, the originator of modern sufficientarianism. On this view, all reasonable distributive

---

4. Roger Crisp, "Equality, Priority, and Compassion," *Ethics* 113, no. 4 (2003): 745–763; Roger Crisp, "Egalitarianism and Compassion," *Ethics* 114, no. 1 (2003): 119–126; Harry Frankfurt, "Equality as a Moral Ideal," *Ethics* 98, no. 1 (1987): 21–43.

5. Casal, "Why Sufficiency Is Not Enough," 307.

claims are satiable and noncomparative; therefore, there is an upper limit to the claims one can make. An ambition is satiable when after a certain amount of the currency is possessed, no more of that currency can satisfy the ambition further. Consider, for instance, my ambition to have $10. An eleventh dollar does not satisfy that ambition further. An ambition is comparative when it does not rely for its satisfaction on the fact that others have less, more, or the same amount of this currency as I possess. In this sense, ambitions do not compete with one another for satisfaction. For instance, if I want one more dollar than you, this is comparative. However, if I want only $10, then the number of dollars you possess is irrelevant from the standpoint of my ambition . If our ambitions were comparative, then satisfying these ambitions may require you to have less than enough. As such, it may not be possible to achieve sufficiency for all, and for this reason it seems unreasonable to insist on comparative ambitions being satisfied for justice to be done.

Frankfurt's original formulation of the sufficiency threshold is as follows:

> To say that a person has enough money is to say that he is content, or it is reasonable for him to be content, with having no more money than he has. And to say this is, in turn, to say something like the following: The person does not (or cannot reasonably) regard whatever (if anything) is unsatisfying or distressing about his life as due to his having too little money.[6]

We need not focus on money as the relevant currency, the thing of which we should have enough. Indeed, later in the paper, Frankfurt focuses on the level of contentment in one's life. Why, then, might a person reasonably be content with the level of welfare or money that he or she possesses? One thought is that it would be unreasonable to demand more. This could be explained by individuals' authentic ambitions or preferences, which may be thought relevant to determining one's share of the appropriate currency.[7] If only some of those ambitions were valid claims that we can press against others, then it would be possible that such ambitions or preferences could be satiable as well. If these ambitions and preferences are noncomparative and satiable once a person has enough, we have no reasons to care about equality or further benefits. This may bring to mind the idea that persons may need enough to pay their rent or feed themselves, but this is an instrumental reason to think that securing enough is important and so cannot help defend a fundamental sufficiency principle. However, unlike rent and nutrition,

---

6. Frankfurt, "Equality as a Moral Ideal," 36.

7. Harry Frankfurt, "Necessity and Desire," *Philosophy and Phenomenological Research* 45, no. 1 (1984): 1–13.

our authentic ambitions or preferences are more plausibly non-instrumental and constitutive of our reasonable contentment and well-being.

This last point can be explained as follows: If I could pay my rent without money, perhaps by providing some service instead, I would not need a sufficient amount of money to pay my rent. However, our authentic ambitions and preferences cannot likewise be detached from our welfare. Moreover, sufficiency need not focus on actual welfare levels but, rather, our opportunity for welfare through resources. On this view, it is possible to be concerned with having enough resources to realize our ambitions, as long as they are satiable and noncomparative, and fail to achieve them for other reasons, such as weakness of will. Note that Frankfurt is concerned with the way in which a deficiency of whatever currency we focus on is the reason for your failure to achieve your aims. Other deficiencies, perhaps those that are in terms of your talents or work ethic, are those that can diminish your welfare in ways that do not concern a theory of distributive justice. As such, this view can be described in either welfarist or non-welfarist terms. That is, it can be described in terms that appeal to how well the individual's life goes for him or her or in other terms that are independent of how well his or her life goes—for instance, how much wealth he or she has accumulated. Because each of these options is available, proponents of the view need not take a stance in long-standing debates between perfectionists and antiperfectionists, who disagree about whether justice may be concerned directly with promoting welfare.

I now discuss the attraction of this view and why we might think noncomparative and satiable ambitions are the only reasonable or relevant demands. An idea that makes sense of preferring noncomparative and satiable ambitions is that insatiable and comparative ambitions cannot be realized by all persons simultaneously. If we think that the entitlements of justice should be compossible (i.e., mutually realizable), and if we think that individuals' authentic ambitions exhaust such claims, then we will be wary of insatiable or comparative ambitions because they will not be compossible. If our ambitions are formulated in ways that make their achievement turn necessarily on the failure of others or on being better than others, then they express a kind of selfishness and disregard for the welfare of others. Consider, for instance, those who care primarily about earning more than their colleagues or those who rely for their own happiness on the unhappiness of others. These sorts of attitudes seem to have no place in a just society. Moreover, the opposite of these attitudes is a kind of mutual regard, respect, and equality. For instance, consider those who would like a pay raise only if others are likewise rewarded or those who can be happy only when others are also happy. These strike us as more noble sentiments, and it is a kind of sufficientarianism that delivers them.

In summary, this focus on noncomparative ambitions enables the upper-limit sufficientarian to claim that the only claims relevant to justice are satiable and noncomparative, and so further benefits are not relevant to justice and should be met with indifference.

Some may remain unpersuaded by this response—for instance, those who believe that preferences need not be satiable to be valid or those who believe that preferences and ambitions are entirely irrelevant to distributive justice, so it is worthwhile to consider an alternative answer to the question.

3.2. The Circumstances of Justice

The circumstances of justice are the material situation in which principles of distributive justice apply. Outside of those circumstances, other moral norms may apply, but not justice. The circumstances of justice are those in which there are not so few resources that no one's claims can be met (extreme scarcity) but not so many that there are no competing claims (superabundance).[8]

It is easy to understand how the "satiable, noncomparative ambitions view" I just explained may be problematic if we accept that principles of justice apply only in the circumstances of justice. If each of our plans requires certain resources to be pursued, and if resources are moderately scarce such that we cannot each have enough, then it appears that it is impossible for our plans, insofar as they give rise to claims of justice for us, to be reconciled with justice. Imagine that a small amount of wood is to be distributed and I have the authentic ambition to play a wooden flute, whereas you have the authentic ambition to go on long walks that require a walking stick. However, the piece of wood cannot be turned into both a flute and a walking stick. Thus, the circumstances of justice make it the case that, even though we both independently chose satiable and noncomparative plans, our ambitions cannot be simultaneously satisfied. However, one could still insist that there is an important difference between plans that we formulate that are noncomparative and satiable and plans that are made comparative by the circumstances of justice. On this view, all plans are made comparative by the circumstances of justice; thus, one could argue that formulating such plans is not especially distasteful and does not entail viewing a person as a competitor or less than equal. When a person formulates a plan that is by *necessity* comparative, because it is in principle comparative, one is viewing that other person as a means or as inferior or as someone to be dominated.

---

8. David Hume, *A Treatise of Human Nature*, Book III, Part II, Section II; John Rawls, *A Theory of Justice*, revised edition (Cambridge, MA: Harvard University Press, 1999), 109–112.

I now consider a separate view. If we take the circumstances of justice seriously, it appears that there are two morally important sufficiency thresholds: one threshold at which resources are too scarce to trigger principles of justice and another at which resources are so abundant that justice no longer applies. We can say that at these points, whether there are enough resources not merely affects which demands of justice apply but also determines whether the demands of justice apply at all. One might think that these thresholds do not determine justice. They tell us when evaluations of justice can properly take place. However, note that we can have a duty of justice to bring about enough resources for distributive justice to apply. Thus, this would play a similar role as the role played by natural duties of justice to set up and maintain the conditions necessary for a just order—in other words, our duties to establish just relations with others.[9] Understood in this way, both thresholds can establish why it is that justice is a self-starting value. If we live in scarcity, we have reasons—reasons to do with the realization of the value of justice—to overcome that scarcity.

Note, however, that according to our definition, these thresholds must be determined in ways that are noncomparative, and that the definition of the circumstances of justice is often in comparative terms. Thus, for example, scarcity is not necessarily avoided when there are 1 million units of resources. This depends on how many people, and needs, there are because scarcity is defined by the absence of enough for everyone and so the more people there are, the more needs there are and the more resources are needed to satisfy those needs. The amount of resources that is necessary to satisfy some claims would not be some fixed level; it would be comparative. The idea of the circumstances of justice being determined by absolute scarcity or abundance would provide a decent explanation of why there may be no distributive reasons or duties over some absolute threshold, as some influential sufficientarians claim.

Having considered some answers that upper-limit sufficientarians can offer to the difficult question they have been asked, I next consider the second major version of sufficientarianism and the ways it may answer the questions that have been asked of it.

4. Headcount Sufficientarianism

Headcount sufficientarianism holds that we should maximize the number of people who have enough.[10] Critics have noted that this view has some very

---

9. See Rawls, *A Theory of Justice*, 98–101.

10. Casal, "Why Sufficiency Is Not Enough," 298, 315–316; Dale Dorsey, "Toward a Theory of the Basic Minimum," *Politics, Philosophy and Economics* 7, no. 4 (2008): 432–445; Edward Page, *Climate Change, Justice and Future Generations* (Cheltenham, UK: Elgar, 2006), 85–95;

counterintuitive implications.[11] Following headcount sufficientarianism will sometimes require benefitting the better off, who are only just below the sufficiency threshold, at the expense of the worse off, who are much further below the threshold. In cases involving some people who are so badly off that they cannot be brought up to the threshold and other people who are only marginally below the threshold, this principle would always recommend benefiting the better off. This type of decision may lead us to reject or question headcount sufficientarianism because it seems to fail to recognize the seriousness of the plight of those most vulnerable—those who can never get enough.

Headcount sufficientarianism seems to contradict two common thoughts underpinning major theories of distributive justice. The first is the idea that the worse off a person is, the more important it is to benefit that person and improve his or her position. This thought does some work in explaining why it is better to help the poor rather than the well-off, and among the poor, the poorest have a stronger claim to assistance. For instance, we might think that it is much more important to help the global poor than to contribute to a friend's drama school tuition. The second thought is that the larger a benefit to a person, the greater the reason to distribute that benefit. This intuition does some work in explaining why if we can give a vaccine, eliminating risk, to someone who faces a very high risk of contracting a disease and someone else who faces a very low risk, then we should give the vaccine to the person who faces the high risk. In many cases, headcount sufficientarianism will favor benefitting the better-off by a small amount, which is sufficient to push them above the threshold, rather than benefitting the worse-off by a large amount, which is insufficient to push them above the threshold.

However, the fact that such a view is open to these counterexamples and contradicts some ideas that underpin much of contemporary normative thought does not settle the matter. Rather, it raises the question of when, if ever, it is appropriate to maximize the number of people who achieve some level of welfare at the expense of various other values. This depends on the importance of benefits that push a person above the threshold rather than benefits that do not push a person above that threshold.

The following question remains:

Q2: Why should we maximize sufficiency at the expense of the least advantaged?

Edward Page, "Justice Between Generations: Investigating a Sufficientarian Approach," *Journal of Global Ethics* 3, no. 1 (2007): 3–20, 11; John Roemer, "Eclectic Distributional Ethics," *Politics, Philosophy and Economics* 3, no. 3 (2004): 267–281.

11. Arneson, "'Good Enough' is not Good Enough," 36–38; Casal, "Why Sufficiency Is Not Enough," 298, 315–316; Roemer, "Eclectic Distributional Ethics."

We can see that the most plausible cases in which maximizing seems appropriate are triage cases. For instance, consider the case of a military doctor who must deal with casualties as they arrive. She will be unable to save some, whereas others will be difficult to save and still others may be fairly easy to save. Rather than investing her time, effort, and resources in those who cannot be saved, or even those who are very costly to save, it makes sense for her to hold back resources and save the least costly ones because she can save many more people that way. This seems like a far more sensible decision procedure than giving her patients equal attention and resources or prioritizing the least advantaged because doing so may minimize the number of lives saved, perhaps saving no one.

We can ask, What are the key features of triage cases that make maximizing the incidence of sufficiency at the expense of benefitting the least advantaged the best thing to do? To answer this question, we should focus on a simple case and we should examine the kinds of claims that the better-off can make and the kinds of claims the worse-off can make. Thus, let us imagine a case in which one person is very badly off and cannot be brought up to some critical threshold, call her Lost Cause, and another person is also badly off but can be brought up to that threshold, call her Savable. Lost Cause is worse off than Savable. As such, she has a stronger claim than Savable in one respect. Being worse off than another beneficiary generally gives us a reason to benefit that person, but this reason is not decisive. It would not be permissible for someone not to pay a debt or meet the terms of a legitimate contract simply because that person was worse off than the person he or she owed.[12] It may also be permissible to benefit the better-off at the expense of the worse-off if by doing so we help a much larger number of people. However, in our case, there are no promises or debts.

One other feature of the claims of the better-off that can trump those of the worse-off concerns the size of the benefit. This is not a wholly uncontroversial claim, but one can support the importance of the size of the benefits, within some range of well-being scores, in the following way. Consider the plight of Amy and Hayley, who are equally well-off. It then becomes possible to offer only one of them a college place. Amy will benefit much more than Hayley from the college place, for various reasons that have to do with her particular interest in college, her intelligence, and her attitude toward work. Hayley would benefit from the college place, but not as much as Amy. If we stipulate that there are no other reasons to give Hayley rather than Amy the place at college, then we should, I think, give Amy the college place. The general reason for this is that Amy would benefit more

---

12. One could argue that no such contract could be valid, but this seems too eccentric a view to take seriously as a general constraint on contract. This is consistent with some inequalities being sufficient to render a contract invalid.

from it. Now, let's change the case so that Hayley is actually slightly worse off than Amy, and the college place would improve her welfare such that she would be at least as well off as Amy. I think in this second case, as long as the size of the benefit to Amy is large, it can still trump the fact that Hayley is worse off, at least assuming that Hayley is neither very much worse off than Amy nor very badly off in absolute terms.

Returning to Lost Cause and Savable, it can be seen that sometimes the size or significance of a benefit can trump the reason why a person is worse off. However, in this case, Lost Cause is very badly off in absolute terms, but so is Savable. Savable and Lost Cause are therefore symmetrically situated with respect to their being very badly off, although one is worse off than the other. This means that Lost Cause can use the reason that she is worse off to support benefitting her, but she cannot use the reason that she is very badly off to support benefitting her because that reason is on both sides of the equation.

What about Savable? What can she use to support her claim to be benefitted? She can say that the size or significance of the benefit, which sees her escape a very bad condition, is sufficient to override the reason of being worse off. It is on the side of the ex post calculation, not the ex ante calculation.

To understand this more clearly, note that the considerations are often associated with efficiency, but they need not only be reducible to efficiency. They could be considerations of justice. In the case of Savable, the benefits she gets do make a major difference to her, but the benefits to Lost Cause do not make a difference with respect to her being very badly off, although they improve her condition slightly. To use the benefit to improve the position of Lost Cause is to use it in a way that is less effective. However, the interesting and important question for the sufficientarian is whether there is some threshold that explains this rather than some general rule about the size of benefits defeating how badly off a person is. If it were simply about benefits of size A being sufficient to override concerns of being worse off by B units, then this rule would apply throughout the distribution and not merely to benefits that secured an above-threshold quality of life. Therefore, if the threshold makes a difference, it must be because being at a certain absolute level (or range) of advantage gives one's claims additional force and not because one stands to benefit greatly. We can now ask, Are there thresholds like this?

In triage cases, it appears that securing a certain level of benefit is a necessary precondition for living a decent life or pursuing other goals, whereas living below it does not. If there is a precondition threshold level of capability, then this condition would work well. It makes sense to maximize the precondition level because below the threshold, one's life is capped at a certain level of welfare—and that welfare level is particularly low. Perhaps this is the difference between a life worth living and a life not worth living, which might be denoted by negative and positive values of welfare.

Thus, we have not provided an argument that can solidly support such thresholds, nor an argument for one particular threshold, but we have seen what the nature of such a threshold must be like and what it must not be like. The consequence of there being a morally relevant threshold cannot be that a benefit of a particular size trumps how badly off the benefit recipient is. Although this is an interesting problem, it is not the essential problem for headcount sufficientarians. The issue for the headcount sufficientarian is to show that only being above the threshold, which opens up many possibilities of gains, is extremely valuable and more so than gains that do not help an individual get above the threshold. I have stated that understanding this threshold as a precondition for not only large benefits but also autonomy or capability may work well. As such, headcount sufficientarianism may, as triage suggests, be a very useful principle in the management of health care. Lives not worth living or of negative value may be particularly supportive of headcount sufficientarian principles because the quality of such lives is so different from that of lives of positive value or that are worth living. It is not simply that one is better than another but that they are very different sorts of life.

However, although it is possible to respond to this question by appealing to triage cases, they do not sit easily with sufficientarianism's commitment to non-instrumental principles. The idea that we should maximize the number of people who have enough to survive can be explained perfectly well by any adequate prioritarian theory that is welfarist because it is reasonable to think that having one's life saved is the only way to promote one's welfare. The unsavable, in particular, cannot have their welfare increased. The difficult-to-save may be worse off than the easier-to-save, but the fact that we can save more people can sometimes override the fact that the most badly off person we could save is not benefitted at all. Some prioritarian views—which claim that the worse off a person is, the more important it is to benefit him or her—can explain this perfectly well, so it is not clear why we would need a sufficientarian view to explain it. A focus on welfare, and life-saving as a contributing factor to welfare, suggests that any sufficiency threshold here is instrumental. This is not to say that thinking about it in sufficientarian terms is not a good idea, because it may draw attention to valuable thresholds; such thresholds cannot be non-instrumental and so do not speak in favor of the necessity of sufficientarianism.

If we are averse to appealing to welfare directly, as many political philosophers are, headcount sufficientarianism becomes more plausible. It might be that having our basic needs met or avoiding severe pain are such important achievements that they should be promoted at the expense of any benefits that fail to achieve them.[13] Thus, we might take this sort of route and defend a headcount sufficientarian view because being above the threshold of pain or need is better than having even slight pain or a slight need. No doubt some will remain unpersuaded by either of these avenues that are open, so it is worthwhile to consider the merits of other sufficientarian views.

5. New Views and New Questions

There are many possible sufficientarian alternatives to upper-limit or headcount sufficientarianism. All of them deny maximizing the number who have enough as the appropriate guidance below the threshold, and all of them deny that the importance of benefits stops at the threshold(s). As such, they avoid the two questions that can be asked of the dominant views, although they face other important questions.

I focus on a few pluralist sufficientarian views, which are pluralist in that they appeal to sufficiency as well as other distributive principles.[14] In addition, they may also appeal to different currencies. Although sufficiency principles, when taken alone, may be implausible, some may be required in the best pluralist account of distributive justice. Securing enough could be one of the many things that matters when evaluating distributions. Utilizing the shift, we can imagine a concern with sufficiency being combined with a concern with equality, responsibility, and rights, and it is worth considering the advantage(s) of having a sufficiency principle among them. The distinct advantage of a sufficiency principle is that it can help explain why we should give special priority or additional weight to persons by virtue of their being very badly off in terms of the relevant currency. Again, if we think there are reasons to be especially morally concerned with those who lack certain opportunities or capacities, that do not apply to those who have them, and that having them does not mark the end of our obligations of justice, then we will have strong reason to think that having less than enough adds weight to claims.

There are two types of pluralist sufficientarian views. One views the rival values or principles as always conflicting but with different weight attached. Thus, equality and sufficiency could both be important distributive principles, but if we can satisfy one more than the other, we may have more reason to do so. I call this "conflicting pluralism." The other pluralist sufficientarian view sees sufficiency as a precondition for some other principle or values. Thus, on this view, sufficiency may need to be secured before equality becomes a relevant demand. I call this

---

13. David V. Axelsen and Lasse Nielsen, "Sufficiency as Freedom from Duress," *Journal of Political Philosophy* 23, no. 4 (2015): 406–426.

14. Some hybrid views are discussed in Casal, "Why Sufficiency Is Not Enough."

"ordered pluralism." Here, I focus on elaborating two pluralist views, and the two variants of them, to illustrate the generally attractive but as yet unchartered territory for sufficientarians.

5.1. Sufficiency and Responsibility

Consider a version of responsibility-sensitive sufficientarianism. Such a view would combine our concern for the badly off and our concern with individual responsibility. This could take either conflicting or ordered forms:[15]

> *Sufficiency as a constraint on responsibility:* No individual should bear costs that would push him or her below a threshold, even if the individual would otherwise be liable to bear those costs.

A drawback of this view is that even very well-off persons could make enormous gambles that, if they do not pay off, those persons would not bear their full consequences. As such, other persons would have to bear the costs of compensating the reckless. Another form of this view, which may be more palatable, would be to ensure that those who are, ex ante, below a threshold cannot be held responsible. The reason for this might be that being in a very bad position currently can render one's decisions to agree to do things, such as to take on dangerous work, nonvoluntarily. A more moderate view may state that whether a person has enough ex post or ex ante should affect our reasons to hold the person responsible for the costs of his or her actions.

Alternatively, we could state that sufficiency, rather than equality, is the relevant benchmark. On this view, no one should have less than enough, except through their own choice or fault:

> *Luck sufficientarianism:* No one should have less than enough through no fault or choice of their own.[16]

This contrasts with the well-known luck egalitarian view that states that no one should have less than anyone else through no fault or choice of their own. This has the advantage of being less demanding, and it could be more easily combined with other principles of justice that provide more efficient distributions.

---

15. For one example, see Andrew Williams, "Liberty, Equality, and Property," in *The Oxford Handbook of Political Theory*, ed. J. Dryzek, B. Honig, and A. Phillips (Oxford: Oxford University Press, 2006), 488–506.

16. This label is given to a view discussed in Kasper Lippert-Rasmussen, "Justice and Bad Luck," *The Stanford Encyclopedia of Philosophy* (Summer 2014 edition), Edward N. Zalta (ed.); http://plato.stanford.edu/archives/sum2014/entries/justice-bad-luck.

5.2. Sufficiency and Self-Ownership

I now consider a final view, which responds to a possible problem that some may have with the upper-limit sufficientarian view. In cases involving benefits that arrive from no one's production, like manna from heaven, it is usually better to give them to someone who will benefit from them than to waste them.[17] Wasting benefits requires a pretty strong justification. Thus, if all people have enough resources, at least, to successfully achieve their satiable noncomparative ambitions, and we still have resources to distribute, why not give someone some more resources? These resources might make their lives more comfortable or allow them to acquire other resources that would make their chances of success even better. Upper-limit sufficientarianism has nothing to say against wasting the resources, except for appealing to some additional aggregative principle. We need at least some positive reason, and not merely the absence of certain claims, to motivate the view that it is permissible to waste the resources.

One such reason may be the costs of providing those benefits. Returning to the hospital case, we might note that hospital staff will be put out by having to provide the additional benefits—for example, cooking better meals and installing, maintaining, and dealing with additional issues caused by having a television, such as monitoring its content and its volume. These costs might provide us with some reason to think that above some threshold the importance of benefitting people may be so trivial that it is not worth imposing the costs on anyone to ensure that they are provided. As currently stated, this view is not satisfactory. First, the costs to others are subject to appraisal by distributive justice, so the diminution of their share of welfare or resources, can be accounted for by principles of distributive justice. Second, the costs to others vary. Thus, insofar as the threshold is going to be non-instrumental, it will constantly change and so sufficiency itself becomes a moving target. It suggests that we should be focusing on maximizing a fundamental currency rather than giving importance to two.

A variation of this view, however, is plausible. If we take the view that individuals have self-ownership rights, and if we believe that apart from manna from heaven, benefits to people can be provided only by taking them from others or otherwise coercing people to produce them, we might think that this would provide a cap on the benefits that can be redistributed.[18] Such a view may appear to preclude distribution at all, but the view can be softened so that only those benefits that are

---

17. Casal, "Why Sufficiency Is Not Enough," 307.

18. One could understand this as amending left-libertarianism with a right to sufficiency rather than equality of the value of natural resources. This would be a rival interpretation of the Lockean proviso to leave "enough and as good." See Hillel Steiner, *An Essay on Rights* (Oxford: Blackwell; 1996).

somehow crucial to living a minimally decent life or other concerns that may be more important than self-ownership rights can override them. Nevertheless, we might think of a sufficiency-constrained self-ownership theory as explaining both why we have no need to benefit people above some point and why we should nevertheless insist on benefitting people up to a point. Because the value of not violating rights or not infringing on them can be viewed as equally serious, no matter how well off the victim is, and the value of benefits can be viewed as diminishing, we have a case of a non-instrumental threshold.[19] This would specify an upper-limit sufficientarian view that could respond to some of the key objections to it. This is not to say that it does not give rise to further worries, but it suggests that there are ways to respond that are at least minimally plausible and so it is a route sufficientarians may wish to take.

In addition, we can make a further claim in defense of this kind of view: It is not committed to maximizing or prioritizing below the threshold. It is, as stated, silent on the issue of how to distribute benefits and burdens below the threshold. Thus, for example, one could hold that we should distribute equally below the threshold where sufficiency for all is not possible by adding some less important concern for equality.

6. Conclusion

Although many have objected to commonly discussed sufficientarian views, there are some adequate responses that can be given. Sufficientarians have a number of lines of arguments available to them with the existing views and also a number of pluralist views that are sufficientarian. The latter views can be extremely diverse and have a number of attractive features. This chapter discussed the promise of views that combine a concern with sufficiency and a concern with self-ownership or responsibility and also the tasks that remain for proponents of them.

Acknowledgments

I thank the editors of this collection, Carina Fourie and Annette Rid, for inviting me to contribute and for several rounds of extremely helpful comments. I also thank the following people with whom I have discussed this chapter or the ideas in it: Nici Mulkeen, Richard Child, Stephanie Collins, Andrew Williams, Fabienne Peter, Matthew Clayton, Zofia Stemplowska, Adam Swift, Victor Tadros, Douglas Bamford, Alex Sutton, David V. Axelsen, and Julie Rose.

---

19. Dale Dorsey, "Equality-Tempered prioritarianism," *Politics, Philosophy & Economics* 13, no. 1 (2014): 45–61.

6

Essentially Enough

ELEMENTS OF A PLAUSIBLE ACCOUNT
OF SUFFICIENTARIANISM

David V. Axelsen and Lasse Nielsen

1. Introduction

In all modern societies, people disagree about how to distribute the benefits and
burdens that arise from their mutual cooperation—that is, the benefits of economic resources, positions of power, and central goods (e.g., access to high-quality
health care, education, and housing) and the burdens of work and risk—all of
which are created through the specialized, societal division of labor (and, to a high
and increasing degree, the *global* division of labor). Theories of distributive justice seek to elucidate such disagreements by establishing principles pointing out
the *just* manner of distributing these benefits and burdens. One such family of
theories claims that justice involves ensuring that everyone has *enough*—so-called
theories of sufficiency (or sufficientarian theories).[1] Sufficientarians, however, are
under heavy fire from proponents of other distributive ideals. Elsewhere, we have
argued that this fire is mistargeted; not only is sufficiency plausible but also, if
understood correctly, it is the proper aim of distributive justice.[2] Here, we build on

1. Harry Frankfurt, "Equality as a Moral Ideal," *Ethics* 98, no. 1 (1987): 21–43; Roger Crisp,
"Equality, Priority, and Compassion," *Ethics* 113, no. 4 (2003): 745–763; Robert Huseby,
"Sufficiency: Restated and Defended," *Journal of Political Philosophy* 18, no. 2 (2010): 178–
197; Liam Shields, "The Prospects for Sufficientarianism," *Utilitas* 24, no. 1 (2012): 101–117;
Yitzhak Benbaji, "The Doctrine of Sufficiency: A Defence," *Utilitas* 17, no. 3 (2005): 310–332.

2. David V. Axelsen and Lasse Nielsen, "Sufficiency as Freedom from Duress," *Journal of
Political Philosophy* 23, no. 4 (2015): 406–426.

these ideas and seek to elaborate on the reasons that lead us to adorn sufficiency
with such high acclaim. We attempt to do so in a relatively general manner—
namely by outlining those elements that must be present in any account of sufficiency, attempting to escape what we take to be the strongest points of criticism
made against such theories.

To thus avoid being struck by the heavy fire under which it has been placed
by its critics, an account of sufficiency must include four main elements. First,
it must be built around a thick concept. In other words, it must rely on a notion
of sufficiency that has both a descriptive and an evaluative component—that, in
itself, provides reasons for why achieving sufficiency is desirable. This will help
sufficientarians escape the very common objection that sufficiency accounts involve an undesirable element of arbitrariness. Second, it must entail an appropriate degree of accuracy so as to avoid being too ambiguous to function as a political
ideal. Third, sufficientarians must employ a relatively high threshold of what constitutes enough, in order to give plausible answers to why inequalities above the
sufficiency threshold are unimportant. Finally, sufficientarians are often attacked
for not being able to accommodate important values such as nondiscrimination,
unfairness, and imprudence. In response to this, we claim that sufficientarians
must embrace a pluralist view of what is important in human lives—what it is
that must be considered in evaluating the justice of a distribution. We propose
an ecumenical view of a flourishing life encompassing three aspects, of which
humans must have enough of each. Finally, we attempt to apply this to the area of
health, thus outlining some thoughts about what a plausible account of sufficiency
in health may contain.

2. Avoiding Ambiguity and Arbitrariness

Sufficiency accounts revolve around a notion of "enough." This concept plays a
double role in being both the threshold up to which people must be brought in the
name of justice and the point above which justice no longer applies (or is of significantly lesser concern). For sufficiency accounts to be plausible, then, they must
give plausible reasons justifying *the positive thesis* that bringing people above some
threshold is especially important and *the negative thesis* that above this threshold
inequalities are irrelevant or, at least, significantly less important.[3]

In an article often considered the big bang of the sufficientarian universe,
Harry Frankfurt formulated a sufficientarian position that holds that "with respect
to economic assets, what is important from the point of view of morality is not that

---

3. Paula Casal, "Why Sufficiency Is Not Enough," *Ethics* 117, no. 2 (2007): 296–326; Shields,
"The Prospects for Sufficientarianism"; Liam Shields, Chapter 5 in this volume.

everyone should have the same but that each should have enough."[4] The doctrine centers on the notion that justice should be concerned with people's *absolute* levels of well-being rather than their relative ones. Thus, he claims, we should care about absolute amounts of economic resources rather than differences in wealth (taking economic resources as a proxy for preference fulfillment).

A clear advantage of Frankfurt's account of sufficiency is that it latches onto a notion that has commonsensical intuitive appeal: Having *enough* economic resources, arguably, relates to a notion the gist of which most people will intuitively grasp. However, Frankfurt's threshold is also an illustration of why sufficientarian theories are often criticized for being too ambiguous or "fuzzy."[5] Thus, it is claimed, sufficientarianism is unable to function as an ideal of distributive justice because it cannot give us clear directions regarding what to do in situations of conflicting claims. The problem is that such principles simply cannot give us political guidance because they rely on excessively vague thresholds—it is simply too difficult to determine when someone has enough. Thus, even if most people intuitively have an idea that someone can possess enough (or not enough) money, the concept is exceedingly ambiguous.

Egalitarians and prioritarians, of course, could likewise be accused of ambiguity because merely stating that people should be equal or that priority should be given to the worst-off is, in itself, ambiguous in the same sense as saying that they should have enough. In those cases, we need to know what it means to be equal (on what dimension and compared to whom?), just as we need to know how to determine who is worst off in order to use these ideals in actual distributional situations. These concepts, however, have been specified to a greater extent than sufficientarianism through decades (if not centuries) of philosophical and societal debate, and so there are several relatively plausible answers available for both egalitarians and prioritarians. However, there is nothing to suggest that ambiguity could not (plausibly) be avoided through further specification by sufficientarians.[6] Thus, ambiguity is not an inherent part of a sufficiency account.[7] Rather, the

---

4. Frankfurt, "Equality as a Moral Ideal."

5. See Casal, "Why Sufficiency Is Not Enough," 313; and Robert Goodin, "Egalitarianism, Fetishistic and Otherwise," *Ethics* 98, no. 1 (1987), 49, respectively.

6. In the words of Frankfurt, "It is far from self-evident, needless to say, precisely what the doctrine of sufficiency means and what applying it entails. But this is hardly a good reason for neglecting the doctrine or for adopting an incorrect doctrine in preference to it" ("Equality as a Moral Ideal," 24).

7. Shlomi Segall, "What Is the Point of Sufficiency?" *Journal of Applied Philosophy* 33, no. 1 (2016): 36–52, seems to think that sufficiency is inherently ambiguous or, at least, that it must rely on other values and that these are ambiguous with regard to determining distributive shares. We claim that the ideal we outline here is not subject to that line of criticism. See

objection (we claim) is better understood as a demand for clarification as to what is *meant* by enough. To accomplish that, a mere appeal to common-sense intuitions is unsatisfying. After all, such intuitions are notoriously vague and their exact meaning is not universally shared. In addition, although they might constitute an adequate standard for everyday rule-of-thumb morality, they cannot function as a principle capable of guiding political action and institutional design. As Ronald Dworkin stated, "Decisions taken in the name of justice must never outstrip an official's ability to account for these decisions in a theory of justice, even when such a theory must compromise some of his intuitions."[8] For this reason, their implications must be relatively clear. Also, many sufficientarians employ thresholds that are simply too ambiguous, of which Frankfurt's is a case in point. More, then, must be said about the threshold if it is to play this political role—to escape ambiguity, sufficientarians must employ a more accurate and institutionally applicable account of what is "enough."

Avoiding ambiguity, however, comes with its own set of dangers. As Casal notes, sufficiency thresholds often become unreasonably arbitrary in the attempt to escape ambiguity.[9] In other words, in trying to set a more accurate threshold with greater potential for political application, sufficientarians often erode the justificatory basis of why having enough is especially important and why it is so much more important than having almost enough. For example, consider a seminal article by Roger Crisp. Crisp builds his sufficientarianism on the requirement (or virtue) of *compassion*.[10] A threshold may be imagined, Crisp holds, below which an impartial and benevolent spectator would feel compassion with whomever was left here. This level constitutes the threshold of sufficiency. In other words, when an impartial spectator, upon placing herself in the shoes of another person, finds that she is no longer moved by compassion to redistribute resources to or increase the welfare of this person, sufficiency has been attained. Now, arguably, this is quite ambiguous (and perhaps even more so than Frankfurt's notion of sufficiency): It is very difficult to determine when someone has enough in this sense—when a person no longer invokes compassion in a benevolent spectator.[11]

---

also Lasse Nielsen, "Sufficiency Grounded as Sufficiently Free: A Reply to Shlomi Segall," *Journal of Applied Philosophy* 33, no. 2 (2016): 202–216.

8. Ronald Dworkin, *Taking Rights Seriously* (London: Bloomsbury, 1977), 162.

9. Casal, "Why Sufficiency Is Not Enough," 313–314. See also Edward Page, "Justice Between Generations: Investigating a Sufficientarian Approach," *Journal of Global Ethics* 3, no. 1 (2007): 15–18.

10. Crisp, "Equality, Priority, and Compassion," 756.

11. It is ambiguous even when taking into account Crisp's clarifications in "Egalitarianism and Compassion," *Ethics* 114, no. 1 (2003): 119–126, that the compassion of the impartial spectator is meant to track only "just claims."

Thus, Crisp suggests, in an attempt to resolve the ambiguity of his impartial spectator's amount of compassion, that "eighty years of high-quality life on this planet is enough, and plausibly more than enough, for any being."[12] As pointed out by Casal, however, this seems to imply that "[a]ccording to Crisp, then, all of humanity could be allowed to die at seventy something for the sake of any nontrivial benefit to somebody just below the threshold."[13] Although Casal unfairly overlooks the clearly probationary nature of Crisp's claim and simplifies his general project, she is correct to highlight the arbitrariness of the general idea.[14] Moreover, whereas the escape from ambiguity calls for more accuracy, avoiding arbitrariness requires employing strong and clear reasons justifying the normative importance of the threshold.

Another way of conceptualizing this problem, we suggest, is that the thresholds employed rely on "thin" concepts. What we mean by this is that saying that someone does not "have enough" or "is in a situation which elicits compassion" does not in itself say something about *why* their situation makes them insufficiently well-off.[15] The concepts on which they rely are "thin," then, because they do not in themselves say what is wrong with insufficiency but, rather, imply that such a situation has some other properties that make it wrong (e.g., not having enough economic resources is not inherently bad or unjust, but the derived lack of opportunities, deprivation, low status, etc. it brings about might be).[16] Rather, both concepts rely on vague descriptions and commonsensical intuitions that, one might say, inform us indirectly—by evoking intuitive associations of *other* reasons—about why a certain state of affairs is above or below the sufficiency threshold. To exemplify, it is not *because* someone's situation is worthy of compassion that we think he or she is a deserving target of distributive justice. Rather, it is the underlying reasons we have for thinking that someone is worthy of compassion that

---

12. Crisp, "Equality, Priority, and Compassion," 762.

13. Casal, "Why Sufficiency Is Not Enough," 313–314.

14. See also Arneson's similar critique of Frankfurt in Richard Arneson, "Egalitarianism and Responsibility," *Journal of Ethics* 3, no. 3 (1997): 225–247; and Page, "Justice Between Generations," 15–16.

15. Of course, compassion is a "thick" concept because saying that an action is compassionate in itself expresses a (positive) evaluation of that action. "Eighty years of high-quality life on this planet," on the contrary, is not.

16. See Bernard Williams, *Ethics and the Limits of Philosophy* (Cambridge, MA: Harvard University Press, 1985), 130, 141–142, 150–152, for a famous distinction between "thin" and "thick" concepts. See also Ronald Dworkin, *Justice for Hedgehogs* (Cambridge, MA: Belknap, 2013), 184, who claims that "thinner concepts draw conclusions but do not themselves suggest much by way of argument."

bring about this intuitive response. However, as mentioned previously, such commonsensical intuitions are too vague to function as distributive principles—these reasons must be fleshed out more.

Furthermore, because these thresholds rely on several underlying normative reasons and have no evaluative content in themselves, specifying their content involves singling out only part of what justifies the threshold in the first place, which will inevitably lead to arbitrariness. Thus, it seems arbitrary to insist on "eighty years of high-quality life" as enough because it is unclear why an impartial spectator would feel compassion for someone living to be seventy-nine but not for someone living to be eighty. However, this, one might say, is partly because of the "thinness" of the concept involved, which is not in itself evaluative and so fleshing out a specific threshold (e.g., 80 years) translates this lack of inherent reasons into a lack of justification. In other words, *part of* what would evoke compassion in an impartial spectator is certainly having a life that is too short. However, this is only a very small part of the reasons underlying this threshold, and so singling it out will inevitably seem arbitrary. Thus, we claim that the problem arises because of the "thinness" of the concepts on which the thresholds rely, which means both that they are ambiguous (because they are not evaluative in themselves) and specifications easily become arbitrary (because their lack of evaluative content will make specifications unable to reflect such content in any satisfying manner).

As mentioned previously, escaping ambiguity requires accuracy, and avoiding arbitrariness entails strong justifications for the placement of the threshold. In the preceding discussion, we suggested that these problems arise due to relying on overly "thin" conceptual thresholds. One way of escaping this, then, seems to be to use a "thicker" threshold, by which we mean one that relies on both descriptive and evaluative elements—one that says something about *when* one is above the threshold and about *why* it is good to attain this level. We sketch such an approach later, but first we discuss another objection often made against sufficientarians—namely that they leave too much outside the scope of justice.

3. Avoiding Underdemandingness

Some sufficientarian accounts cope better with the problem of ambiguity and arbitrariness than others. Most notably, accounts based on some notion of basic needs[17] seem more proficient in elaborating the specific content of the threshold,

---

17. David Miller, *National Responsibility and Global Justice* (Oxford: Oxford University Press, 2007), Chap. 7; Michael Blake, "Distributive Justice, State Coercion, and Autonomy," *Philosophy & Public Affairs* 30, no. 3 (2001): 257–296; Henry Shue, *Basic Rights* (Princeton, NJ: Princeton University Press, 1980).

while still maintaining its normative relevance, than the accounts mentioned previously. Note that basic needs are a "thick" concept in that having one's basic needs satisfied is not only descriptive of one's situation but also in itself evaluative and thus provides reasons for why the emergence of this situation is positive (namely that one's biological existence is secured and is safe from imme- diate, standard threats). This fact alone does not fully rescue sufficientarianism as a distributive ideal, however. Although basic needs accounts do rather well in justifying what is so critically important about reaching the threshold, they face problems with explaining why inequalities above the threshold are unimportant (or significantly less important) to justice. More precisely, they face problems of underdemandingness—of requiring implausibly little of us and only capturing a minimal part of what matters to justice.[18] Next, we consider such a critique.

In substantiating the compassion-based sufficiency account described previ- ously, Roger Crisp points to a hypothetical example known as the Beverly Hills case in which we are asked to choose between distributing fine wine to either a group of rich people or a group of super-rich people. Crisp argues that egalitar- ians and prioritarians are both committed to prioritizing the rich in this case, and he deems this implausible, claiming that distributional differences at such high levels are not a matter of justice.[19] Even if we grant this assumption, however, as Casal notes, it is far less plausible not to be concerned by inequality between the super-rich and the people who have just barely enough.[20] This is the case if we un- derstand Crisp's notion of compassion in a minimal sense—as one in which the benevolent spectator's compassion is only triggered at very low levels of well-being (which is what Casal hints at). It is even more clearly the case if we set the level at basic need fulfillment as depicted previously. Thus, just having your basic needs met when others are super-rich does seem to ground a justice-based claim for redistribution, and claiming otherwise seems to imply an overly underdemanding notion of distributive justice. In other words, setting a fairly low threshold makes it difficult to justify the negative thesis—that above the threshold, inequalities are unimportant (or significantly less important). Although the fulfillment of basic needs is built around a thick notion of sufficiency, justice simply requires more. Thus, in addition to the elements mentioned previously, ideals of sufficiency should avoid underdemandingness.

---

18. See Casal, "Why Sufficiency Is Not Enough," 315–316. See also Nils Holtug's critique of David Miller's global sufficientarianism: "The Cosmopolitan Strikes Back: A Critical Discussion of Miller on Nationality and Global Equality," *Ethics & Global Politics* 4, no. 3 (2011), 158–160.

19. Crisp, "Equality, Priority, and Compassion," 755.

20. Casal, "Why Sufficiency Is Not Enough," 311.

Some political theories with a sufficientarian outlook succeed in avoiding underdemandingness by turning to a threshold based on autonomy.[21] Such thresholds seem intuitively to fare better in regard to underdemandingness than basic needs-based accounts, both due to the obvious fact that being autonomous demands more than just having one's basic needs met and, more important, the commonsensical intuitive force in the statement that claims of justice are significantly less relevant once people are above a certain level at which they able to act autonomously. Note again that this is a "thick" concept having both a descriptive and an evaluative component (that someone has achieved autonomy in itself gives us reason to evaluate his or her situation positively). However, one can be autonomous—free to act in accordance with one's own plans—in many different areas of life. Most would agree, however, that we need some type of objective standard to determine whether people can really be said to be acting autonomously. We need to avoid, for example, considering that people's autonomy is hampered by false consciousness, lack of information, adaptive preferences, or other factors, which may disrupt the manner in which people form preferences and act upon them.[22] There are different ways of doing so, but one promising suggestion involves understanding autonomy in a less subjective sense—namely as connected to ideas of a *flourishing* or *successful* life. Whereas autonomy more generally is concerned with allowing people to live in accordance with their chosen conception of the good life, a flourishing life may be viewed as a more objective subset of such conceptions. This means that justice should be concerned with enabling people to live autonomous lives from within this subset and that the scope of justice is appropriately delimited to a concern with the dimensions of human life that must be available in order for humans to flourish. Martha Nussbaum has provided an extensively elaborated notion of what is entailed in a flourishing life—or in having the opportunities for doing so. Leaning on Aristotle's theory of the human good, she describes 10 central human capabilities that enable people to live a flourishing life.[23] Such a threshold would, obviously, be set at a significantly higher level than mere fulfillment of basic needs.

As we have argued elsewhere, the threshold can, indeed, be convincingly formulated in a way that leans on the concept of leading a successful life.[24] For the

21. Joseph Raz, *The Morality of Freedom* (Oxford: Oxford University Press, 1986), 390–395. See also Blake, "Distributive Justice, State Coercion, and Autonomy," and Nielsen, "Sufficiency Grounded as Sufficiently Free."

22. For a discussion about mistakes and preferences, see Hugh Lazenby, "Mistakes and the Continuity Test," *Politics, Philosophy, and Economics* 15, no. 2 (2016): 190-205.

23. Martha Nussbaum, *Women and Human Development* (New York: Cambridge University Press, 2000) 70–77.

24. Axelsen and Nielsen, "Sufficiency as Freedom from Duress."

purpose of this chapter, we merely note that understanding "enough" as having the relevant opportunities for a successful or flourishing life could live up to the criteria described previously (without thereby ruling out that other thresholds might also fulfill these desiderata). First, it latches onto a "thick" concept in that "flourishing" (and success) includes an evaluative element—that someone has a flourishing life (or the opportunities to lead one) is in itself a positive evaluation of the person's situation and thus provides reasons for affirming the positive thesis (that it is important to achieve sufficiency). In this way, it also avoids arbitrariness by supplying strong reasons for the placement of the threshold—namely the importance of human flourishing. Second, it is not as ambiguous as "having enough economic resources" or "being unworthy of impersonally experienced compassion," but it latches onto a comparatively well-elaborated and intuitively appealing concept of the flourishing or successful life (which contains both an objective standard and latches onto a long tradition in philosophy running from Aristotle to Nussbaum of how to understand the flourishing life by which it may be informed). Finally, it avoids underdemandingness by setting a relatively high threshold, thus making more plausible the claim that inequalities above the threshold are irrelevant. We return to this proposal later and henceforth refer to this type of threshold as based on the value of a *flourishing life*. First, however, we discuss some other considerations of which sufficientarians must be wary.

4. Avoiding Blindness to Important Values

Sufficiency, as we have seen, has been met with many objections. Sufficientarians, however, often find the previously mentioned points of criticism unconvincing—to them, one might say, the threshold is not ambiguous or arbitrary in the sense implied by egalitarians and prioritarians (but, rather, intuitively convincing). There is one objection, however, that sufficientarians generally take on board and to which they seek to shape their principles. That is the claim that sufficientarianism is blind to a range of important values, about which it is implausible to claim that they are beyond the scope of justice. Thus, for example, sufficientarianism has been charged with being unable to see the wrongness of unfairness and discrimination.[25] To clarify, because sufficientarians claim that justice is served once everyone has reached the threshold, they are accused of being blind to (hypothetical) situations in which everyone is above the threshold and one group or individual is then treated unreasonably (but still left sufficiently well off).

---

25. For such lines of criticism, see Casal, "Why Sufficiency Is Not Enough," 315; Larry Temkin, "Equality, Priority, or What?" *Economics and Philosophy* 19 (2003): 61–87; Arneson, "Egalitarianism and Responsibility."

One way in which sufficientarians have usually attempted to incorporate this critique is by adopting a broader basis for their threshold by appealing to things that are valuable *apart* from achieving sufficiency, such as respect or moral equality.[26] Another way is to claim that instances of unfairness, discrimination, or other wrongs are not insignificant but just less significant above the threshold—this is what Liam Shields pioneeringly refers to as "the shift thesis."[27] Third, sufficientarians have often resorted to hybrid models, in which sufficientarianism is coupled with another distributive ideal such as prioritarianism or luck egalitarianism. Such hybrid views, then, apply more than one distributive principle when evaluating the justice of different distributions (e.g., sufficiency coupled with responsibility-sensitive equality above the threshold). In such views, sufficiency is often seen as a secondary part of the ideal—as something that tempers or softens the primary ideals and thus mainly relies on nonsufficientarian reasoning.[28]

Although these solutions all point in the direction of important ways that sufficiency may take the problem of blindness to other important values into account, they all do so at the cost of incurring two further problems. First, they reopen the door to ambiguity about how to understand what constitutes enough, which, as discussed previously, sufficientarians are compelled to avoid. Note that the problem is not that the location of the threshold necessarily becomes less clear (it might, for example, be placed at the rather unambiguous level of basic need satisfaction) but, rather, that the reasons behind the threshold are rendered more ambiguous. Thus, further questions arise about which of the values dominate, how and when this is the case, and, most important, why. Why, one would want to know, should we care so much about responsibility above a certain threshold and not at all below it? Thus, in important ways, the sufficientarian reasoning on which the threshold is founded is compromised and rendered more ambiguous—but this time at the level of weighing different principles against each other.[29] This may, of course, be helped by a "thickening" of the concepts involved in defining the threshold, as mentioned previously. Thus, it would involve accounting for the connection between the different distributive principles and how their importance

---

26. See Frankfurt, "Equality and Respect," *Social Research*, 64, no. 1, (1997): 3–15.

27. See Shields, "The Prospects for Sufficientarianism," 108; Liam Shields, Chapter 5 in this volume.

28. See, for example, Casal, "Why Sufficiency Is Not Enough," 318–323; Shlomi Segall, *Health, Luck, and Justice* (Princeton, NJ: Princeton University Press, 2010), 68–72.

29. For the reverse claim that sufficiency may clash with luck egalitarianism, see Lasse Nielsen and David V. Axelsen, "Three Strikes Out: Objections to Shlomi Segall's Luck Egalitarian Justice in Health," *Ethical Perspectives* 19, no. 2, (2012): 311–315.

is related. This, however, is yet to be done. Importantly, hybrid accounts also involve a second danger: They lose the important and strongly political dimension that comes from focusing only on those who do not have enough. Consider the following example, which is offered by Benbaji (and which is structurally similar to the Beverly Hills example mentioned previously):

> Think of Bill Gates and Warren Buffet, and suppose that they are extremely well off. Would the fact that Buffet is much less well off than Gates be a reason to prefer benefiting Buffet to benefiting Gates? I find it utterly implausible to suppose that any priority at all should be assigned to helping a worse off person rather than a better off one when both persons are extremely well off."[30]

The point is, of course, that prioritarians or egalitarians would be committed to saying that we have *some reason* to prioritize benefitting Buffet over Gates (because he is least well-off and to further equality, respectively). This is, arguably, the case for all the sufficientarian hybrid positions described previously (including the "shift" version by Shields). However, by doing so, we claim, they lose one of the main attractions of ideals of sufficiency—namely that they reject this focus entirely. Not only do they think the Buffet/Gates example is beyond the scope of justice; they also carry with them an inherently political dimension in stating, "Do not look to claims made above the threshold; such claims do not deserve the attention of political philosophers."[31] This claim is a strong one in a world in which too many people have too little and in which many who have more than enough still find reason to make claims on others—and leaving behind this value, we argue, is leaving behind the inherently political focus that is special to sufficiency. Hybrid sufficientarians might object that they can (and do) incorporate this claim by saying that such inequalities do matter, but they are so much more insignificant than insufficiencies. However, this misses the mark. Sufficiency, we take it, holds a specific potential in embracing a certain way of doing political philosophy, which takes actually occurring (as opposed to possible) injustices as its point of departure. They involve the claim that there are certain things with which political philosophy should not concern itself—not just because they are comparatively unimportant but also because admitting them into the scope of justice in any form distorts and devalues the notion of justice. This, we take it, is an important but

30. Benbaji, "The Doctrine of Sufficiency," 315.

31. See also Benbaji's spirited claim to this effect in "The Doctrine of Sufficiency," 315–316, and David V. Axelsen, *Global Redistributive Obligations in the Face of Severe Poverty* (Aarhus, Denmark: Politica, 2014), 27–28.

often overlooked message conveyed by the Buffet/Gates example, the Beverly Hills case by Crisp, and the claim by Frankfurt that such discussions tend to "divert attention from considerations of greater moral importance than equality."[32] It is this inherently political dimension that hybrid accounts applying different distributive principles above and below the threshold stand to lose. Of course, this leaves open the question of whether it is possible to evade blindness to important values such as avoiding discrimination and unfair treatment in our account of sufficiency without incurring these troublesome flaws.

Previously, we argued that a threshold based on the value of a flourishing life may serve as a plausible candidate for sufficiency. So far, however, it is not clear how such a notion of sufficiency may oppose discrimination and unfair treatment—after all, it seems that setting the threshold at the level of a flourishing life would still leave open the possibility of placing unfair burdens on or discriminating against someone who is above this level. This, we claim, is due to an overly monistic view of sufficiency. This, of course, is the claim made by the other sufficientarian approaches mentioned previously that attempt to integrate other distributive principles into their ideal. As discussed previously, however, this leads to debilitating problems of reintroducing ambiguity and neglecting the focus on current insufficiencies. Instead, we claim, sufficiency should embrace *aspect* pluralism—that is, ensuring that sufficiency is secured in different aspects of human life.[33] In other words, a life that is flourishing has several key aspects, and sufficiency must be achieved in *all of* and *each of* these—but without compromising the sufficientarian focus.

5. Aspect Pluralism

Aspect pluralism, as we call it here, is founded on the idea that the most important aspects of a human life "are not commensurable in terms of any single quantitative standard."[34] As mentioned previously, the notion of a flourishing life, which we take to be a plausible candidate for a sufficiency threshold, entails that justice is delimited to a concern with the aspects of human life in which humans may

32. See Frankfurt, "Equality as a Moral Ideal," 23. It might also be worth noticing the parallels with a central element in the theories of many social egalitarians—for example, Elizabeth Anderson, "What Is the Point of Equality?" *Ethics* 209, no. 2 (1999): 287–337, and Jonathan Wolff, "Fairness, Respect, and the Egalitarian Ethos," *Philosophy & Public Affairs* 27 no. 2, (1998): 97–122.

33. By choosing the word "aspect," we are deliberately not taking a stand on the currency of distributive justice.

34. Martha Nussbaum, *Frontiers of Justice: Disability, Nationality, Species Membership* (Cambridge, MA: Harvard University Press, 2007), 166. See also Amartya Sen, *Inequality Reexamined* (Oxford: Oxford University Press, 1995), 46–49.

flourish. It is a matter of some disagreement, however, which exact aspects should be included in such a pluralist ideal.[35] We shall not attempt to settle this here in any final sense.[36] As we argued previously, we must be able to give a thick account of the sufficiency threshold that can give non-arbitrary answers about when and why someone does or does not have enough. Because our purpose in this chapter is to elaborate on the theoretical elements needed for any sufficientarian account to serve as a distributive ideal for political guidance, and not to propose a specific sufficiency ideal, we propose three general aspects that we believe any plausible account of human flourishing must include and that we take to be relatively "ecumenical." For someone to be sufficiently well-off and to be able to lead a flourishing life, then, he or she must have enough in each of these three overall aspects:

1. *Aspects related to biological and physical human needs*: These are the aspects of enjoying basic commodities that every human being needs. They are mainly biological and physical requirements that humans necessarily have, such as nourishment, clean air, health care, housing, and physical and emotional security. At the outset, these aspects are related to survival and basic needs, and they make up the platform from which one may pursue a flourishing, human life.

2. *Aspects related to fundamental interests of a human agent*: These are aspects needed to shape, reshape, and pursue valuable ends. They include being able to imagine, think, reflect critically, and evaluate normatively; being educated and informed in basic functional and technical skills; the ability to understand the implications of decisions and actions for one's life; being able to enjoy natural life; being able to work (in a broad sense); having well-developed emotional capacities; and feeling emotionally affiliated with other human beings.

3. *Aspects related to fundamental interests of a social being*: These are aspects needed for pursuing one's valuable ends within a community. These include the aspects of political freedoms, such as the freedom to vote, the freedom of assembly and association, and the freedom from discrimination and oppression, but also access to some form of market in which one can trade on fair terms with others, enjoying a sufficiently high societal status, not to be dominated by others, etc.[37]

---

35. See, for example, Rutger Claassen and Marcus Düwell, "The Foundations of Capability Theory: Comparing Nussbaum and Gewirth," *Ethical Theory and Moral Practice* 16, no. 3 (2013): 493–510.

36. For a discussion of this issue, see Lasse Nielsen & David V. Axelsen, "Capabilitarian Sufficiency: Capabilities and Social Justice," *Journal of Human Development and Capabilities* (doi: 10.1080/19452829.2016.1145632).

37. For an enlightening analysis of the distinction between basic needs and fundamental interests, see Fabian Schuppert, "Distinguishing Basic Needs and Fundamental Interests," *Critical Review of International Social and Political Philosophy* 16, no. 1 (2013): 24–44. Also,

These aspects, we claim, all constitute vital elements for living a flourishing life. Thus, all three must be secured to a sufficient degree. Note that this fleshed-out conception of a flourishing life meets the criteria described previously in that it escapes ambiguity, due to being fairly accurate in determining the guiding threshold level, and it escapes arbitrariness by being "thick." Recall also that our purpose here is not to propose a specific sufficiency ideal for political guidance but only to lay out the necessary elements for any plausible sufficientarian theory. Thus, the three aspects outlined previously should not be taken as an alternative to other pluralist ideals (such as the one proposed by Nussbaum) but, rather, as outlining a plausible conception of what must be present in all such ideals. Second, it avoids underdemandingness by suggesting a relatively high, threefold threshold. Finally, it avoids the problem of blindness to other important values. It does so by emphasizing the plurality of the aspects involved, which differ not only in their contribution to the good life but also in their distributive logics.

Thus, with regard to aspects related to the fundamental interests of a social being, their just distribution requires a concern with relative shares. In other words, in order to evaluate whether someone has enough with regard to these aspects, we must not only consider their absolute level but also how much they have compared to others. At first, this seems to run against the general sufficientarian idea involved in the negative thesis that inequalities above the threshold are unimportant. However, this is not the case. The reason why we must be concerned with relative holding is that aspects related to the fundamental interests of a social being have strong relational and positional aspects, meaning that one's relative place in the distribution has a major impact on one's absolute capabilities to succeed. Arguably, discrimination is a case of just that—that is, it runs against the fundamental interests of a social being. Thus, when someone above the threshold is discriminated against, he or she is made worse off—and insufficiently badly off—because he or she, and not others, suffers from discrimination. To take a broader example, which may also be said to include cases of discrimination, it seems plausible that societal status be understood as a relational or positional good. In other words, the problem is that a lower status conveys a message of lesser worth in absolute terms. Also, this message is disrespectful because treating one group as having less worth is failing to respond to their humanity with impartiality and failing to respond properly to the equal importance of the success of each human life (as mentioned previously).[38] Finally, the feeling that accompanies

---

for a distinction between the freedom to exchange in itself and trade on capitalist markets as we know them, see Chapter 1 in Amartya Sen, *Development as Freedom* (Oxford: Oxford University Press, 1999). Finally, for a distinctly capabilitarian proposal fleshed out within this framework, see Nielsen & Axelsen, "Capabilitarian Sufficiency."

38. This point is inspired by Frankfurt, "Equality and Respect."

discrimination is a serious threat to the self-respect of the discriminated. Such circumstances would severely hinder any normal person in his or her pursuit of a flourishing life; thus, a relatively low status or being the subject of discrimination brings the person below the absolute threshold. In this way, a pluralist account of sufficiency can capture many of the values to which other sufficiency accounts are normally blind.

With respect to other aspects, however, it seems more reasonable that distributional procedures should be designed so that everyone acquires a decent absolute level, and that relative positions do not matter in themselves. This is generally true for aspects that are not intrinsically relational or positional. This is the case for most aspects related to biological and physical human needs, such as health, housing, and nutrition. It is not in itself a concern of justice that someone is more capable than others in these areas as long as everyone fares well enough. Certainly, everyone needs some level of these to succeed (which is what makes them basic). However, it seems wrong to state that people need equal levels to be able to lead flourishing lives. For example, one is not in any reasonable way unable to live a flourishing life merely because one's health is less perfect than that of others.[39] Thus, inequalities in health *tout court* are not problematic, but only insofar as they simultaneously create inequalities in aspects with relational or positional aspects because this leaves people with an absolutely insufficient access to a successful human life. One might, of course, claim that this relation is inevitable—that inequalities always bring about such problems—and we agree that inequalities are often problematic for these reasons. Importantly, however, how problematic such inequalities are depends on the degree to which they affect positional capabilities. This is even more clearly the case for aspects related to fundamental interests of a human agent, which seem notoriously drawn in both directions.[40] However, it seems both normatively and empirically dubious to state that inequalities are equally important and for the same reasons with respect to these three overall categories of aspects of human lives.

The way in which we propose to avoid blindness to important values, then, is by embracing an aspect pluralist view of a flourishing life. This, we claim, avoids the two worries addressed previously, to which many ideals of sufficiency succumb when attempting to include the important values proposed by other theorists. Thus, the values are incorporated without opening the door to ambiguity (rather, the account has been thickened) and dismissing matters above the threshold as outside the scope of justice; thus, the sufficientarian focus on the injustices of our current world is retained.

---

39. Nielsen and Axelsen, "Three Strikes Out."

40. In "Capabilitarian Sufficiency," Nielsen & Axelsen characterize and discuss these as *quasi-positional capabilities*.

To make these points more clear, it is worth examining more closely a specific application of an ideal that includes the elements outlined previously. In the following, we attempt to do so with respect to health.

6. Sufficiency and Health

Sufficientarians should care about health for several reasons. First, some level of health functioning is objectively important for everyone's ability to lead a flourishing life. Second, health plays an important role in enabling access to other central aspects of life.[41] Health, then, is a suitable case for clarifying the plural aspects of a flourishing life and, consequently, being sensitive to the various distributional logics that apply to the different central aspects.

Imagine the society of Hailithos, in which your health massively impacts other important aspects of your life. First, your societal status is largely determined by how healthy you are; people treat you as a superior person if you are in good shape, disease-free, and entirely without handicaps, whereas you are looked down upon if you are obese, ill, and have a body that does not function well in other respects. Second, people of great health have more of a say in political matters and get access to better schools because people listen more when they speak and instinctively afford them privileges. Assume, on this background, two people (who are representative of two larger groups in Hailithos), Agate and Belle. Agate's health level is adequate but nothing compared to Belle's super-health (let us further assume that the difference is due to factors beyond their control). Because health translates directly into societal status and other important aspects in Hailithos, although Agate enjoys a sufficiently high level of health in itself, she has low status, inadequate political opportunities, and is generally met with scorn and disrespect due to her health being relatively lower than that of Belle (due to the positional nature of this capability). Thus, she must live with a feeling of inferiority and lesser worth vis-à-vis others and a sense of being looked down upon, as Elizabeth Anderson reminds us.[42] This clearly constitutes considerable pressure against Agate's possibilities for living a flourishing life. Recall that this is not because Agate has insufficient health but, rather, because her *relative* level of health determines her relative social status and communal opportunities, which—due to their strong relational and positional aspects—settles her absolute position.

The point of this example is not to say that health has intrinsic positional aspects and should be distributed equally. Instead, we believe that, as a matter of fact

---

41. Lasse Nielsen, "Why Health Matters to Justice: A Capability Theory Perspective," *Ethical Theory and Moral Practice* 18, no. 2 (2015): 403–415.

42. Anderson, "What Is the Point of Equality?" 313.

of actual societies, health distributions should almost exclusively be focused on ensuring that everyone has enough in absolute terms. The point, rather, is that in all actual societies, health has some of the tendencies, which was demonstrated in extreme form in the example of Hailithos. Thus, when considering what it means to ensure that people have a sufficient level of health (or access to health care), we must be aware of how health influences aspects that have strong positional or relational aspects—how it influences people's societal status, their opportunities to influence collective decisions, their job opportunities, etc.—besides, of course, being concerned with ensuring that people are healthy *enough*.

One way of alleviating insufficiencies brought about by the influence on positional or relational aspects would be to redistribute health care from Belle to Agate, and in this manner bring Agate above the threshold regarding status and other opportunities by way of the derived effect of health on this capability. However, in cases in which redistribution is not so straightforward (and we take it that this is often the case for redistributing health from one person or group to another), this might involve a significant amount of waste and inefficiency—if, for example, making Agate's societal status sufficiently high requires making Belle less healthy so that it becomes equally status-endowing to that of Agate. In such circumstances, a strategy of ring-fencing may be employed to lessen the effect of health on other aspects to avoid leveling down.[43] We might, so to speak, cut the bonds that connect the two by undermining the norms and values that make low health be viewed as a special mark of status. Furthermore, because it is actually insufficiency of status and not health that puts Agate's capabilities under pressure, ring-fencing will help target the problem more head-on. Of course, whether ring-fencing ought to be preferred will depend on the feasibility of breaking the causal link and the relative costs and gains involved.[44]

A related point is made by Wolff and de-Shalit, who show that many disadvantages have a tendency to "cluster."[45] In other words, low levels of one aspect often have strong and unexpected negative effects on other aspects, and this seems especially pertinent with regard to health. Ring-fencing might help limit this unpredictability and facilitate greater control when alleviating people's disadvantages.

7. Conclusion

A plausible account of sufficiency must avoid four dangers: It must avoid ambiguity, arbitrariness, underdemandingness, and blindness to other important values

---

43. Regarding ring-fencing, see also Matthew Johnson, "Towards a Theory of Cultural Evaluation," *Critical Review of Social and Political Philosophy* 17, no. 2 (2014): 145–167.

44. In Harry Brighouse and Adam Swift, "Equality, Priority, and Positional Goods," *Ethics* 116, no. 3 (2006): 488–491, the authors suggest a similar strategy.

45. Wolff and de-Shalit, *Disadvantage* (Oxford: Oxford University Press, 2007), 122–127.

besides sufficiency. To do so, a sufficiency account must be built around a "thick" concept and avoid ambiguity so as to be able to function as a political principle, it must not set the threshold at too low a level, and it must embrace aspect pluralism. We suggested that such a threshold may be constructed around the value of a flourishing life, which involves ensuring that people are adequately well-off in (at least) three separate aspects of human life.

Acknowledgments

We are very grateful to the editors of this volume, Carina Fourie and Annette Rid, as well as Tom Parr, Clare Burgum, and Liam Shields, for thorough and insightful comments on an earlier draft of this chapter.

PART III

Sufficiency, Health, and Health Care Justice

7

Intergenerational Justice, Sufficiency, and Health

Axel Gosseries

1. Introduction

Does sufficientarianism have a distinctive message to deliver on matters of inter-generational justice in relation to health? This chapter aims to answer this question. It is limited in three ways. It focuses on a single type of theory of justice, namely sufficientarianism. It is concerned with intergenerational justice, which is only one dimension of justice, and even more precisely with justice between birth cohorts, with the latter focusing on one of the understandings of the word "generation." Finally, it limits itself to one object of justice—that is, health and health care.

The distinction between birth cohorts and age groups is key here. "Birth cohort" and "age group" are two meanings of "generation." A birth cohort is a set of people born between date x and date y (e.g., all those born in 1970), whereas an age group is a set of people sharing the same age, regardless of the period at stake. For instance, those who were 40 years old in 1722 and those who are 40 years old in 2016 belong to the same age group while clearly not belonging to the same birth cohort. Whenever we are concerned about justice between birth cohorts, we are concerned about whether (individuals from) different cohorts treat each other fairly—for example, whether the cohort born between 1970 and 1980 does what it owes the previous or the next one. When we wonder about the demands of justice between age groups, we ask ourselves what an age group owes another—for example, what people in their 40s owe pensioners and children.

Most of us share intergenerational justice concerns. We wonder what we owe future generations in terms of natural and cultural heritage—for example, in terms of climate justice and of educational effort, in terms of nuclear waste management and of financial sustainability for our pension schemes, in terms of biodiversity conservation and of democratic institutions, and so on. Insofar as health care is concerned, the "care" aspect may suggest that we primarily frame issues in terms of justice between *age groups*, with age being associated with stronger dependency (infants and elderly people) or with the incidence of specific pathologies (diseases that primarily affect children, late adults, elderly people, etc.). However, we focus here on health and health care issues from the angle of justice between *birth cohorts*.

Admittedly, there are specific challenges to claims of justice between birth cohorts. Insofar as obligations toward future people are concerned, such challenges typically include doubts as to whether people who do not exist yet could have rights or the non-identity objection to which we return later.[1] Also, reasons to care about justice between birth cohorts are roughly of the same nature as those one may invoke to ground concerns of, for example, global justice. For instance, a "chronopolitan" will typically adopt as a starting point the view that people should be treated impartially, regardless of their *date* of birth, just as a cosmopolitan in debates about global justice will tend to consider a person's *place* of birth as an unjustified ground for disadvantage. If major disadvantages are associated with our date of birth, an impartialist will call for a justice-driven response. Such advantages and disadvantages do arise, and they are significant. For instance, the average life expectancy at birth in a European country such as Belgium evolved from 46.52 years in 1900 to 77.78 years in 2000.[2] Similarly, there has been a significant increase in years of schooling in the same country during roughly the same period, evolving from 5.36 years on average in 1921 to 10.04 years on average in 2001.[3] Thus, for most theories of justice, concerns of justice between birth cohorts make sense and are significant.[4]

As mentioned previously, I do not deal here with sufficientarian justice *between age groups*. Let me briefly discuss the main issues in this respect.[5] The question

1. See Axel Gosseries, "On Future Generations' Future Rights," *Journal of Political Philosophy* 16, no. 4 (2008): 450–464.

2. Sources: "Human Mortality Database" (https://www.mortality.org), University of California (Berkeley, CA), and Max Planck Institute for Demographic Research (Germany). See also https://data.oecd.org/healthstat/life-expectancy-at-birth.htm.

3. David De la Croix and Vincent Vandenberghe, "Human Capital as a Factor of Growth and Employment at the Regional Level: The Case of Belgium," Report to the European Commission, Employment and Social Affairs, 2004, p. 10.

4. For a comparative overview, see Axel Gosseries, "Theories of Intergenerational Justice: A Synopsis," *Surveys and Perspectives Integrating Environment and Society* 1, no. 1 (2008): 61–71.

5. For further developments, see Axel Gosseries, "What Makes Age Discrimination Special? A Philosophical Look at the ECJ Case Law," *Netherlands Journal of Legal Philosophy* 43, no. 1 (2014): 59–80.

arising with respect to age groups and health/health care is typically the follow-ing: "Should access to treatment x be subject to an upper and/or lower age limit?" This leads us to ask to what extent an age limit differs from gender or "racial" criteria. The key distinctive feature in this respect is that *we all age*, which has no equivalent in the cases of gender and race. What follows at the normative level? At least two types of arguments, both relevant to health care.

First, there is the "complete life" argument that claims that age limits tend to be unproblematic both because we should take people's complete lives as the rel-evant units of ethical concern and because age limits generally do not lead to dif-ferential treatment over people's complete lives. The problem is that, in practice, the latter (factual) claim is often violated. Moreover, sufficientarians will tend to have a specific approach to the argument's normative premise, in two ways.[6] They might claim that equality over complete lives is not enough and that sufficiency should be guaranteed *all along* people's lives, continuously. This might be espe-cially relevant for certain types of health care—for example, pain medicine. They might also give a sufficientarian interpretation of what is required over complete lives, claiming, for instance, that we should make sure that as many as possible reach a minimum, sufficient number of years of existence, a life span threshold beyond which the nature of what justice requires would change.

The defensive "complete life" argument claims that there is often nothing wrong with age limits. There is also a set of arguments that claim that there can be something good about age limits. These arguments tend to focus on two types of dimensions: efficiency and equality. A typical *equality-oriented* argument—that can easily be given a sufficientarian form—is that upper age limits tend to shift resources toward young people, increasing equality over complete lives. For in-stance, not reimbursing or even not providing access to certain life-saving health services (e.g., organ donation) beyond a given age shifts health resources toward younger patients. This might equalize life expectancies.[7] Typical *efficiency-oriented* arguments for using age limits include the efficiency of using age as a proxy in order to save on information-gathering costs (e.g., a proxy for the ability to con-sent to certain forms of treatment) and/or of using age limits as ways of structur-ing our lives in an efficient way. Consider compulsory education until a certain age to ensure that people study before they start working, or compulsory vaccina-tion before a certain age to ensure that people get a vaccine as early as possible. For most sufficientarians, both types of reasons may be relevant. Equalizing life

---

6. Gosseries, "What Makes Age Discrimination Special?" 67–68.

7. See Marc Fleurbaey, Marie-Louise Leroux, and Grégory Ponthière, "Compensating the Dead," *Journal of Mathematical Economics* 51 (C) (2014): 28–41.

expectancies matters to the extent that it allows more people to reach the suffi-ciency level, framed in terms of sufficient life expectancy. Efficiency matters to the extent that it increases our ability to level up more people to the sufficiency level.

Hence, although I do not address issues of justice between age groups in this chapter, they are crucial to health and health care. They require us to scrutinize the numerous age criteria on which health care regimes rely. They also invite us to understand the nature of obligations that adults have toward children and that midlife adults have toward the elderly, especially insofar as informal care is concerned.

Note more generally that connecting justice between age groups with justice between birth cohorts is not straightforward. Some may adopt a view on justice between age groups that rejects the complete life view, the latter being key for justice between birth cohorts.[8] Alternatively, one may understand age-specific rights and duties as a mere *translation* of whole life duties and rights. Finally, we might understand their relationship as one of *compatibility* rather than *derivation*. Age-specific rights and duties should be compatible with rights and duties deriv-ing from justice between cohorts, in the same way as rights and duties deriving from justice between birth cohorts should be compatible with the definition of our global rights and duties, and vice versa.

I proceed in three steps. First, what sufficientarianism requires in general in the intergenerational realm is discussed. I also examine whether there are spe-cifically intergenerational defenses of sufficientarianism. I do not focus on health at this first stage and will understand generations as "birth cohorts" all along. Second, I discuss health issues. I try to determine whether some health issues are especially of intergenerational interest. Third, I discuss what a *non-isolationist* ap-proach tells us about intergenerational justice in health and health care.

2. Sufficientarianism and Birth Cohorts

2.1. Three Distinctive Features

Let me first identify whether and how the intergenerational demands of sufficien-tarianism may differ from those of other theories of justice. I take as a starting point a generalist sufficientarian view extending itself to the realm of justice be-tween birth cohorts. Its metric can be of a "basic needs" or of a "basic capabilities" type, although it could be welfarist too (discussed later). Consider four formula-tions, the first three of which are clearly sufficientarian:

---

8. Dennis McKerlie, *Justice Between the Young and the Old* (Oxford: Oxford University Press, 2013), Chap. 4.

Pinchot (1910): "It recognizes the right of the present generation to use what it needs and all it needs of the natural resources now available, but [also] recognizes equally our obligation so to use what we need that our descendants shall not be deprived of what they need."[9]

Brundtland (1987): Development is sustainable if it "meets the needs of the present without compromising the ability of future generations to meet their own needs."[10]

Daly (1996): "The basic needs of the present should always take precedence over the basic needs of the future, but the basic needs of the future should take precedence over the extravagant luxury of the present."[11]

Sen (2014): "The idea of sustainable development can be broadened from the formulations proposed by Brundtland and Solow to encompass the preservation and expansion of the substantive freedoms and capabilities of people today without compromising the capability of future generations to have similar or more freedoms."[12]

The Pinchot/Brundtland formulations share the same spirit, whereas that of Daly departs from intergenerational impartiality unless we can argue that there are good reasons to discount the moral importance of future people's needs.[13] Sen's proposal differs in various ways from those of Pinchot and Brundtland: The *criterion* differs because it calls not only for the preservation but also for the expansion of substantive freedoms and capabilities (for people today but also, as a result, for people tomorrow); the metric differs too because it replaces a concern for basic needs with a broader concern for freedom and capabilities. A sufficientarian could adopt one of these formulations to characterize his or her intergenerational views.

---

9. Gifford Pinchot, *The Fight for Conservation* (New York: Doubleday, Page, and Company, 1910), 80, cited in Richard Howarth, "Towards an Operational Sustainability Criterion," *Ecological Economics* 63 (2007): 656.

10. World Commission on the Environment and Development, *Our Common Future* (Oxford: Oxford University Press, 1987), 53 (often referred to as the *Brundtland Report*, after its Chair's name).

11. Herman Daly, *Beyond Growth. The Economics of Sustainable Development* (Boston: Beacon Press, 1996), 36.

12. Amartya Sen, "Global Warming Is Just One of Many Environmental Threats That Demand Our Attention," *The New Republic* (August 22, 2014).

13. See, for example, Luc Van Liedekerke, "Discounting the Future. John Rawls and Derek Parfit's Critique of the Discount Rate," *Ethical Perspectives* 11, no. 1 (2004): 72–83; Gregory Ponthière, "Should We Discount Future Generations' Welfare? A Survey of the "Pure" Discount Rate Debate," Liège: CREPP Working Paper, 2003.

Here, I note three features of sufficientarianism. First, a sufficientarian view defines what we owe the next generation partly independently from what we inherited, or from what we ended up having ourselves through a mix of inheritance, work, and natural circumstances specific to our period of existence (as suggested by Sen's formulation). This potentially leads to a set of properties on which we cannot expand here.[14] In contrast, for a typical *cleronomic* view—meaning roughly "ruled by inheritance" in Greek—it is what we inherit from the previous generation that sets the standard for what we owe the next one. Egalitarianism, for instance, can be framed in those terms (see Table 7.2). In Brundtland's case, the basic needs metric sets the target *in part* independently from that—in part only, because under Brundtland's definition, the amount of what we inherited is indirectly taken into account through a concern for the current generation's ability to ensure the coverage of its own basic needs associated with the effort necessary to provide for the next generation's basic needs. If very little were bequeathed to us, the chances are significant that our efforts to provide for the basic needs of the next generation would threaten our own ability to cover our own basic needs.

Admittedly, whereas Brundtland's definition is only moderately non-cleronomic, a sufficientarian could adopt a *strictly non-cleronomic* view, totally disregarding what was inherited and, as a result, what efforts would be required from the current generation to guarantee sufficient conditions for covering the next generation's basic needs. Would such a strictly non-cleronomic view not violate the requirement that we should treat members of different cohorts impartially? Does it not disregard the costs on the current generation, potentially bringing it below the sufficiency threshold? The answer depends on the extent to which the possibility of having children is included in the set of basic needs for each individual. For if resources were insufficient to guarantee that the basic needs of the next generation be covered, we could decide to reproduce less.[15] In this case, we would be able to adjust our effort in a manner compatible with the coverage of our own basic needs through adjusting our reproduction rate, possibly to a level equal to zero if resources are radically scarce. In contrast, if we believe that any plausible sufficientarian view should include the basic right to a reproduction rate that is above zero, as well as the means associated to it, sufficientarianism should be *moderately* non-cleronomic.

Although Sen is often viewed as a sufficientarian due to his insistence on basic capabilities, the account of sustainability that he provides us with here is arguably

---

14. Axel Gosseries, "A Justiça Intergeracional e a Metáfora do Refúgio de Montanha," *Philosophica (Lisbon)* 38 (2011): 121–141.

15. For a sufficientarian case for a duty to reproduce, see Anca Gheaus, "Could There Ever be a Duty to Have Children?" in *Permissible Progeny?* ed. Samantha Brennan, Sarah Hannan, and Richard Vernon (New York: Oxford University Press, 2015).

Table 7.1 The Cleronomicity of Various Views

	Cleronomic	Noncleronomic
Strict	Egalitarianism	Sufficientarianism without guaranteed reproductive right
Moderate	Sen's suggestion	Brundtland's sufficientarianism

not sufficientarian. However, Sen's formulation ("of people today") suggests another way in which a non-sufficientarian could be *moderately cleronomic*—as opposed to *strictly non-cleronomic* or *moderately non-cleronomic*. Such a view would adopt as a reference point neither an independent standard (e.g., objective conditions for basic needs satisfaction) nor what we inherited (as is the case for most theories, such as egalitarian ones). It would focus instead on what we ended up having benefited from in terms of opportunities *by the end of our life*, which involves a mix of inheritance and the fruits of *our own* labor. This is another option that is not explored here.[16] However, it helps the reader to understand the distinctiveness of a sufficientarian approach. The claim is that any sufficientarian view applied to the intergenerational realm should fit within one of the two rows of the right column of Table 7.1.

A second important feature of sufficientarianism comes to light when we consider how non-sufficientarian views deal with generational savings and dissavings. *Generational savings* obtain whenever a birth cohort transfers more (per head) to the next one than what it inherited. *Generational dissavings* obtain whenever a birth cohort transfers less (per head) to the next one than what it inherited. A *utilitarian* theory of justice aims at maximizing the total amount of well-being of a relevant group—here the members of current and future generations altogether. It will typically defend a *duty of generational savings*, for the purposes of the intergenerational maximization of welfare.[17] The driving intuition is that under certain conditions, one unit of *x* invested in a productive way today will allow for much more consumption and well-being in the future than if it were consumed today. Unless they relax a requirement of intergenerational impartiality, utilitarians will tend to require an indefinite sacrifice of earlier generations to the benefit of later ones.

A *leximin egalitarian* view differs from a utilitarian one in that it is more distributive. Rather than maximizing the total amount of *x* within a given population, it aims at maximizing the amount of *x* that the least well-off enjoys, and then for

---

16. I am also unable to explore here what the equivalent of the cleronomic intuition would amount to in terms of global justice.

17. On what follows, see Gosseries, "Theories of Intergenerational Justice."

Table 7.2 The "Savings/Dissavings" Lens: Sufficientarianism
and Two of Its Alternatives

	Generational Dissavings	Generational Savings
Utilitarianism	Prohibited	Compulsory
Leximin egalitarianism	Prohibited	Prohibited
Sufficientarianism	Authorized unless insufficient for basic needs of future generation(s)	Authorized unless insufficient for basic needs of current generation

the second least well-off, for the third least well-off, and so on, within the reference population. It will *prohibit* both generational dissavings and generational savings. The driving intuition underlying this surprising prohibition on savings is that savings entail an opportunity cost for the (early) least well-off. This is incompatible with the leximination of the least well-off's expectations across generations.[18]

As to sufficientarianism, it will typically *authorize* both dissavings and savings provided that we remain above the sufficiency level. The theory therefore differs substantially from the other ones. If we want to adopt policies through which one generation wants to tighten its belts to render the next generation much richer than itself, there is no objection in principle as long as such efforts do not bring anyone below the sufficiency level. Similarly, a generation that wishes to spoil most of what it inherited is allowed to do so provided that it leaves enough to its descendants to cover for their basic needs. Table 7.2 summarizes the three views and their prescriptions in terms of generational dissavings and savings.

In addition to the two distinctive features emphasized so far—namely moderate non-cleronomicity and the authorization (within limits) on both generational dissavings and savings—characteristics of the metrics that sufficientarians tend to adopt might be of relevance here as well. For general purposes, the core of some of the main theories of justice can be presented as a mix of the following: a *criterion* ("maximizing the total amount of *x*," "maximizing the least well-off's level of *x*," "equalizing *x* for all," "guaranteeing a minimum of *x* to all," etc.) and a *metric* (or currency) (with *x* standing for "basic capabilities," "welfare," "opportunity for welfare," etc.).

We previously focused on the criterion. Regarding the metric, it can be more or less *preference-sensitive*—that is, take into account people's actual (or filtered) preferences as opposed to trying to adopt "objective" standards such as the daily intake

18. For further developments, see Frédéric Gaspart and Axel Gosseries, "Are Generational Savings Unjust?" *Politics, Philosophy & Economics* 6, no. 2 (2007): 193–217.

of calories that an average person needs. It can also be more or less *responsibility-sensitive*—that is, only aim at equalizing, maximizing, and so on the level of x that is independent of people's (problematic) choices. Equalizing welfare differs from equalizing opportunity for welfare. One label that usually refers to such responsibility-sensitivity is "luck" (as in "luck egalitarianism," "luck leximin egalitarianism," "luck utilitarianism," "luck sufficientarianism," etc.).

Sufficientarians tend to adopt a metric that is less preference-sensitive, such as basic needs. It is not that sufficientarianism should necessarily abandon a preference-sensitive approach. It is rather that, if distributive duties are more limited, such preference-insensitivity remains more easily compatible with the liberal concern for respecting the variety of conceptions of the good life. Sufficientarians also tend to adopt a *responsibility-insensitive* metric.[19] For some, this is the very reason for adopting a sufficientarian perspective. Again, such responsibility-insensitivity is not too burdensome on duty-holders because distributive duties are supposedly more limited than for other distributive views. Also, a sufficientarian defending a responsibility-sensitive metric might be subject to the "harshness objection" to an especially strong degree, at least if there are no demands of justice above the sufficiency threshold. The idea is that it would be too harsh on a person with some of her basic needs unmet to claim that we do not owe her distributive transfers because she is responsible for her situation. Very few would thus defend luck sufficientarianism.[20]

Do such preference-insensitivity and responsibility-insensitivity have any interesting implications in the intergenerational realm? As to the former, one important feature of intergenerational relations is that the content of the next generation's preferences is not independent from the decisions of the current generation. Through informal and formal education, each cohort has a significant impact on the preference-formation process of the next one. This means that to some extent, if the view were strictly based on each generation's actual preferences, each of them could decide to soften its intergenerational obligations through inculcating easy-to-satisfy preferences into the next generation. The move toward a less preference-sensitive metric is therefore a strength in this respect.[21]

---

19. See Axel Gosseries, "Qu'est-ce que le suffisantisme?" *Philosophiques* 38, no. 2 (2011): 472–475.

20. See, however, Cécile Fabre, *Justice in a Changing World* (Cambridge, UK: Polity Press, 2007), 37 ("not to be left below the sufficiency threshold *for reasons which are outside their control*—such as race, gender, disability") (italics added).

21. See Danielle Zwarthoed, "Creating Frugal Citizens: The Liberal Egalitarian Case for Teaching Frugality," *Theory and Research in Education* 13 (2015): 286–307.

Regarding responsibility-insensitivity, it often refers to whether the potential beneficiary of a social transfer should be held responsible for his disadvantaged situation. One less often discussed aspect is whether the difficulties that a duty-holder experiences in achieving such transfers should also be considered. Interestingly, a plain non-cleronomic view will tend to disregard the difficulties that a generation may have in securing the conditions for sufficiency for the next generation. Each generation should meet the target, regardless of how much it received from its predecessors and how much bad luck it experienced during its own existence. As indicated previously, sufficientarians can instead endorse a moderate non-cleronomic view, taking into account the impact of the current generation's efforts on its own ability to meet its basic needs. It can do so without necessarily shifting to a responsibility-sensitive metric.

In contrast, a responsibility-sensitive view that takes responsibility seriously, including on the duty-holder side, may actually tend to support a stronger degree of cleronomicity. However, the link between taking what we inherited as a reference point and limiting the inheritance preservation efforts of the current generation is not totally straightforward. Moreover, insofar as the beneficiaries of potential social transfers are concerned, imagine that our predecessors have underinvested in a manner considered problematic. If they run short of resources by the end of their lives, sufficientarians will still guarantee that the basic needs of these predecessors will be covered through ascending transfers from the current generation to the previous one. This may entail significant efforts for the currently active generation.

2.2. Two Specific Defenses

Later, I return to whether the three features just identified—moderate non-cleronomy, qualified authorization to save and dissave, and preference- and responsibility-insensitivity—carry any implications in the realm of health and health care. I have just shown how sufficientarianism differs from other theories of justice in the intergenerational realm. Let me now discuss two specific ways in which sufficientarianism can be defended in this realm. Rather than asking ourselves *what* sufficientarianism entails, we ask ourselves *why* we should adopt it. The two possible defenses presented here are special in the sense that they could be endorsed by authors who do not necessarily adopt sufficientarianism as a general theory of justice in the domestic and/or intragenerational realm. Note that each of these strategies leads to a different definition and understanding of the nature of the sufficiency threshold.

The first strategy is Rawlsian and amounts to defending "institutional sufficientarianism." It rests on the factual assumption that a certain amount of resources are necessary to enable institutions to protect basic freedoms. This is distinct from a political sufficientarianism à la Elizabeth Anderson ("democratic egalitarianism").[22] The idea is not (only) that each individual should reach a minimum threshold in order to be able to function as a citizen in a democratic regime. It is (rather) that the institutional setting needs resources to protect the citizens' basic freedoms.

What is the context of this defense of accumulation *up to a certain threshold?* Rawls is worried about the fact that compulsory savings—as defended by utilitarians—violate the demands of justice. The most plausible reason to worry about it is that an accumulation path does not allow for making sure that the least well-off be as well off as the least well-off under any alternative path. Whenever a generation transfers more to the next one than what it inherited, an opportunity cost for the least well-off members of the current generation follows. If there is a surplus, why not direct it to the least well-off members of our generation rather than to the next generation? The idea is not one of generational partiality here. Rather, if each generation were to direct its "surplus" (compared to what it inherited) at the least well-off in its generation, we would end up with an intergenerational path compatible with the demands of maximin/leximin.[23] At the same time, without any form of accumulation, at least at the beginning of mankind's evolution, we would not dispose of enough resources to support basic institutions. Rawls' proposal amounts to limiting the violation of maximin as much as possible to what is necessary (and *sufficient*) to support such institutions. Hence the label "institutional sufficientarianism," which relies on the priority of liberty to justify a temporary violation of the demands of leximin/maximin egalitarianism during an accumulation phase.[24]

How does this type of "institutional sufficientarianism" connect with more standard "substantive sufficientarianism" (e.g., of a basic needs type)? First, one may be more radical than Rawls. Instead of allowing for both savings and dissavings once the demands of institutional sufficiency are met, one could advocate a prohibition on both savings and dissavings (i.e., strict rule) once accumulation has allowed us to reach an institutional sufficiency threshold (see Table 7.2). The reference point for such a "neither save, nor dissave" rule will be what we inherited from the previous generation. Combined with the definition of the institutional threshold, it follows that in full compliance, steady state would amount de facto to sticking to this institutional sufficiency threshold forever—again, without

---

22. Elizabeth Anderson, "What Is the Point of Equality?" *Ethics* 109, no. 2 (1999): 287–337.

23. For further developments, see Axel Gosseries, "Nations, Generations and Climate Justice," *Global Policy* 5, no. 1 (2014): 96–102; Axel Gosseries, "Reply to My Critics," *Diacritica* 28, no. 2 (2014): 343–348.

24. Gosseries, "Reply to My Critics."

necessarily endorsing sufficientarianism in general. Second, there does not seem to be a full overlap between resources that are needed to support basic-freedom-protecting institutions and resources that are needed to support basic needs of individuals. It seems that resources necessary to support the latter are more extensive than resources to support the former because not all basic needs are basic-freedom-related.

There is another pathway that does not require endorsing sufficientarianism in general. It responds to the non-identity problem. The latter arises as soon as an allegedly harmful action is also a necessary condition for a person's existence.[25] An example is when a child who is the result of cloning claims that such cloning was wrongful to her. In such cases, a standard person-affecting concept of harm delivers the following conclusion: If we cannot show that the alternative state of this very person would have been better for her than her current state, she cannot claim to have been harmed. If the person would otherwise not have existed, there is no alternative state for that person. As a result, no harm resulting from the allegedly harmful action—a necessary condition for this person's very existence—follows. A variety of responses have been envisaged. One of them consists of substituting a threshold-based concept of harm to the standard comparative-to-counterfactual concept that I just presented. Under such an alternative, threshold-based understanding of harm, a person would be harmed not if her current condition is worse than her condition in the absence of the allegedly harmful action. Instead, she is harmed if her current condition is simply "bad"—that is, worse than an independently defined threshold. This response to the non-identity challenge may then lead in turn to adopting sufficientarianism as a theory of intergenerational justice because our intergenerational relationships are extensively affected by the non-identity problem.[26]

As in the case of "institutional sufficientarianism," the challenge is how to relate such "harm threshold sufficientarianism" with a standard substantive sufficientarianism (e.g., of the basic needs type). A dilemma obtains: If the harm threshold is higher than what a "life worth living" requires, we would consider "bad" some lives that would be perfectly worth living. For example, claiming that harm would not be avoided unless the beings we bring to life can have the capacity to be "fully functioning members of society"[27] is setting the standard too high for a life "worth living." On the other hand, if such a low threshold serves as a reference

---

25. Derek Parfit, *Reasons and Persons* (Oxford: Oxford University Press, 1984), Chap. 16.

26. Lukas Meyer and Dominic Roser, "Enough for the Future," in *Intergenerational Justice*, ed. A. Gosseries and L. Meyer (Oxford: Oxford University Press, 2009), 220–249.

27. Edward Page, "Justice Between Generations: Investigating a Sufficientarian Approach," *Journal of Global Ethics* 3, no. 1 (2007): 17. Compare with David Copp (1998), cited in Page, "Justice Between Generations" 17 ("Matters of basic need are things anyone would require in some quantity and in some form in order to avoid a blighted and harmed life").

point not only for the definition of harm but also for the definition of our inter-generational distributive duties in general, it sounds as if this harm-derived form of sufficientarianism would define far too minimalistic intergenerational obliga-tions, arguably lower than what basic needs sufficientarianism would require. In other words, if basic needs coverage corresponds to a higher standard than one of a life "merely" worth living, the type of life-worth-living sufficientarianism that one may derive as a response to the non-identity problem will be less demanding than what standard sufficientarianism requires. Avoiding that the life of the next generation be harmful in this sense is quite a minimalistic goal indeed.

What follows is that although in the intergenerational sphere, there may be specific reasons to defend "institutional sufficientarianism" or "life-worth-living sufficientarianism" without endorsing sufficientarianism in general,[28] such thresholds are likely to be too low to serve as a reference point for plain suf-ficientarians. As a result, these defenses cannot plausibly support a robust suf-ficientarian account of intergenerational justice. Extending standard substantive sufficientarianism to the intergenerational realm remains the best avenue to de-velop an intergenerational sufficientarian view.

3. Health Policy Implications: The Isolationist Approach

It is one thing to present a general theory of intergenerational justice and to point at some of its distinctive features. It is another to identify what (if anything) it has to say in a given sector about the distribution of specific goods. One might be tempted to adopt an isolationist (or good-specific) approach here[29]—that is, view

---

28. A third reason for why non-sufficientarians may want to endorse intergenerational suf-ficientarianism is invoked by Fabre: "The difficulty which population size poses for luck egalitarians is one reason why some people of a strongly egalitarian bent are tempted to adopt a sufficientist view of our obligations to our successors. ... Deciding how much to save [to ensure that our successors have enough resources not to be utterly destitute] is *much easier* than working out how much to save to ensure that our successors each have an equal share" (Cécile Fabre, *Justice in a Changing World*, 36–37; italics added). However, even under a constant population scenario, it is unclear why setting the level of basic needs and specifying what it requires (including in terms of reproductive rights) is *much easier* than assessing what our generation inherited under the relevant metrics. Also, when the popula-tion fluctuates, we have to adapt the level of generational transfers accordingly, both under an egalitarian view and under a sufficientarian view.

29. See Axel Gosseries, "Are Seniority Privileges Unfair?" *Economics & Philosophy* 20, no. 2 (2004): 298–301 (articulating "good-specific" analysis and "all-things-considered" analysis in the employment sector); Simon Caney, "Just Emissions," *Philosophy & Public Affairs* 40, no. 4 (2012): 259 (introducing the "method of isolation" and the "method of integration" in the climate context); Andreas Albertsen and Carl Knight, "A Framework for Luck Egalitarianism

the distribution of a good or set of goods as if they were the only goods we had to distribute between people—and here between generations—applying our general principle to such goods. Consider a situation in which several goods should be distributed across generations. Imagine that we do not know anything about whether the distribution of other non-health-related goods is fair or not. For instance, we do not know whether there is a significant public debt, whether we are emitting a large amount of CO_2, whether educational technology is flourishing, whether extreme poverty is likely to shrink, and so on. We only have knowledge about specific health-related goods. We would then simply apply intergenerational sufficientarianism to such goods/issues and provide policy advice accordingly.

One advantage of "isolationism" is that it is more likely to deliver faster, operational recommendations than an integrated (or "all-goods-considered") approach, the latter being more data-intensive. However, operationality does not necessarily go hand in hand with rightness (see Section 4). Moreover, in the case of health care, the literature on the social determinants of health reminds us of the difficulty involved in isolating health-related issues from health-unrelated ones.[30] In the list mentioned previously, CO_2 emissions, poverty, and education all have significant health impacts. However, let me assume for the time being that isolationism is right and consider three policy issues.

3.1. Drug Patent Length

Incentivizing medical research raises various issues. One concerns the research versus curing alternative: Should we devote funds to finding new cures rather than more fully implement existing ones? Medical research is an investment. It entails net costs for the drug-developing generations and net benefits for the post-development generations. In contrast, implementing existing cures entails net benefits to the present generation too. From a sufficientarian perspective, assuming that we have enough technology today to allow most people to lead a life of sufficient length and quality, public funding should probably give priority to curing people through existing drugs and to transferring the existing knowledge to the next generations rather than to research on new drugs.

However, although sufficientarians are less likely than, for example, utilitarians to support the public funding of extensive medical research, they are more

in Health and Healthcare," *Journal of Medical Ethics* 41, no. 2 (2015): 166 (on "isolationism" and "integrationism" in health and health care).

30. Richard Wilkinson and Michael Marmot, eds., *Social Determinants of Heath: The Solid Facts*, 2nd ed. (Copenhagen: WHO Europe, 2003): 31.

likely than others to allow people to invest in medical research privately. This is so because sufficientarianism typically caps duties of justice more than do other theories of justice, which would lead to a lesser fiscal pressure, for example. Moreover, for pathologies for which medical research is needed to bring people to sufficiency, sufficientarians will also support public funding for research.

The question then arises as to how to best design incentives for such research. Let me discuss one ingredient of such a scheme: patent length. It is sometimes suggested that a shorter patent duration would be fairer. Of course, shorter patent length might reduce investment. However, holding the amount of investment constant, if a return on investment needs to be achieved over a shorter period, prices per unit are likely to be higher, ceteris paribus, which will hinder access for the least well-off. Let us consider, hypothetically, a patent that deals with a life-saving drug against a disease that affects mostly younger people, making it especially relevant to sufficientarians. Consider a two-periods world, with each cohort living through one period only. We also assume that patent holders fully adjust drug prices to patent length. If the patent period is longer, the drug will be cheaper from the beginning. Table 7.3 shows this synoptically. Shortening patent length increases the differential between younger people getting sick during period 1 and those who would get sick during period 2. Members of cohort 1 will have costly access to the drug, whereas access will be free for members of cohort 2. Everything else being equal, and given the assumptions stated above, we could conclude that shortening patent length is intergenerationally unfair. Making it longer would increase access during period 1 and make access more equal between period 1 and period 2 while still allowing for the same return of investment, spread across a longer period of time.

Actually, the situation is slightly more complex. In theory, if access could be fully funded during period 1 through private or public funds by the first generation to guarantee sufficiency to all—and leaving aside here the other possibility that the drug would address health problems that do not tend to bring people below sufficiency—sufficientarians could be indifferent between both patent lengths. As such, the fact that the two generations would unequally fund the drug development, or the fact that such funding/access distribution would move us away from the demands of leximin egalitarianism, is of no concern for sufficientarians

Table 7.3 Drug Prices Under Two Patent Length Scenarios

	Period 1	Period 2
Short patent length	High price	Free
Long patent length	Low price	Low price

as long as sufficiency is met by both generations. However, in real-life conditions, such funding/access distribution will tend to affect the first generation's ability to meet the sufficiency threshold. This is so whenever the patented drug is able to bring at least some people above the sufficiency threshold and when actual public funds tend to be too limited to bring all above sufficiency. In such cases, sufficientarians will share the concern of, for example, leximin egalitarians and might advocate longer patent lengths under the conditions identified previously.

3.2. Controlling Versus Eradicating Infectious Diseases

Consider a second health issue with an interesting temporal dimension: the choice between controlling an infectious disease and eradicating it. There are two relevant features associated with intergenerational justice here. The first one is relatively standard for any investment decision. Although eradication may be extremely beneficial in the long term, all the costs are concentrated on the pre-eradication generation(s). By way of illustration, consider the eradication of smallpox:

> Very roughly, a one-time cost of about US$ 100 million saved the world about US$ 1.35 billion a year. Using a discount rate of 3%, this implies a benefit–cost ratio for global eradication of about 450:1. Smallpox eradication was an extraordinarily good deal for the world."[31]

If eradication were not to lead to immediate benefits for the current generations, there might be room for spreading the costs through running a compensatory debt in one way or another. Note, however, that in the smallpox case, and despite a large discount rate of 3% here,[32] even the eradication generation seems to have benefited in net terms because of the significant size of the short-term benefits— assuming Barrett's figures are correct.

Although smallpox eradication seems to provide us ex post with a clear case of intergenerational benefits, including for the generation incurring most of the costs, it has also remained a unique case. Polio may be another example, although we have not reached full eradication yet.[33] We need to consider cases in which low

---

31. Scott Barrett, "Eradication Versus Control: The Economics of Global Infectious Disease Policies," *Bulletin of the World Health Organization* 82, no. 9 (2004): 684.

32. By "large," I mean larger than what seems defensible on sound philosophical premises.

33. The Global Polio Eradication Initiative has managed to reduce the number of cases from 350,000 in 1988 to 416 in 2013. Source: http://www.polioeradication.org. See also Kimberly Thompson and Radboud Duintjer Tebbens, "Eradication Versus Control for Poliomyelitis: An Economic Analysis," *Lancet* 369 (2007): 1363–1371.

cost control in perpetuity is an option, cases in which animal reservoirs are difficult to eliminate, and cases in which political circumstances are such that eradication might fail. In short, aiming at eradication is not always the most efficient path, even against the background of a large number of future generations. We should keep this in mind, especially in light of theories of justice that are primarily distributive rather than aggregative, and in a context in which it might not always be possible to pass part of the eradication costs onto future generations—for example, because of budgetary golden rules that limit authorized annual deficits and national debt levels.[34]

Eradication is interesting for another reason—that is, its *irreversibility*. One of the features of intergenerational relations is the dependency on intermediary generations, associated with our near complete inability to enforce policies beyond our death.[35] If we want to transfer something to several generations in the future (e.g., a language, some values, a renewable resource, institutions that we think are right, or the composition of a useful drug), we depend on the action and abstention of intermediary generations. In order to reduce such a dependency, we may want to try to increase the irreversibility of our choices. We render constitutional provisions rigid to a certain point. We make sure that certain types of long-term radioactive waste are difficult to retrieve from deep repositories. Eradicating a disease can be interpreted through the same prism. Not only does it allow for preventing the disease from spreading again but also it protects future generations from the possible carelessness of intermediary ones. This intergenerational dependency/enforcement is related to the analogous enforcement challenge raised by infectious diseases. Barrett states, "The international system is not well suited to implementing interventions that require enforcement, but this failing helps to make eradication an attractive policy goal."[36]

3.3. Antibiotic Resistance

Consider a third case with an interesting temporal structure. The effectiveness of antibiotic drugs tends to decrease with time. It is thus comparable to a certain extent to a non-renewable resource that shrinks over time, putting future generations in a disadvantaged position. There are interesting peculiarities.[37] First, contrary to the

34. See, as well, James Wilson, "The Ethics of Disease Eradication," *Vaccine* 52 (2014): 7179–7183.

35. See Axel Gosseries, "Les générations, le fleuve et l'océan," *Philosophiques* 42, no. 1 (2015): section 2 (discussing the implications of generational "period-lockedness").

36. Barrett, "Eradication Versus Control," 686.

37. This paragraph draws extensively on Jasper Littmann, *Antibiotic Resistance and Distributive Justice* (PhD thesis) (London: University College London), Chap. 3.

depletion of a fish stock due to overfishing, the problem with antibiotic effectiveness degradation may result from both overprescription (increasing resistance) and underprescription (increasing transmission). It is thus more complex than usual resource depletion cases because there are both negative (higher resistance) and positive (lesser transmission) externalities associated with a given level of prescription.[38] Second, there is a limited degree of renewability of antibiotic effectiveness, although in the long term the effectiveness of an antibiotic drug should more realistically be presented as nonrenewable.[39] Temporary or partial drug bans may allow some effectiveness to recover, provided that we manage to keep the underprescription problem under control. However, this may lead to sacrificing certain generations to the benefit of others. Third, we should definitely envisage in a case such as this one the development of both new drug substitutes and prophylactic strategies aimed at reducing transmission and hence reducing the need for such antibiotic drugs in the first place. Antibiotic resistance, given its temporal dimension, is thus typically of interest to an intergenerational approach. The unwise use of antibiotics or the lack of substitution (with other drugs or with alternative nondrug solutions) can be framed as unfair between birth cohorts ceteris paribus.

3.4. Discussion

Having presented three examples, two tasks are in order. First, we need to compare the structure of the three examples (hereinafter referred to as "patent," "eradication," and "resistance," respectively). Second, we can try to generalize what sufficientarians have to say about them and whether there is anything specific about this theory compared to other views.

Let me begin with the first task. The three situations are cases involving *investment* and its associated distribution of costs and benefits across time. Patent royalties reimburse an investment followed by health benefits and free access in the post-patent period. The eradication effort is followed by very significant benefits in the post-eradication period. The case of resistance is slightly different. Investment in substitution drugs is required, but as a compensation of depletion from which we benefit, regardless of whether or not under- and overprescription obtain. Resistance is mainly a depletion problem (to which we can respond in part by investment), whereas patent and eradication do not necessarily presuppose any depletion. In the patent and the resistance cases, there is a link between drug use and investing in drug development. However, the nature of this link differs. In the patent case, drug use renders resources unavailable for drug development. In the

---

38. Littmann, *Antibiotic Resistance and Distributive Justice*, 59–60.

39. Littmann, *Antibiotic Resistance and Distributive Justice*, 66.

resistance case, (inappropriate) drug use renders alternative drug development necessary. Finally, the efficiency aspect differs in the three cases. In the way we discussed them, the patent and the resistance cases mainly raise distributive issues, without any significant efficiency dimension. In the patent case, we took development costs as given. In the resistance case, although drug use can be more or less efficient, slowing down the problem, the long-term depletion issue remains. In contrast, in the eradication case, the efficiency gains can be huge in the long term, and the possible tension between efficiency and fairness is central.

That being said, can we say anything general about the way in which sufficientarians would approach such issues, despite their differences? We can make the following statement: If the health problem at stake affects our ability to guarantee sufficiency for all ("sufficiency-relevance" in Table 7.4), sufficientarians will tend to support investment while keeping an eye on the fact that the costs of such an investment should not jeopardize the ability of the investing generations to reach sufficiency themselves. Thus, all depends on the particular patent, the particular disease one wants to eradicate or particular antibiotic, and whether the investment at stake jeopardizes the ability of the investing generation to reach sufficiency. This echoes Brundtland's moderate non-cleronomic approach that cares about sufficiency both in the future and in the present, as well as Rawls' concern about an accumulation phase because of its costs for the least well-off.

In contrast, if the drug is not about a sufficiency-relevant disease ("sufficiency-irrelevance" in Table 7.4), the crucial question will be about the impact of its costs. If it leads to an investment incompatible with guaranteeing sufficiency for all for the members of the investing generation ("sufficiency-aversion" in Table 7.4), then the investment should not take place. In the reverse case, the investment should be allowed by sufficientarians, unless they complement their view with other concerns of justice (combined sufficientarianism), in which case the answer will be less clear. Table 7.4 summarizes the four general cases just discussed along the two axes: Is the health treatment at stake sufficiency-relevant or sufficiency-irrelevant for the generation(s) that will potentially benefit from it? Is the investment sufficiency-averse or sufficiency-compatible for the investing generation?

Table 7.4 Does Sufficientarianism Allow, Require, or Prohibit a Given Health Investment?

Costs for the Investing Generation/Nature of the Health Treatment	Sufficiency-Relevant	Sufficiency-Irrelevant
Sufficiency-averse	Trade-off	Prohibited
Sufficiency-compatible	Compulsory	Allowed

What follows for our three examples? Table 7.4 gives us an indication about patent lengths, depending on whether or not the short patent length scenario would entail costs on the patent-bearing generation that are sufficiency-averse. Regarding eradication, it is likely that, given the type of disease at stake, we will find ourselves in one of the two boxes in the sufficiency-relevant column, depending on the impact of the eradication costs. With regard to resistance, because it is less of an investment problem than primarily a depletion one, we should simply ask ourselves whether or not this depletion is sufficiency-relevant. If it is, then we will find ourselves again in one of the two boxes of in the sufficiency-relevant column.

In short, isolationist sufficientarians will tend to deliver a message that is roughly in line with the one of isolationist leximin egalitarians (although of a more discrete type), except for the bottom right box in Table 7.4. Leximin egalitarians will tend to look at the bottom right box in Table 7.4 in terms of trade-off, as they would for the top left box, with the aim of maximizing the situation of the least well-off, of the second least well-off, and so on, for whichever generation of which they are part.

4. Isolationism, Substitutability, and Sufficientarianism

There are two key difficulties with isolationism: *limited separability* and *substitutability*. Regarding separability, most of the possible focus points of an isolationist approach to justice have extensive ramifications. This is true for education, climate, housing, employment, and so on. It is clearly the case with health, too, as the literature on the determinants of health emphasizes. In short, what belongs to the realm of health extends very far and overlaps with other domains of justice and social life.

Substitutability is a more serious problem than limited separability, however. Substitutability is an issue for both intragenerational and intergenerational justice. For most theories of intergenerational justice, some degree of substitutability is in order, within the basket of "goods" that justice requires us to transfer to the next generation. For instance, unless we consider that non-renewable resources should never be consumed by any generation, it makes sense to allow for some substitution of such resources with technology—broadly understood. Moreover, substitutions may also take place within types of goods (e.g., "within" health). Even for someone claiming that no substitution should be allowed whenever health is at stake ("health is sacred"), there might still be room for substitution within the health domain. Among two treatments for different diseases that have the same impact with regard to quality-adjusted life-years, one generation might invest in one treatment, whereas another generation would rather invest in the other one and include it in the basket of goods it aims to provide for the next generation. Hence, we need at least some degree of substitutability. Now, if substitution is needed—and allowed—requirements of justice in health cannot be assessed in isolation, independently of how the individuals or generations at stake fare in other respects. For instance, an egalitarian may have no problem with someone being disadvantaged in health terms if he or she is advantaged to the same extent in other respects.

Here, I do not explore the extent to which having to abandon isolationism is a challenge to theorists of justice concerned about relevance for public policy. One may of course want to object that an isolationist approach would at the very least constitute a step in the right direction. However, not even that is true. Even in a simplified setting involving only two patients who are potential recipients of a single treatment, equalizing health inequalities may sometimes deepen inequalities, all things considered, through improving the situation of the patient who is already the most advantaged one in overall respects. Moreover, the same situation may arise with respect to costs on health service providers. Here, an intergenerational approach is of interest. We have seen that some views consider that giving more to the next generation is not necessarily fair. Hence, giving more of each good will not necessarily further fairness because it might be unfairly burdensome on providers. For a strict equivalence view, giving more of one good will then only be fair if we give less of another good to the next generation. For such views that are concerned with the fairness of the investment burden, the critique of isolationism will amount to saying, "If you do not know everything, you know nothing." In other words, if you do not map all transfers, you cannot determine whether a given transfer contributes to a fairer overall distribution or whether it diverts us from it. This is obviously very demanding for policymakers concerned about fairness.

Our question here is more specific: Does sufficientarianism allow for less substitutability, leading to a lesser gap between an isolationist and an integrationist approach? Insofar as sufficientarianism is concerned, what is key is the *threshold* level.[40] The lower the threshold, the lesser the substitutability. Of course, better food or warmer clothes may compensate for having the worst shelter. However, from a certain level of each of these goods onwards, the daily need for it becomes

40. I am leaving aside here another dimension—that is, whether there is a case for specialism ("health is special") that could support some degree of isolationism. See, for example, Shlomi Segall, "Is Health (Really) Special? Health Policy Between Rawlsian and Luck Egalitarian Justice," *Journal of Applied Philosophy* 27, no. 4 (2010): 344–358; Lasse Nielsen, "Why Health Matters to Justice: A Capability Theory Perspective," *Ethical Theory and Moral Practice* 18, no. 2 (2014): 403–415.

incompressible. No matter how well insulated your house is, you will still need to eat something if you want to survive. If we accept the idea that below a certain level onwards, no further substitutability is possible anymore, it might be argued that sufficientarianism allows for less substitutability, which entails that isolationist sufficientarianism might make some sense, even for those with integrationist views in general. This may have to do with the "list" feature characteristic of a basic needs approach—that is, the fact that some basic needs or basic capabilities theorists list them as qualitatively distinct items that should all be met.[41] However, it has even more to do with the threshold level than with whether the selected metric is more or less preference-sensitive (welfarist vs. basic needs sufficientarianism).[42]

Moreover, in addition to this general feature, when applied to the intergenerational realm, sufficientarianism is sensitive to the burdens of investment for the current generation to the extent that they might bring those bearing the burden of accumulation below sufficiency. This is clear in the Pinchot/Brundtland definition. As a result, as for the strict equivalence views, it is not obvious that guaranteeing better health care for the next generation necessarily goes in the right direction if the costs of health care bring the members of the current generation below the sufficiency threshold. If sufficientarianism were strictly cleronomic as opposed to moderately so, an isolationist approach would be even more relevant because the costs to the current generation of better health in the future would be fully discounted. However, the opportunity cost of having invested in health for our ability to cover other non-health-related basic needs of the next generation would still have to be taken into account, even for a strictly cleronomic approach.

Thus, we can conclude that although an isolationist approach may provide us with some direction, it is as such insufficient if we take substitutability seriously. This should be taken all the more seriously if we consider that sufficientarianism should not have too low a threshold.

5. Conclusion

In this chapter, I stressed first the need to distinguish two dimensions of intergenerational justice—that is, justice between members of different age groups and justice between people from different birth cohorts. I focused on the latter. I explored the specific features that sufficientarian intergenerational justice exhibits. I emphasized moderate non-cleronomicity, a qualified authorization to generationally save and dissave provided that the sufficiency level of the generations

41. See, in this volume, the chapters by David V. Axelsen and Lasse Nielsen (Chapter 6), Efrat Ram-Tiktin (Chapter 8), and Carina Fourie (Chapter 10).

42. I am indebted to Carl Knight for an interesting exchange on this topic.

at stake can be met, and some implications of two of the typical features of a sufficientarian metrics (lesser preference-sensitivity and lesser responsibility-sensitivity). I also briefly presented two alternative defenses of intergenerational sufficientarianism that would not imply endorsing sufficientarianism in general, concluding that they have limited plausibility.

I then moved on to implementing such a general approach in the health/ health care context. I did so with isolationist lenses first. Through the three examples (patent length, eradication vs. control, and antibiotic resistance), I illustrated and generalized what intergenerational sufficientarianism would entail, as summarized in Table 7.4. Such isolationist analysis is of course of some relevance, and it exhibits slightly distinct features from other approaches. However, some modesty is in order because even for a sufficientarian, an integrationist approach means that we cannot decide on health policy without taking into account how the generations at stake are expected to fare under the various scenarios in respects other than health. This is why we should resolutely continue to ensure that rules of thumb and proposals derived from theories of justice are relevant for real-life policy while remaining modest about the directions we advocate. Being sufficientarian, especially if the threshold is not implausibly low, does not immunize one from this task.

Acknowledgments

I thank Andreas Albertsen, David de la Croix, Nir Eyal, Carina Fourie, Richard Howarth, Carl Knight, Jasper Littmann, Alain Marciano, Tim Meijers, Lasse Nielsen, Toby Ord, Annette Rid, Ester Rizzi, Nicholas Vrousalis, James Wilson, Dan Wikler, and Danielle Zwarthoed. Apologies for not being able to do full justice to their very rich set of comments. I also acknowledge funding from the projects ARC 09/14-018 "Sustainability" (Communauté française de Belgique) and ESF ENRI "Rights to a Green Future" (European Science Foundation), as well as support from the Czech Academy of Science through a Franz Weyr Fellowship.

8

Basic Human Functional Capabilities as the Currency of Sufficientarian Distribution in Health Care

Efrat Ram-Tiktin

1. Outline of the Sufficiency of Capabilities Account

What would be a just way of allocating health care resources? Addressing this question requires a distinction between two subquestions: (1) What is the currency of justice in health care? (2) What is a just scheme of allocation—equality, utility, priority, sufficiency, or something else?

The purpose of this chapter is to present portions of my account of a just distribution of health care, namely the sufficiency of basic human functional capabilities (or sufficiency of capabilities (SOC) for brevity). Because a thorough discussion of the entire theory is impossible in the space of one chapter, my strategy is to present parts of it as a set of basic presumptions and to provide argumentation for two topics. First, I address the nature of the good being distributed, in answer to the first question presented previously. Second, I argue for a sufficientarian principle in prioritizing patients—that is, that a fair amount of health care is required to guarantee them the ability to live a good human life and pursue their life plans. I do not provide a thorough discussion of egalitarianism and prioritarianism, which are a matter for a different chapter. My goal is more modest—to show why, when considering the distribution of health care, justice requires no more than sufficiency.

The SOC account is based on the following assumptions:[1]

1. Justice is a political concept that describes the moral conduct of the basic institutions of a state. In other words, natural differences among individuals (e.g., the level or diversity of capabilities) are not a matter of justice in themselves. They become a matter of justice only when state institutions operate in such a way that makes those differences affect individuals' well-being and opportunities.

2. Contrary to John Rawls, who thought that there is one set of distributing principles for different kinds of goods,[2] I endorse Michael Walzer's position. Walzer claims that there are different "spheres of justice," each constituted by different social goods, or different sets of goods, and in each one of these spheres there are different criteria and distributing arrangements that are appropriate for the distribution of the good(s) in question.[3] He states that the criteria for distributing a good must derive from the particular nature of the good in question in a given society at a given time: "[G]oods don't just appear in the hands of distributive agents who do with them as they like. ... Rather, goods with their meanings—because of their meaning—are the crucial medium of social relations." Walzer argues that if we have an understanding of the good, and what meaning it has for the members of a given society, we gain an understanding "how, by whom, and for what reasons it ought to be distributed."[4] For example, health, education, and political participation are distinct social goods that constitute different distributive spheres. The just distribution of each one of them must be in accordance with society's shared conception about the goods' meanings and purpose. Following Walzer, I hold the position that not only will different social goods (e.g., health, education, and political participation) be allocated differently in different cultures but also, even in a given society, each one of the goods will be allocated according to the different principles derived from the specific meaning of each good.

---

1. A full discussion of these assumptions is presented in Efrat Ram-Tiktin, "Distributive Justice in Healthcare" (PhD dissertation, Bar-Ilan University, 2009).

2. Rawls listed five primary social goods: basic liberties, freedom of movement and free choice of occupation, powers and prerogatives of offices, income and wealth, and social bases of self-respect. John Rawls, *A Theory of Justice* (Cambridge, MA: Harvard University Press, 1999).

3. Michael Walzer, *Spheres of Justice* (Oxford: Robertson, 1983).

4. Walzer, *Spheres*, 9.

3. A just pattern of distribution of health care services is sufficiency, not equality or priority. In other words, just health care distribution is achieved when people have a sufficient level of capabilities required to live a good life and not when we aim for equality (each individual has an equal level of capabilities) or when we follow prioritarian concerns (giving priority to those who are worse off regardless of how badly off they are).[5]

4. The currency of justice in the distribution of health care is capabilities. Following Sen's and Nussbaum's extensive discussion of capabilities,[6] I hold the position that capabilities more accurately reflect the relative position of individuals in a given society, the extent of freedom individuals are able to enjoy, and their ability to pursue their life plans and live a good human life than do resources, opportunities, or welfare.

As stated previously, I do not provide argumentation for these assumptions. However, a short explanation regarding the sphere of health is required. My account addresses the just allocation of health *care* (we allocate health care services, not health per se), but the relevant sphere is health. The thing that we value is health, and health care is only instrumentally valuable as long as it promotes health. Health is a broader notion than health care and relates to the multiple variables that affect human health, such as housing, education, road safety, and access to clean water, air, food, and so on. Health care, by contrast, relates to different kinds of intervention for the purposes of curing, preventing, rehabilitating, and so on. Within the sphere of health, different questions of resource allocation arise. One central question is the following: Given scarcity of resources, what is the most just way to promote a population's overall state of health? For example, would it be by improving children's access to education or providing them with a

---

5. I present a sufficientarian principle. Because my discussion does not address the dispute over sufficientarianism (e.g., how can one set a non-arbitrary threshold, what argumentation can be presented against Richard Arneson's "threshold fetishism" objection, etc.), I present the sufficiency view as a basic assumption.

6. Amartya Sen, "Equality of What?" in *The Tanner Lectures on Human Values: Vol. 1*, ed. Sterling M. McMurrin (Salt Lake City, UT: University of Utah Press, 1980), 197–220; Amartya Sen, *Commodities and Capabilities* (Amsterdam: North Holland, 1985); Amartya Sen, "Justice: Means Versus Freedom," *Philosophy and Public Affairs* 19, no. 2 (1990): 111–121; Martha C. Nussbaum, "Nature, Function, and Capability: Aristotle on Political Distribution," *Oxford Studies in Ancient Philosophy* Suppl. Vol. (1988): 145–184; Martha C. Nussbaum, "Human Functioning and Social Justice," *Political Theory* 20, no. 2 (1992): 202–246; Martha C. Nussbaum, *Women and Human Development—The Capability Approach* (New York: Cambridge University Press, 2000); Martha C. Nussbaum, *Frontiers of Justice: Disability, Nationality, Species Membership* (Cambridge, MA: Harvard University Press, 2006).

safe and clean environment, or perhaps by ensuring equal access to quality and affordable medical care?[7] Promoting a population's health requires the involvement of different institutions of the state, not just the medical institutions.

SOC addresses a narrower and more focused question within that sphere: What would be a just scheme of resource allocation with respect to health care? How should we prioritize groups of patients that differ in size, severity of illness, and potential gains they might enjoy if provided with the right treatment? Addressing this question is necessary for the policy planner who wishes to formulate a fair health policy for patients. Unlike the promotion of health, which requires the involvement of multiple state institutions, the allocation of health care resources is provided by medical institutions alone. My purpose in this chapter is to address the narrow question of just allocation of health care via these institutions. It is important to stress that I am not denying the importance of other health determinants on health justice. They are simply beyond the scope of SOC in health care and therefore will not be addressed here.

In relation to assumptions 2 and 4, I base my account on a specific understanding of the concept of "health." In the relevant literature, there is an ongoing debate about how we should define the terms "health" and "illness."[8] My aim here is not to present a full discussion of the subject, which would divert from the focus of the current chapter, but to describe in general my view of these terms.[9] It is necessary to get a general understanding regarding the health sphere and the currency of justice in health care that will be specified in Section 2.

---

7. For discussion of the various factors that affect human health, see Michael G. Marmot and Richard G. Wilkinson, eds., *Social Determinants of Health* (New York: Oxford University Press, 1999); Richard G. Wilkinson, *Unhealthy Societies* (London: Routledge, 1996); Norman Daniels, *Just Health: Meeting Health Needs Fairly* (Cambridge, UK: Cambridge University Press, 2008).

8. There are two rival views in the literature. The biostatistical view is presented by Christopher Boorse. See Christopher Boorse, "A Rebuttal on Health," in *What Is Disease? Biomedical Ethics Reviews*, ed. James M. Humber and Robert F. Almeder (Totowa, NJ: Humana Press, 1997); Christopher Boorse, "On the Distinction Between Disease and Illness," *Philosophy and Public Affairs* 5, no. 1 (1975): 57–62; Christopher Boorse, "Health as a Theoretical Concept," *Philosophy of Science* 44, no. 4 (1977): 554–573. The Holistic view is presented by Lennart Nordenfelt. See Lennart Nordenfelt, "Concepts of Health and Their Consequences for Health Care," *Theoretical Medicine* 14, no. 4 (1993): 277–281; Lennart Nordenfelt, "On the Relevance and Importance of the Notion of Disease," *Theoretical Medicine* 14, no. 1 (1993): 15–26; Lennart Nordenfelt, *Quality of Life, Health and Happiness* (Aldershot, UK: Avebury, 1993); Lennart Nordenfelt, *On the Nature of Health—An Action-Theoretic Approach* (Dordrecht, The Netherlands: Springer, 1995); Lennart Nordenfelt, *Health, Science, and Ordinary Language* (Amsterdam: Rodopi, 2001).

9. The relative strengths and weaknesses of these views are discussed in Ram-Tiktin, "Distributive Justice," 154–165.

1.2. Definitions of Health and Illness

Health is a value-laden concept, although it has a value-free element as its basis. When reflecting on the concept of health, physiological and psychological (cognitive and emotional) functional capabilities are brought to mind. These capabilities have value-free elements related to their biological aspects. They also have value-laden elements expressed in accordance with social meanings (mores, values, traditions, and regularities) that determine in which situations biological functions can be considered to be either in order or defective. Infertility is a very clear example of the value-free and value-laden nature of physiological capability. Infertility is a condition of biological dysfunction. From this perspective, infertility is a value-free condition, a result of normatively neutral facts. Whether and to what extent infertility is considered an impairment is related to a given society's understanding of the impact of infertility on individuals' lives. If, in a given society, conception is an important goal, then that society will consider infertility to be an impairment. By contrast, if a given society understands self-realization as the ability to reach one's maximum career potential, infertility may become a significant advantage.

Therefore, in my view, two levels must be differentiated: the physiological and social–cultural–political levels. The physiological level is neutral, presenting natural facts that, in themselves, have no normative meaning. Normative meaning is attached to those facts only when one moves from the physiological to the social–cultural–political level. Because of the necessary distinction between the two levels, I suggest using different concepts for each level:

The Physiological Level

Malady:[10] Any deviation from the normal structure or function typical to the individual's species and reference class (sex and age) that creates a reduction in his or her physiological and/or psychological function.[11]

---

10. The term "malady" was suggested by Clouser, Culver, and Gert as a general and relatively neutral concept. Other terms, such as "injury," "disease," "disorder," and "trauma," have specific connotations regarding the individual's condition and how it was caused. On the other hand, "malady" is less informative and therefore "useful as a beginning point for labeling a phenomenon, without being diverted into one or another connotation." Danner K. Clouser, Charles M. Culver, and Bernard Gert, "Malady," in *What Is Disease? Biomedical Ethics Review*, ed. James M. Humber and Robert. F. Almeder (Totowa, NJ: Humana Press, 1997), 212. The definition of malady provided previously is mine.

11. Although the words "deviation" and "reduction" may seem value-laden, we should consider them at the physiological level to be normatively neutral. At the physiological level, everything is value-free. Cells, tissues, hormones, etc., *in themselves* carry no normative judgments. When I say that there is deviation or reduction in an organism's functioning (e.g., the secretion level of a hormone or oxygen saturation), I am describing deviation from the

Intactness: The absence of malady or the presence of a normal species structure and function relevant to the reference class.

In both definitions, "normal" refers to the species' statistical normality. For example, the statistical normality of the human heart rate in a state of rest is 60–100 beats per minute (for humans ages 8 years or older).

The Social–Cultural–Political Level

Illness: A structural and/or functional change that negatively affects the physiological and/or psychological capabilities of an individual to advance his or her goals within his or her social environment.

Health: An expression of physiological and psychological capabilities that advance an individual's goals within his or her social environment.

Given these definitions, the currency of justice in health *care* is made up of basic human functional capabilities (BHFCs). In other words, to evaluate individuals' abilities to achieve their goals and life plans, one needs to focus on their BHFCs and not on their level of wealth or welfare.

Building on these assumptions, I present an account of distributive justice in health care. In the following section, I specify the goods in question—that is, the list of BHFCs that are the concern of justice in health care. In Section 3, I present my version of sufficiency, specify the reason I find that claims of injustice can be presented only by those who are located beneath the sufficiency threshold of BHFCs, and show how we should delineate the threshold. The allocation principle for the prioritization of patients located beneath the sufficiency threshold is presented in Section 4.

2. The Currency of Justice in Health Care

As claimed previously, the currency of justice in health care is BHFCs. My proposed account could be considered as an elaboration and modification of the Sen–Nussbaum capability approach. Nussbaum's general theory of justice relates to multiple aspects of life.[12] Therefore, her list of 10 central human capabilities is too extensive for the purpose of a theory of distributive justice in health care. Sridhar Venkatapuram develops the Sen–Nussbaum capability approach to health,

---

statistical norm of the organism's species. It is a neutral description (of level or function of the cell, tissue, hormone, etc.) in relation to the statistical norm of the species.

12. Nussbaum, "Human Functioning"; *Women and Human Development; Frontiers.*

describing the capability to be healthy as "a person's ability to achieve or exercise a cluster of basic capabilities and functions, and each at a level that constitutes a life worthy of equal human dignity in the modern world."[13] The capability to be healthy is a meta-capability—that is, the capability to achieve or exercise Nussbaum's 10 central human capabilities. As a meta-capability, it relates to different aspects and factors affecting human health, including individual genetic disposition; exposure to external pathogenic factors; various factors affecting individual levels of nutrition (e.g., gender, age, freedom from parasites, and social and familial norms); education in and awareness of health hazards and family planning; and access to clean water, food, air, and medical care.

Although Venkatapuram's account provides an important contribution to the literature on health justice and the capability approach in general, given its extensive understanding of the capability to be healthy, it cannot provide guidance for the policy planner who has the specific task of determining a just distribution of health care for different groups of patients with various types of malfunctions and levels of health. As mentioned previously, this is the aim of my proposed account. Although I acknowledge the effect of multiple factors on human health, my account addresses a very specific issue: the just distribution of health care. To this end, it is necessary to specify the currency of health care distribution. In other words, although Venkatapuram's account is an application of the Sen–Nussbaum capability approach to health, it is still a very broad account. It can propose an understanding of justice in health in general, but it cannot provide guidance for patients' prioritization. To do that, we must look for specific functional capabilities that underlie our ability to function, and the use of a meta-capability is too vague to be useful in this matter. The list of BHFCs presented later may be regarded as a *partial* specification of the various capabilities included in Venkatapuram's meta-capability to be healthy. This specification focuses on the capabilities relevant to the distribution of health care (and not on how we improve or sustain a population's health in general).

The identification of BHFCs must start from the terms "malady" and "intactness," which define the normatively neutral level. This strategy will guarantee that possible socially valuable capabilities, such as the capability to fly or to be extremely immune to diseases, are not included in what is "normal" and therefore not required by the state to guarantee an individual's health. I identify nine key systems of physiological and psychological capabilities that are required for the individual to achieve a good and prosperous life. They are as follows:

---

13. Sridhar Venkatapuram, *Health Justice: An Argument from the Capabilities Approach* (Cambridge, UK: Polity, 2011), 143.

1. Thinking and emotions: The capability to perform different modes of thinking; the ability to experience a range of feelings toward the self and others; the capability to form meaningful relations with others; and the ability to understand one's own feelings and thoughts and express them to others.

2. Senses: The ability to use all five senses in order to access the world and thus enjoy and acquire new knowledge about external phenomena.

3. Circulation: The capability of blood and essential components to circulate to different parts of the body—for example, the ability to provide oxygen to tissues with the required frequency and for different levels of activity.

4. Respiration: The capability to supply the right dosage of oxygen to cells and expel CO_2.

5. Digestion and metabolism: The capability to eat the various kinds of food that are needed for the human body. This includes the ability to digest, absorb essential materials, and excrete waste.

6. Movement and balance: The ability to crawl and stand straight at different developmental stages according to the species' functional pattern. It also includes the ability to move four limbs in accordance with the range of movement typical for the species.

7. Immunity and excretion: The capability of the body to protect itself from foreign factors (antigens), to identify a substance as foreign and produce antibodies, to remember a foreign substance (immunological memory), to excrete dangerous by-products, and so on.

8. Fertility: The ability to reproduce, which involves the abilities to create sex cells, transfer those cells, and set the required conditions for successful fertilization. In women of a fertile age, it is also the capability to create and maintain optimal conditions for the development of the fetus until its successful delivery.

The first eight systems are under the constant control of the ninth system:

9. Hormonal control: The capability to produce different hormones required for either activation or suppression of bodily processes, according to need and circumstance, in appropriate frequency and quantity.

The previous description does not reflect the standard classification of human physiology as presented in anatomy textbooks. The purpose of this classification is to distinguish among capability systems that are responsible for different functions. Each system represents a group of capabilities related to a particular function. For example, system 7—immunity and excretion—refers to the immune system (leukocytes, bone marrow, lymph glands, etc.) but also to the urinary system (kidneys, bladder, etc.) and to the digestive system (liver, intestines, and cecum). The variable that differentiates system 7 is its functional end. Consequently, the classification here is artificial, and there are interactions and mutual influences among the different capability systems, such as between circulation and respiration.

In full function, the nine systems characterize a state of intactness and not a state of health, which is a social–cultural–political concept. These systems may characterize a state of health when they are applied to certain social–cultural–political circumstances, which determine whether neutral variables at the physiological level receive normative meaning at the social–political level. For example, a person with an enzyme defect such as G6PD[14] would be described as deviating from the normal human metabolic capability of digesting broad beans. However, the person will be characterized as having an impairment or an illness only in societies in which broad beans are a dominant component of nutrition (as they are, for example, in Egypt) and not in societies that consume other primary sources of protein (because of cultural norms or agricultural conditions).

The previously mentioned nine systems formulate the currency of justice in health care. In other words, these are the capabilities that health institutions have a duty to treat, restore, or compensate to the threshold level in cases in which deviations from normal human functioning reduce patients' ability to advance their goals in their social environment. The BHFCs are a necessary but insufficient condition for people's ability to exercise their positive freedom and live a good human life. Without them, people lack the basic capabilities required for full human functioning—but even with them, other conditions are required to enable people to achieve their goals, such as political rights and liberties.

Three basic qualifications can be derived from the previous paragraph. First, although some capabilities are more crucial than others (breathing is more important for our existence than the ability to consume broad beans), each capability system is important in itself. The fact that someone has a higher capability in one system does not invalidate his or her claim for justice if there is some functional shortcoming in another capability system. Consider the physicist Stephen Hawking, for example. Although he is much more intelligent than most people (capability system 1), he has a valid claim to medical care for his impaired capabilities in other systems because of his illness. Second, in each capability system, the obligation is to ensure capabilities, and not actual functions, in order to guarantee autonomy of the individual. It is the individual's decision whether he or she wishes to exercise a given capability so that it becomes a developed and successful

---

14. G6PD is an X-linked recessive heredity disease characterized by abnormally low levels of glucouse-6-phosphate-dehydrogenase (G6PD). G6PD deficiency may lead to nonimmune hemolytic anemia if exposure to certain chemicals or medication occurs.

function.[15] Third, the health institutions' obligation is to ensure that individuals have, to the furthest extent possible, a sufficient level of these capabilities and not to guarantee an equal state of health. As the informed reader has probably noticed, these three basic qualifications are presented by Nussbaum in her capabilities approach.[16] Here, I follow her rationale and adapt it to the distribution of health care.

The last qualification leads us to Section 3, in which I argue for my version of sufficientarianism and explain how the sufficiency threshold should be delineated.

3. Sufficientarian Distribution in Health Care

As stated in Section 1, just allocation of health care should be guided by sufficientarian concerns, trying to achieve sufficiency of BHFCs for patients. Although I present some argumentation in favor of sufficiency, the discussion does not replace the need for further argumentation in favor of sufficientarianism. At the end of this section, I discuss how we should delineate the sufficiency threshold of capabilities in health care.

Paula Casal[17] distinguishes between two theses of sufficientarianism. According to the *positive thesis*, there is something morally significant about the sufficiency threshold, and there is greater moral value in benefiting those beneath the threshold than there is in benefiting those who are above it. The *negative thesis* of sufficientarianism rules out the relevance of other patterns of distribution (i.e., the pattern of distribution above the threshold has no moral significance).

My version of sufficiency endorses only the positive thesis. I believe that, above the threshold, there is moral importance to the pattern of distribution and it could be equality, priority, or utility; it depends on the nature of the good in question. I have presented my view on that matter elsewhere.[18]

I begin by clarifying how my version of sufficiency differentiates itself from egalitarianism and prioritarianism.[19] First, unlike egalitarianism, sufficiency does

---

15. Some of our physiological and psychological capabilities are involuntary. Here, I refer to complex voluntary capabilities such as running, talking, eating, and conceiving, the performance of which is dependent on human will.

16. Nussbaum, *Frontiers.*

17. Paula Casal, "Why Sufficiency Is Not Enough," *Ethics* 117 (2007): 297–304.

18. Efrat Ram-Tiktin, "The Right to Health Care as a Right to Basic Human Functional Capabilities," *Ethical Theory and Moral Practice* 15, no. 3 (2012): 347–349.

19. The informed reader will notice that this version differs from other versions of sufficiency, such as Roger Crisp's "Equality, Priority and Compassion," *Ethics* 113 (2003): 755–763, and Yitzhak Benbaji, "Sufficiency or Priority?" *European Journal of Philosophy* 14, no. 3 (2006): 338–344. However, because differences were presented in Ram-Tiktin, *Distributive Justice*, 194–202, I do not discuss them here.

not attribute any value to substantive principles of equality, only to formal principles of equality. Equality as impartiality is a formal principle of equality that "reflects the view that all people must be treated impartially" and can be found in any
theory of justice (including utilitarianism and libertarianism).[20] Sufficientarians
reject substantive principles of equality, such as Temkin's *equality as comparability*,
according to which "it is bad for some to be worse off than others through no fault
or choice of their own."[21] According to my positive thesis of sufficientarianism,
equal distribution of health care services and resources is possible above or below
the threshold, but it will be according to formal principles of equality and not substantive ones. For example, if beneath the threshold there is a group of patients
suffering from a similar impairment, they should be given an equal treatment.

Prioritarians, unlike egalitarians, are not concerned with relative positions.
Whereas egalitarians are concerned with how one individual's level of health (or
welfare or resources) compares to that of another, prioritarians "are concerned
only with people's absolute levels"[22] or what "they might have been."[23] The second
clarification is that my version of sufficientarianism, unlike prioritarianism (but
similar to egalitarianism), takes into account the relative position of an individual
compared to other individuals who inhabit his or her social environment.

Third, unlike egalitarianism and prioritarianism, according to my version of
sufficientarianism, it is both possible and crucial to mark a critical threshold reflecting the moral distinction between those who have the ability to live a good
human life and those who do not because they lack certain BHFCs. The threshold
distinguishes between those who are beneath the threshold and can present legitimate claims of injustice and those who are at or above the threshold and cannot
present legitimate claims. In the following discussion, I elaborate on the differences between them.

What can we say regarding the value of equality in the sphere of health and
in the distribution of health care? The question of whether equal health has intrinsic value is important, but it is not really my concern here. My account addresses the distribution of health care or, more accurately, of BHFCs. Thus, the
question should be: Does equal distribution of BHFCs have intrinsic value? Is it
good in itself regardless of its possible effects? To crystallize the different concerns

---

20. Larry Temkin, "Inequality: A Complex, Individualistic, and Comparative Notion,"
Philosophical Issues 11 (2001): 327–353.

21. Temkin, "Inequality," 330. This view is connected to Temkin's *Justice as Comparative
Fairness*.

22. Derek Parfit, *Equality or Priority? The Lindley Lecture* (Lawrence, KS: University of
Kansas, 1995), 23.

23. Parfit, *Equality*, 22.

egalitarians, prioritarians, and sufficientarians have regarding the value of equal BHFCs, consider the scenario discussed next.

Let us assume that one person, Goliath, is in perfect health. All of his BHFCs are far above the sufficiency level (i.e., in the top values of normal human function statistics). Another person, David, is in good shape, although not in such perfect condition as Goliath. In other words, all of his BHFCs are below the median of normal human function statistics but still above the sufficiency level. Does equality of BHFCs have intrinsic value? Would it be sound to claim that it is bad for David to be worse off than Goliath, through no fault or choice of his own? To answer this question, we need to ask the following: In what *meaningful* way is David worse off than Goliath, if David has BHFCs and he does not have any functional disadvantage? What is "bad" in this state of affairs? As long as David has a sufficient level of BHFCs, it is difficult to see what is bad about the situation. Being at the same level of health as Goliath is not good in itself. In other words, equality has no intrinsic value regarding BHFCs. If it did, it might see value in policies of leveling down the health condition of the better-offs (i.e., causing them impairment) while not improving the health of the worse-offs. In addition, although equality of BHFCs might coincidentally have instrumental value, it would not be the reason we should pursue it. In the Goliath–David case, I suspect that society's sense of solidarity would not be affected in any way if David's BHFCs were at the same level as Goliath's, nor would other important goals be realized, such as increasing individuals' fraternity, maintaining democratic institution, or anything else. Would David's sense of self-esteem improve if he had the same level of BHFCs as Goliath? Not necessarily—it depends on his personality and preferences. He might envy Goliath for his perfect endowments, or he might be satisfied with his own capacities (quickness, resourcefulness, musical talents, etc.). In any case, David's personal response is not our concern in health care justice. Taking into account individuals' preferences would lead to the well-known problem of expensive tastes.[24] Our limited concern is to ensure that David has sufficient BHFCs required to advance his life plans in his social environment while taking into account what he can reasonably expect society to provide him with or compensate him for.[25]

---

24. According to some views, if an individual's level of welfare is low, then she would not be entitled to compensation if her low level of well-being is the result of *freely* chosen tastes (desires and preferences) that are expensive or difficult to provide. See, for example, Ronald Dworkin, *Sovereign Virtue: The Theory and Practice of Equality* (Cambridge, MA: Harvard University Press, 2000), 289–296.

25. I discuss the problem of expensive taste in health care elsewhere. Efrat Ram-Tiktin, "Fair Equality of Opportunity Versus Sufficiency of Capabilities in Healthcare" (manuscript available from the author).

Prioritarians deny the intrinsic value of equality. Parfit states that the only value equality might have is in giving priority to the worse-off. He writes; "[B]enefiting people matters more the worse off these people are."[26] Prioritarians would say that we should benefit David not because he is worse off than Goliath (recall that prioritarians do not care for relative positions) but because David is worse off than he might have been. I am not persuaded by this claim because I do not see the moral value of nonessential benefits. Once someone lacks one of the BHFCs or has some of them to a very minimal degree, so it cannot be developed to functional ability, providing her treatment or compensation would be an essential benefit and would carry a moral value. Therefore, such a person has a legitimate and justified claim for health care resources. However, once someone has BHFCs (i.e., she is at a sufficient level required for the development of a functional ability, as in the case of David) but these are at a lower level than those of another, the provision of a benefit might be desirable to her but not an essential benefit that has moral value. Contrary to Parfit's priority view that rejects distinguishing the better-off from the worse-off by means of a threshold level,[27] a sufficientarian position holds the view that such a threshold could and should be delineated. The threshold marks and differentiates those whose lives are burdened and difficult, and it indicates that benefiting them is morally required, as opposed to those who are above the threshold and who lack legitimate claims for health care resources. Providing intervention that would provide greater functional abilities to someone who already has them in the range of norm values is not a requirement of justice. Such a benefit could be regarded as an enhancement, and to that I do not object. However, it is important to stress that this kind of benefit is an enhancement and not a medical treatment for the worse-off. Enhancement is a type of desirable intervention above the sufficiency threshold, and it may have moral value once we have already provided treatment (to the extent that it is possible) for those beneath the threshold.[28]

3.1. Setting the Threshold

Arguing for sufficientarianism without offering a way to mark the threshold that makes a moral distinction between the well-off and the worse-off is problematic (at least at the practical level). Here, I suggest that the delineation of the BHFCs threshold requires two steps. The first involves examining the range of

26. Parfit, *Equality*, 19.

27. Parfit, *Equality*, 18.

28. For discussion of the issue of prioritizing enhancement and other interventions above the threshold, see Ram-Tiktin, "The Right to Health Care," 347–349.

the physiological variables that characterize normal human levels of functioning. The second involves considering when deviation from normal values creates a burden on individuals' abilities to fulfill their life plans in their social environment.

The following examples will clarify the concept of impaired capability:

1. Normal levels of thyroxin are 64–154 nanomoles/liter (nmol/l). Low levels of thyroxin (<64 nmol/l) lead to hypothyroidism, the symptoms of which include low pulse rate, constipation, depression, and dementia. High levels of thyroxin (>154 nmol/l) lead to hyperthyroidism, causing (among others) an elevated pulse rate, high blood pressure, diarrhea, and weakness. In these cases, only values within the normal range have positive normative meaning.
2. Normal levels of sperm cell count in adult males are 20–150 million sperm cells/ml. Levels lower than 20 million might indicate infertility. In this case, only values lower than the norm will receive negative normative meaning if fertility in males is valuable in a given society.

As is evident, sometimes a single value defines the sufficiency threshold, as in the case of sperm cell count; at other times, a range of values defines the sufficiency threshold, as in the case of thyroxin. *A condition of insufficiency is one in which deviation from normal values narrows individuals' ability to pursue their life plans and live a good human life.*

Such a characterization of the threshold, however, seems too coarse. It lacks sensitivity to different levels of malfunction, and it assumes that once people are located beneath the threshold, it is morally irrelevant how far they fall beneath the threshold. Therefore, a more careful deliberation is required. When we consider people located beneath the sufficiency threshold, we should distinguish between two fundamental levels of severity. We can mark certain capabilities that differentiate human lives from nonhuman lives and label them as "personhood-making capacities."[29] Hence, there are those who are located below or who might fall below what we can mark as the *personhood threshold* (PT). Beneath PT, according to some views, life is hardly worth living because people in this range of capabilities lack essential features of human life (e.g., consciousness or the ability to breathe without mechanical assistance). In addition, there are those who are located beneath the sufficiency threshold (i.e., the BHFCs threshold) but above the PT, for whom decent human existence is not possible because they experience various disadvantages but still have essential features of human life.

---

29. This lower threshold is mentioned in Nussbaum, "Human Functioning," 221; and Benbaji, "Sufficiency or Priority?" 339–340.

These two thresholds differ in a fundamental way. The PT is universal and is not affected by social conditions or norms. Wherever humans are found, in order to be considered to have the essential features of being human, they must have personhood-making capacities. On the other hand, the BHFCs threshold is relative to social conditions (e.g., level of wealth and technological advancement) and norms (influenced by local history and traditional values). The BHFCs threshold is principled and abstract, not specific or concrete. There are negative and positive aspects to such a characterization. The negative aspect is that the account could have been more practical and easier for implementation had I presented an explicit and obvious threshold—one not open to interpretation and additional social debate. The positive aspect is that a principled–abstract characterization of the threshold is flexible and can fit different cultures and times.

A careful reading of Nussbaum shows that my route is not entirely different from hers. In her early work, she writes explicitly on two distinct thresholds:

> A threshold of capability to function, beneath which a life will be so impoverished that it will not be human at all, and a somewhat higher threshold, beneath which those characteristic functions are available in such a reduced way that, although we may judge the form of life a human one, we will not think it a *good* human life.[30]

For the formulation of public policy, Nussbaum focuses on the higher threshold—the good-enough human life threshold—which determines what kinds of things citizens are entitled to demand from their governments. However, that goal may be unrealistic because there are individuals beneath the threshold who could never reach the threshold level, no matter how many resources are expended in an effort to improve their functional capabilities. The severely mentally ill, the cognitively challenged, and the terminally ill could never reach the good-enough human life threshold Nussbaum has in mind. Nussbaum firmly asserts that we should use only one threshold, and she provides two convincing arguments. The first is a strategic argument: If we set a lower threshold, medical institutions would make little effort to improve the well-being of those individuals residing below it. The second argument is normative: One threshold for everyone reminds us of the dignity we must preserve for the mentally, cognitively, or terminally ill. It obliges us to view them as equal members of the human community, entitled to a good human life despite their impairments.[31]

---

30. Nussbaum, "Human Functioning," 221.

31. Nussbaum, *Frontiers*, 190–193.

Nevertheless, she never provides suggestions as to where that threshold should be delineated, because "there is a continuum here, and it is always going to be difficult to say where ... [it] should be located."[32] In addition, she writes,

> The approach ... specifies this threshold only in a general and approximate way, both because I hold that the threshold level may shift in subtle ways over time, and because I hold that the appropriate threshold level of capability may, at the margins, be differently set by different societies in accordance with their histories and circumstances.[33]

Therefore, Nussbaum acknowledges that cultural and social differences might affect the exact location of the threshold. According to SOC, in allocating health care services, we should take into consideration the PT and the BHFCs thresholds, as I argue in the following section. The PT is a universal threshold. It characterizes the most fundamental level of human capabilities required for an organism to be considered as having the essential features of being human. The BHFCs threshold, however, is relative to social traditions and values, levels of wealth, technology, and so on, but it must be uniform for all members of a given society. In that respect, I fully accept Nussbaum's strategic and normative arguments. My disagreement with her resides on two matters. First, social policy should not be informed only by the "good-enough human life" threshold but also by the PT and BHFCs threshold in order to reflect our different concerns to different severity levels of those who lack BHFCs. Second, I contend, it is impossible to talk about an (almost) universal good-enough human life threshold that Nussbaum has in mind. This conclusion is unavoidable because, in line with Walzer, I take the position that justice is relative to social values, traditions, levels of wealth, etc. In addition, as I claimed previously, the BHFCs threshold is relative to social conditions and norms. As an example, consider Israel's health policy regarding the provision and subsidization of in vitro fertilization (IVF) compared to that of other European countries. During 2008, the number of IVF treatments provided in Israel was 3945 per 1 million. This is 1.47 times more than in Belgium, the western European country that provided the greatest number of IVF treatments that year (2687 per 1 million).[34] Israel's pro-natal policy (and the higher threshold it sets regarding women's reproductive capabilities) reflects the country's unique

---

32. Nussbaum, "Human Functioning," 221.

33. Nussbaum, *Frontiers*, 180.

34. The State Comptroller of Israel, *Annual Report 63c* (May 8, 2013): 935 [in Hebrew], accessed May 1, 2014, http://www.mevaker.gov.il/he/Reports/Pages/114.aspx.

perspective regarding the desirability of IVF that is rooted (among other things) in its history and dominant religious beliefs.[35]

4. Setting Priorities Between Competing Claims Beneath the Threshold

As I claimed previously, health care policy should be informed by both the PT and BHFCs thresholds. That raises a problem of macro allocation—the prioritization of different groups of patients located at different levels beneath the two thresholds. Persons just above the PT, who might possibly fall below that threshold, have a stronger claim to resources because of a preeminent moral urgency to preserve their capacities to function as human beings. Thus, when we want to prioritize patients beneath the BHFCs threshold, we should grant greater priority to those located further beneath the threshold, especially those beneath the PT.[36]

However, my version of sufficientarianism is non-absolute. In other words, the worst-off are not automatically given first priority because there are other variables that should be taken into consideration in prioritizing patients, such as the size of the potential benefits and the number of people beneath the threshold who would benefit. Our commitment is not to aggregate benefits beneath the threshold, as a utilitarian position would recommend. Sufficiency is concerned with bringing people as close to the BHFCs threshold as possible because being beneath the threshold implies that they are worse off in a morally relevant way.

Assume that with a given amount of money, we could benefit only one out of two groups of patients. Group A consists of 10 patients, and they are worse off than the patients in group B, which consists of 100 patients. If we choose to benefit group A, each individual will gain significant improvement (instead of dying at the age of 40 years, they will each gain an additional 7 years of a good quality of life). If we choose to benefit group B, each individual will gain a relatively less significant benefit (1 additional year of living, and they would die at the age of 51 years). The aggregate benefit to group A is 70 years of living. The aggregated benefit to group B is 100 years of living. Sufficientarian concern is not to maximize the numbers of years gained but, rather, to improve individuals' condition if they happen to be beneath the threshold because of the moral imperative to benefit the worse-off who

---

35. I want to emphasize that I am not claiming that Israel's pro-natal policy is justified or that it is not. I am simply providing an example of how cultural differences lead to different thresholds.

36. As indicated, below the BHFCs threshold, I apply prioritarian concerns (it is morally more important to give priority to the worse-off). However, because I insist on the moral significance of the threshold that differentiates between the worse-offs and the better-offs, the principle I will soon present cannot be regarded as a prioritarian principle.

lack the ability to live a good human life. Therefore, if significant improvement can be provided to one small group of patients, it should be done, even if the improvement in their capabilities will not bring them above the BHFCs threshold, or even if the alternative could produce a greater aggregate utility (by providing small benefits to a large number of beneficiaries in a different group).

These concerns—to give priority to the worse-off beneath the threshold and to prioritize significant benefits over more trivial ones—require further discussion. How would we determine the severity level of patients' illnesses (how far they are beneath the BHFCs or the PT threshold) and how would we evaluate the size or the significance of benefits?

The advantage of the SOC lies in the notion of capabilities that can help us to determine when and why a person is worse off and when the benefit is significant.[37] I propose two criteria for determining the severity of an individual's condition. The first is the number of BHFCs systems that are or will be negatively affected. According to my account, all nine capability systems are important because they reflect normal human functioning and are required for an individual to achieve a flourishing life. The more capability systems that are negatively affected, the more an individual's ability to function decreases. The second criterion is the extent of the decrease in each of the capability systems, which determines the individual's position under the BHFCs threshold (the greater the decrease, the lower an individual's position beneath the threshold). Therefore, the severity of an individual's condition is directly proportional to the number of capability systems negatively affected and the extent of the decrease in each capability.

Because the severity of an individual's condition is determined by these criteria, they should be used to value the size or the significance of the benefit. The benefit is more significant as more capability systems are repaired or compensated for and the greater the degree of improvement in each capability system.

The previous discussion is summarized in the following two statements:

1. There is a greater moral importance to benefitting the worse-off, as long as the potential benefit to them is not trivial.
2. Allocation policy beneath the threshold should grant greater moral importance to the size of the benefit of each individual (in each group), and not to the aggregate benefit of many, as long as the size of the benefit to each individual is significant.

---

37. For an extended discussion, see Ram-Tiktin, "Equality of Opportunity."

These two statements underlie the prioritization principle:

> *Number and benefit-size weighted sufficiency*: When allocating health care re-
> sources, priority should be given to individuals below the BHFCs thresh-
> old. Below the threshold, benefiting people matters more the worse off
> such people are (beneath the PT or BHFCs threshold), the greater the size
> of the benefit in question, and the more there are of such people. The size
> of the benefit is more important than the number of beneficiaries.

Patient prioritization is far more complicated and includes additional considerations such as cost-effectiveness calculations and the relative importance and
weight of different kinds of benefits (e.g., the value of prevention of death vs. prevention of various degrees of handicaps). However, these considerations exceed
the scope of this chapter and so will be addressed elsewhere.

5. Conclusion

SOC is an account of distributive justice in health care that deals with one issue
of justice within the health sphere. It is built on several theoretical frameworks,
such as Walzer's spheres of justice, the Sen–Nussbaum capability approach, and
Frankfurt's doctrine of sufficiency. In developing a theory of distributive justice
in health care, I identified nine key systems of BHFCs that are the currency of
justice within health care. I argued that, at least in relation to health care, we
should not care about equality and that we have good reason to reject a prioritarian view. I stated that if we believe in equality or priority, we should strive to
eliminate health disparities whenever they are visited upon people, even if the
individuals in question are in a reasonable state of health. However, according
to the sufficiency viewpoint, legitimate claims for health care can be presented
only by individuals who are located (or who might fall) beneath the PT or BHFCs
thresholds.

The interpretation I suggested for the doctrine of sufficiency is non-absolute.
For this reason, we should not give ultimate priority to those located below the
BHFCs threshold (or even PT), or to the greatest possible number of beneficiaries,
but also take into consideration the size of the benefit. The doctrine of sufficiency
is obligated to guarantee that individuals have enough to live a good human life,
and if we can provide significant improvement to members of one small group of
patients, we should do that, even if the aggregate improvement in their capabilities is smaller than the aggregate improvement to a larger group of patients (when
each one of them gains a smaller benefit). The advantage of SOC is that by using

the notion of capabilities, we can explain when and why one person is worse off than another and when we should consider a benefit significant.

Acknowledgments

I express my deep gratitude to the editors of this volume, Carina Fourie and Annette Rid, for their insightful and thought-provoking comments that enabled me to crystallize my thoughts and arguments. In addition, I thank Noam Zohar, Ruth Faden, and David Enoch for their helpful oral and written comments and suggestions on previous drafts of this chapter.

9

Disability, Disease, and Health Sufficiency

Sean Aas and David Wasserman

1. Introduction

Health *sufficientarianism* holds that insofar as health matters to social justice, what matters is that everyone have *enough* health—not, per *health egalitarianism*, that everyone be equally healthy or, per *health prioritarianism*, that the *least healthy* or otherwise least-advantaged should be as healthy as they can be. Each of these accounts of health justice requires some account of what health is, insofar as it matters to justice. Sufficientarian accounts face an additional burden: They have to state not just what makes someone *more or less healthy* than someone else but also what makes someone *healthy enough* for the purposes of justice.

In this chapter, we take up the last task, developing an account of health that is best suited for health justice and that is better than rival accounts in meeting the additional burden facing a sufficientarian account of health justice.

Our key examples, developed in the first section, derive from the case of disability. Following and extending a "social model" of disability, we argue that some disadvantages apparently caused by biomedical abnormality are actually due primarily to unjust societal responses to biological difference.[1] People whose bodies disadvantage them only in this socially mediated manner, we claim, are not *unhealthy* in any way that matters to health justice: Their claims are claims to environmental or social modification, not to biomedical intervention. Claims

---

1. David Wasserman et al., "Disability: Definitions, Models, Experience," in *The Stanford Encyclopedia of Philosophy*, ed. Edward N. Zalta (2013), accessed March 3, 2015, http://plato. stanford.edu/archives/fall2013/entries/disability.

to biomedical intervention enter in only when there is something about the body itself that causes or threatens to cause harm. What is required for health sufficiency, indeed for any theory of health justice, is some way of understanding "health" that helps us to distinguish health-relevant from health-irrelevant differences in biological functioning.

In Section 2, we argue that many existing accounts are not helpful here—and that this is especially worrying for sufficientarian theories of health justice. "Biostatistical" accounts threaten to make all disability unhealthy, whereas "goal-oriented" accounts make it impossible to say anything general about whether and to what extent a given impairment generates health-justice claims.[2] In Section 3, we draw on suggestions by Ron Amundson and Peter Hucklenbroich to develop a novel "harm-oriented" account that does better than biostatistical and goal-oriented views on these counts.[3] On our harm-oriented account, to be more or less healthy is to be more or less free from "disease processes"—roughly, processes that cause or threaten to cause certain harms: premature death, pain, or life-disrupting loss of function.

The result of all this is not an argument for health sufficientarianism over other conceptions of health justice. Our hope, however, is that our analysis of health can show what demands a health sufficiency approach will place on society—not to normalize biological differences or give everyone the ability to do more of whatever they might want but, rather, simply to do its best to ensure that no one has to worry that their lives will be ruined by disease.

2. The Social Model of Disability and the Proper Domain of Health (Care)

In this section, we make two related points about disability, health, and well-being. These points, we argue, are critical in fashioning a definition of health appropriate for a sufficiency approach to justice in health care.

First, in order to restrict the domain of health in a way that a *health* sufficiency approach requires, we need to recognize that much of the disadvantage in many disabilities arises from an inhospitable physical and social environment and is best alleviated by environmental and social changes

2. Christopher Boorse, "Health as a Theoretical Concept," *Philosophy of Science* 44, no. 4 (1977): 542–573; Lennart Nordenfeldt, *On the Nature of Health* (New York: Springer, 1995).

3. Ron Amundson, "Disability, Handicap, and the Environment," *Journal of Social Philosophy* 23, no. 1 (1992): 105–119; Peter Hucklenbroich, "'Disease Entity' as the Key Theoretical Concept of Medicine," *Journal of Medicine and Philosophy* 39, no. 6 (2014): 609–633.

rather than biomedical intervention—for example, by ensuring the avail-ability of Braille texts and keyboards, voice-based Windows programs, sign-language interpreters and visual smoke detectors, ramps and elevators in buildings, and paved paths in parks. The role of environmental factors in causing disadvantage is emphasized by proponents of social models of disability—those who maintain that the disadvantages associated with disability are exclusively or primarily produced not by bodily differences but, rather, by unaccommodating social environments. The importance of social and environmental factors, however, is also recognized by philoso-phers concerned with the impact of health conditions on well-being. For example, in questioning whether it is possible to separately assess health-related quality of life, John Broome observes that the quality of life of people with disabilities depends heavily on nonhealth factors: "Asthma is less bad if you if you are well-housed, mental handicap is less bad in supportive communities, deafness is less bad if you have access to the Internet."[4]

Second, there is a clear sense in which people with some disabilities can be healthy: Many people with major sensory and motor disabilities, such as blindness, deafness, and paraplegia, go through life with no more pain, discomfort, disrup-tion, or (further) loss of function than most nondisabled people, and they require no more medical attention. Indeed, some are athletes in peak condition; others are artists and actors in peak form, unhampered by significant health problems.

Both these points are important for carving out a distinct domain for health and setting a feasible sufficiency threshold. Recognizing the social causes of disability-related disadvantage places many of the justice claims of people with disabilities outside the domain of health. Recognizing that many people with disabilities are, or can be, fit, high-functioning, and free of pain, discomfort, and nonroutine med-ical needs places them above any plausible health-sufficiency threshold.

These points expose prima facie difficulties for one of the most detailed proposals for health care sufficiency thus far presented, Efrat Ram-Tiktin's sufficiency of capabilities account.[5] Her account seeks to maintain a "separate sphere" for the distribution of health care, distinct from other goods subject to the demands of justice. It takes the basic "currency" of justice in health care to be capabilities, specifically nine enumerated basic human functional capabilities

4. John Broome, "Measuring the Burden of Disease by Aggregating Well-Being," in *Summary Measures of Population Health: Concepts, Ethics, Measurement and Applications*, ed. Christopher J. L. Murray, Joshua A. Salomon, Colin D. Mathers, and Alan D. Lopez (Geneva: World Health Organization, 2002), 95.

5. Efrat Ram-Tiktin, "The Right to Health Care as a Right to Basic Human Functional Capabilities," *Ethical Theory and Moral Practice* 15, no. 3 (2012): 337–351.

(BHFCs).[6] These BHFCs, Ram-Tiktin argues, are only a subset of all the capabilities that suffice for human flourishing; their possession is necessary but not sufficient for people's ability to exercise their positive freedom and live a good human life.

In her chapter in this volume (Chapter 8), Ram-Tiktin emphasizes that possession of the BHFCs is required for *intactness* but not (necessarily) for health. The former is a value-free concept, whereas the latter is a value-laden sociocultural concept.[7] BHFC deficiencies presumably underwrite claims for health care only in an environment in which they are disadvantageous or deleterious. Ram-Tiktin gives the example of an enzyme deficiency that causes problems only in a society in which broad beans are a diet staple. In such a society, that deficiency would prevent the individual from achieving his or her goals and would place the individual below the threshold level. It is the duty of health institutions to raise individuals to that threshold when they can and to compensate individuals when they cannot.

We focus initially on Ram-Tiktin's proposal not only because it is a carefully developed account of health sufficiency but also because it seeks to treat health as a separate sphere of justice. She criticizes, as we will do, other normative accounts of health for failing to distinguish health from other domains of well-being or capability. We argue, however, that by neglecting the role of the physical and social environment in disadvantaging people with disabilities, her account is open to a version of the same objection.

Among Ram-Tiktin's nine BHFCs, two deserve special scrutiny from a disability perspectve: *senses*, which she defines as the ability to use all five senses and thus acquire new knowledge about the external world, and *movement and balance*, including the ability to move all four limbs with a species-typical range of motion. The inclusion of these capabilities on the list makes it prima facie implausible that the BHFCs are necessary for health. It is not clear that being able to see, hear, or walk is necessary for "health" in a sense that would give people lacking those functions a claim to their acquisition as a matter of justice. (In Section 4, we offer an account of health which vindicates the intuition that being blind, deaf, or paraplegic is not per se unhealthy.)

Ram-Tiktin might deny that this is an implication of her view. She might claim that the absence of sight, hearing, or full mobility need not place people who lack those capabilities below the threshold of sufficient health or give them a claim to treatment or compensation. A successful individual with a disability can "advance [his or her] goals in his or her social environment."[8] For that reason, they have no sufficiency-based

6. See Efrat Ram-Tiktin's chapter in this volume (Chapter 8).

7. Ram-Tiktin, "The Right to Health Care," 341f8.

8. Ibid., 340.

claim to health care resources. Also, although they may not be "intact," that does not mean they are unhealthy, which is a sociocultural determination.

But if so, the BHFCs cannot be necessary to living "a good human life"[9] as Ram-Tiktin claims, in any sense of that phrase that can define a sufficiency threshold. Moreover, the application of Ram-Tiktin's scheme would yield counterintuitive results. Consider two individuals who are both blind and otherwise healthy. They live in different societies, one of which has comprehensive Braille text services and voice- and keyboard-based Internet access; the other has little of either. Many blind people who would be able to advance their goals in the first social environment would be unable to do so in the second. (We can imagine similarly contrasting environments for deaf or paraplegic individuals.) It seems odd, if not perverse, to claim that the blind individual in the first society is more healthy than her counterpart in the second or that the latter, and only the latter, has a claim to *health care* resources that the former lacks. The latter individual, we maintain, has a claim to exactly what the former individual already has: the *social* resources that will enable her to read and communicate like her sighted peers. On views like that of Ram-Tiktin, the health of an individual could not be assessed for sufficiency purposes by a medical examination; it would require not just a medical but also a social assessment. Rather than preserving separate spheres of justice, Tiktin's scheme undermines them by allowing injustices in the distribution of social resources to give rise to claims of injustice in the distribution of health care resources. (We are not denying that it would make practical sense to push for sight-restoring treatments in a state whose bureaucracy generously provided health care resources but adamantly refused to provide what the Americans with Disabilities Act calls "reasonable accommodation."[10] However, recourse to health care would not negate the social injustice.)

We therefore need an understanding of health that more plausibly identifies health care needs for purposes of threshold and priority setting and that better preserves a separate sphere for health. That understanding of health should allow for the possibility that someone might be as "healthy" as he or she has any claim on others to be, although (1) this person lacks physiologically normal function in some body part or other and (2) this lack of function contributes in some way to harm. Our thesis, instead, is that harms related to the state of the body do not detract from health unless they are harms of the right kind and caused in the right way. The most prominent existing accounts of health, we argue in the next section, are unhelpful here.

---

9. Ibid., 338.

10. Americans with Disabilities Act of 1990, Public Law 101–336, §§3, 108th Congress, 2nd session (July 26, 1990).

3. Naturalistic and Normative Accounts of Health and Health Sufficiency

In this section, we argue that two prominent approaches to the concept of "health" are mostly unhelpful for the purposes of a sufficientarian account of health justice. "Naturalist" accounts of health in terms of statistically normal physiological function make "health" too demanding: Anyone who has an impairment, on these accounts, is not healthy, no matter whether or why this impairment affects the person's life. Goal-oriented "normative" accounts of health, which make health a matter of having a body suited to achieving one's goals, can be too demanding in a different way: Someone might be "unhealthy" in these terms because she wants to do unusually demanding activities, such as winning marathons. Both "naturalist" and "normative" accounts have trouble distinguishing dysfunction or harm caused by the body itself from dysfunction or harm more properly attributable to society. Both, therefore, suggest a health sufficiency standard that is overdemanding in another way: demanding that we devote health resources to addressing non-health problems.

These criticisms are not arguments against these accounts qua explanations of the concept of health used in clinical practice or biomedical science. Our claim here is not that these accounts get "health" wrong but, rather, that the extent to which we are "healthy" in their terms does not track the force of our claims to health resources. The onus here, then, is less on theorists of "health" than on theorists of health justice. If, as we argue, existing accounts of health say that people with impairments are unhealthy to the extent they are impaired, then people with impairments would have the same place in health justice as people with more conventional illnesses. However, as we argue below, the social model of disability teaches us that the right response to impairment is often different from the right response to paradigm illness: accommodation and inclusion rather than medical intervention. All theorists of health justice, including (indeed, we argue, *especially including*) sufficientarian theorists, require some way of distinguishing those departures from biological normality that generate claims on health resources from those that do not.

So how should we understand the "health" in "health justice"? "Health" is often said to be, simply, the "absence of disease." If this is so, then to define health we need only define "disease." One approach would be simply to define by extension—to list the diseases and define health as their comprehensive absence.

Such an expansive list of disease conditions is provided, for example, by the American Medical Association's *Nomenclature of Diseases and Operations*.[11] As Ron

---

11. National Conference on Medical Nomenclature et al., eds., *Standard Nomenclature of Diseases and Operations*. (New York: McGraw-Hill, 1961).

Amundson observes, its list is "extraordinarily long," including not only what Christopher Boorse calls "paradigm objects of medical concern," such as malaria and cancer, but also static conditions such as color blindness, missing limbs, and supernumerary digits and injuries such as stab and gunshot wounds and animal bites.[12] As Amundson notes, an account of health posed solely in terms of such a list confuses symptoms with causes of symptoms and, more generally, lacks an organizing principle. An eclectic, one-dimensional list is therefore of limited relevance in discussing normative issues such as those concerning health justice. We do not know whether having or lacking an item on a pathologist's list matters to justice unless we know why some things, but not others, are on that list. What we need is some sense of *why* pathologists include stable sensory impairments such as congenital blindness on the same list as lung cancer or Ebola virus; only then can we judge the relevance of biomedical health to distributive justice.

3.1. A Naturalist Account of Health

Throughout the years, Christopher Boorse has developed a sophisticated philosophy of biomedical science, which is meant to provide just this sort of explanation: An account not only of *which* biological conditions are diseases, or (to use his preferred term) "pathologies," but also of *why* those conditions are diseased or pathological.[13] Boorse's basic idea is that a pathology is a failure of some part of an organism to make its normal contribution to that organism's ability to accomplish certain species-typical goals. Perhaps despite appearances, this definition of pathology has no obviously ineliminable normative terminology. The "goals" in question are simply survival and reproduction. A "failure" of a part to contribute to functioning is similarly non-normative; it is simply a matter of its not promoting the achievement of these goals as effectively as those parts tend to do, in physiologically normal human beings.

Boorse has claimed that the normatively aseptic character of his account is advantageous for the purposes of biomedical ethics.[14] With a clear, scientifically valid definition of health in hand, he says, we can get on to thinking about whether, why, and how health is best protected and promoted. We are not so sure. The phenomenon of "healthy disability," suggested above, calls into question the adequacy

---

12. Amundson, "Disability, Handicap, and the Environment," 105; Boorse, "Health as a Theoretical Concept," 945.

13. Boorse, "Health as a Theoretical Concept," 945, originally; for further development, see Christopher Boorse, "A Rebuttal on Health," in *What Is Disease?* ed. James M. Humber and Robert F. Almeder (Totowa, NJ: Humana Press, 1997).

14. Boorse, "A Rebuttal on Health," 98f.

of Boorse's account as an analysis of the "health" in "health justice." Cases from disability show that Boorsean biomedical health is distinct from the sorts of health status that matter to justice in at least two ways.

First, the Boorsean focus on health as the absence of part-"dysfunction" does not distinguish between those who function less well "on the whole" as a result of dysfunctional parts and those who do not. Thus, for instance, blindness as a dysfunction of the visual system detracts from Boorsean health just as much whether it significantly impedes a person's life or not. Someone who has always been blind but has developed skills or abilities that allow him to function fully in his society (skill at using a cane and Braille, enhanced hearing, echolocation, etc.) is as unhealthy on Boorse's account, ceteris paribus, as someone who is having significant trouble adapting to a recent loss of sight. The *actual* adaptations or accommodations are irrelevant to whether human beings without sight have *normally* been less able to survive and reproduce than others as a result of their blindness. Now, we are not sure whether Boorse is correct that biomedical science could not recognize that people such as the former are "healthy." However, we are sure that the poorly adapted blind person has a stronger claim to health care, such as occupational rehabilitation, than the well-adapted one. Boorse's account does not help us distinguish these claims.

Second, considering now only people who do function poorly on the whole because of part-dysfunction, Boorse's account fails to distinguish between those with claims to biomedical assistance and those with claims to social and environmental reconstruction—thereby neglecting a key insight from the social model of disability. Even when impairment is associated with a decrement of a body's ability to function, it may not be the impairment itself to which this decrement should be attributed. Consider, for example, a scheme for allocating scarce life-saving resources that gave lower priority to people with disabilities on the assumption that their lives, if prolonged, would be of lower quality than those of nondisabled people. If such a scheme were adopted in a time of pandemic, people with a variety of disabilities would have worse prospects for survival and reproduction as an indirect result of their disabilities. This, we believe, would be unjust. However, this injustice does not arise from the failure to treat the disabilities before the pandemic. If the disabled people in question were well-adapted, then there may have been no injustice in the lack of prior treatment. What is unjust is not the failure to raise them to (or closer to) Boorsean health by fixing their dysfunctional parts but, rather, invidious discrimination against them based on false beliefs about the relevance of their part-function to their flourishing as a whole.[15] Boorse's account is unhelpful in this kind of debate. It suggests

---

15. That discrimination may also be based on the questionable moral view that one's level of well-being is relevant to one's priority for the allocation of life-saving resources—that is, *even*

that all part-dysfunction is equally relevant to health, failing to distinguish cases in which the associated disadvantage is a matter of health justice from cases in which it is a matter of accessibility and inclusion.

This is especially troublesome for sufficientarian accounts of health justice. It is difficult to comprehend how such an account could adopt a Boorsean theory of health without generating unreasonable demands on health resources. Take any significantly impaired person who is well adapted to his or her impairments—a successful physicist, for example, who is unable to move much of his body but interacts fluently using technological aids. Assume that his condition is stable in the sense that no further loss of function is expected to occur and no health resources are required to sustain him at his current level of functioning. He has a body that departs radically from species-typical functioning—much more radically than, for example, the body of a construction worker with a painfully dislocated shoulder. However, the latter seems to have a stronger claim on health resources than the former.

This difference cannot be explained by a difference in their health. However, it is difficult to comprehend how else a *health sufficientarian*, in particular, could explain it. A maximizing approach to health justice can appeal to the enormously greater efficiencies involved in using scarce resources to treat the easily treatable shoulder condition. A prioritarian approach can maintain that what matters is that the ailing construction worker is worse off overall than the flourishing physicist. However, a sufficientarian seems stuck saying that both are below the same health threshold—and thus that both have claims to be raised above it and the physicist would have a stronger claim because he was farther below it. Treating health justice in terms of restoring normal function gives the suffering construction worker a weaker claim to inexpensive treatment than the physicist has to much more expensive treatment.

Sufficientarians could attempt to resolve this prima facie problem in various ways. Rather than canvass these, we simply pursue one such response in Section 4. Our approach is to delineate a conception of health on which people well-adjusted to nonprogressive, nonpainful, non-life-shortening impairments do not have claims in health justice at all and a fortiori no implausible claims to useless, nonbeneficial health interventions.

---

if disability entailed a decrement in well-being, it might still be objectionable to discriminate against the disabled in the way that QALY- and DALY-based health policies sometimes do. Cf. John Harris, "QALYfying the Value of Life," *Journal of Medical Ethics* 13, no. 3 (1987): 117–123; Paul Menzel et al., "Toward a Broader View of Values in Cost-Effectiveness Analysis of Health," *The Hastings Center Report* 29, no. 3 (1999): 7.

3.2. Instrumental Normative Accounts of Health

Against Boorsean *naturalists* about health, *normativists* maintain that the absence of health must be "bad" by definition. Different normative theories of health understand the badness of ill health in different ways. *Goal-oriented* or *instrumental* views are, or can be, normatively *maximalist*; they treat health as a matter of having a body suitable to achieving one's goals, whatever they might be. *Harm-oriented* views are normatively *minimalist* and *non-instrumental*; they treat health not in terms of goal achievement but harm avoidance. Being healthy is a matter of *not* being harmed, in a certain way, by the state of one's body.

Normative theories, in general, are prima facie more promising for the purposes of health justice than Boorse-style naturalist theories. After all, making health valuable by definition promises to help explain why people have claims to be healthy. However, in this section, we argue that existing normative theories are poorly suited to ground plausible claims about health justice. In particular, (1)goal-oriented theories have difficulties defining a generalizable standard of bodily functioning as a threshold for health sufficiency, whereas (2) existing harm-oriented accounts fail to adequately distinguish health-relevant harms from harms that are not relevant to health per se.

The analysis of health in goal-oriented terms was first developed by Lennart Nordenfelt, who defined health as the ability of an individual to reach her "vital goals"—that is, those goals whose achievement is individually necessary and jointly sufficient for minimal happiness.[16] On this account, the relationship between disability and health depends on the goals that are considered vital or central and on the role of typical functions in achieving them. This is responsive to some of the arguments offered previously: For example, some impairments will hinder the pursuit of some goals, other impairments will have no effect, and some will enhance the pursuit of some goals. Thus, for example, someone devoted passionately and exclusively to oenology might be a better wine taster if blind than if sighted. Thus, this account straightforwardly allows for the possibility of disability without ill health.

Still, any attempt to use Nordenfeldt's account of health in a sufficientarian approach to health justice would face other serious challenges. "Vital goals" as Nordenfeldt defines them are highly variable between individuals; they include general species-wide aims such as Boorse's "survival and reproduction," but they also include much more idiosyncratic goals. Nordenfeldt states, for instance, that an ambitious athlete having a bad day, unable to perform his best, is not healthy that day, even if his body can still perform better athletically than the bodies of

---

16. Nordenfeldt, *On the Nature of Health*.

most others.[17] A Nordenfeldtian sufficiency approach to health justice would have to either (1) assert that such people have forceful claims to health resources or (2) restrict the range of "vital goals" that are relevant to whether someone is "healthy enough" for justice. We believe that option 1 is deeply implausible as a claim about justice. Option 2 is more promising, but it raises difficult issues about how to restrict "vital goals." What is required is some *general* account of aims more-or-less universally relevant to both health and health justice.

Some concerns about this sort of generality arise in Sridhar Venkatapuram's account, which modifies that of Nordenfelt.[18] Venkatapuram replaces Nordenfelt's mix of universal and personal vital goals with the "basic capabilities for minimal happiness" enumerated by Martha Nussbaum.[19] Unlike Ram-Tiktin, he does not select a subset of those capabilities as relevant to health. Venkatapuram maintains that what is important is "the idea of health as the capability to achieve a cluster of basic capabilities and functionings."[20] Although the avoidance of disease and impairments remains one of those basic capabilities, health involves the acquisition of all of them. Far from denying that this conception resembles the much-ridiculed 1948 World Health Organization definition of health as "a state of complete physical, mental, and social well-being," Venkatapuram accepts a modified version of that definition, albeit one that refers only to a capability for *minimal* well-being.[21] Nor does he shirk from the practical implications of this conception: "Health policy and expertise will have to encompass all the determinants of the core human capabilities that constitute a minimally decent life."[22]

A goal-oriented approach, taken to Venkatapuram's extreme, gives health unbounded jurisdiction by attenuating its connection with the body and with medical interventions. One can certainly stipulate that to be healthy, one must be able to acquire the capabilities for play, meaningful social affiliations, and control of one's political environment. However, it involves a radical departure from common understanding to state that someone who simply lacks the opportunity to play, form close friendships, or avoid political upheavals in her country is thereby unhealthy

---

17. Ibid., 71.

18. Sridhar Venkatapuram, "Health, Vital Goals, and Central Human Capabilities," *Bioethics* 27, no. 5 (2013): 271–279.

19. Martha C. Nussbaum, *Women and Human Development: The Capabilities Approach* (New York: Cambridge University Press, 2000).

20. Venkatapuram, "Health, Vital Goals," 277.

21. World Health Organization, "Constitution of the World Health Organization" (1948), http://www.who.int/governance/eb/who_constitution_en.pdf.

22. Venkatapuram, "Health, Vital Goals," 278.

when this lack does not come from the biofunctional state of her body at all (although all three may create *risks* to health in a conventional sense).[23]

This "health imperialism" is particularly worrying from the perspective of disability. As noted previously, it is important for disabled people to distinguish disadvantages due to the functional status of their bodies from disadvantages due to stigmatization and exclusion.[24] An account such as that of Venkatapuram does no better than Boorse's account in explicating a distinction between disadvantage elicited by biomedical atypicalities and disadvantage more generally; thus, Venkatapuram, like Boorse, ignores information that policymakers and activists need in order to understand the particular kinds of injustice to which disabled people are so often subjected. Claiming that people with disabilities are denied their right to health in this expansive sense makes their complaints no different than those of poor people denied adequate resources for education, housing, and physical security. However, despite commonalities, the injustices faced by people with disabilities have distinctive features. Injustice against disabilities involves a particular form of discrimination: the stigmatization of physical and mental difference perceived as abnormalities or defects, and deliberate or negligent exclusion by practices that fail to accommodate those differences.[25]

To avoid these problems, proponents of sufficientarian accounts of health justice should want a normative account of health that appeals to a much less expansive set of values. In particular, they would be well advised to focus on health as a bodily status that precludes certain *harms* rather than on health understood as having a body that allows the achievement of positive goals. If, as sufficientarians maintain, we have forceful claims to the resources we need in order to have a certain sort of body, there had better be something seriously wrong if we do not have a body of this sort.

As mentioned previously, some existing normative accounts take this harm-oriented form. Jerome Wakefield, for instance, has proposed a hybrid

---

23. Henry Richardson suggests that Venkatapuram's definition of health could be narrowed to avoid this problem of unlimited jurisdiction if it were limited to the nonvoluntary bodily preconditions for realizing the basic human capabilities enumerated by Nussbaum. Henry S. Richardson, "Capabilities and the Definition of Health: Comments on Venkatapuram," *Bioethics* 30, no. 1 (2016): 1–7. Although such a limitation would improve on Venkatapuram's account by "embodying" it, it would still need to explain how social and environmental factors affected whether a nonvoluntarily bodily state or function was in fact a precondition for realizing the capabilities.

24. Amundson, "Disability, Handicap, and the Environment"; Wasserman et al., "Disability."

25. Disability injustice is to be distinguished from racial and gender injustice by way of this constitutive connection to perceptions concerning *normality* and *function*; although Black people and women are disadvantaged on account of prevailing beliefs about their bodies, their bodies are not regarded as *abnormal* or *dysfunctional* (although perhaps as inferior).

normative–naturalist view that takes health to be the absence of harmful deviations from Boorse-style species-typical functioning.[26] This avoids the health imperialism of some goal-oriented normative approaches; not every process that
leads to harm entails ill health—only processes that go by way of biomedical
pathology count.

Wakefield's view, however, inherits some deficits from its naturalist forebears.
Even if it denies that disability per se is harmful, it will have a difficult time distinguishing importantly different cases in which disability does lead to harm. Indeed,
it faces precisely the same problems as Boorse's account in distinguishing health-
relevant harms from health-irrelevant harms. As formulated, it implies that any
time a Boorsean biomedical pathology is a causal condition of harm, there is a
deficit in health. However, we have argued, this is false—or at least false for the
purposes of health justice. If a failure to function normally harms, not intrinsically but only because of an unjust social response, complaints against this harm
are not claims to restore "health" but, rather, for example, claims to stop invidious
discrimination against those with biostatistically atypical bodies.

In summary, a health-sufficientarian (or indeed any theorist of health justice)
should be sympathetic to "normativist" claims that health can be understood as
having a body suited to achieving certain goods or (better) preventing certain bads.
However, existing normative accounts are not sufficiently careful in specifying
what counts as a bad to be prevented or what counts as having a body suited to
preventing it. As a result, they fail to account for the distinctiveness of health as
a domain or sphere of justice, conflating disadvantage due solely or primarily to
bodily conditions with disadvantage due solely or primarily to societal responses
to health-neutral bodily differences.

These accounts are especially problematic for sufficientarian approaches to
health. Recall the two blind people we discussed while criticizing Ram-Tiktin's
version. The one in a Braille-rich society would fall comfortably above the health
threshold, and the one in a Braille-poor society would fall far below it, despite their
identical bodily conditions. As we argued, the latter does not seem to be suffering
from a lack of health resources but, rather, the social resources for greater accessibility and inclusion. This is admittedly a problem for maximizing and prioritarian
approaches as well; all three approaches treat the second individual as having a
claim of justice to health care resources.

---

26. Jerome Wakefield, "The Concept of Mental Disorder," *American Psychologist* 47
(1992): 373–388. Wakefield's account also differs from that of Boorse in understanding biological "normality" in evolutionary rather than statistical terms; a part functions "normally"
if it does what it was selected to do, not if it makes a statistically average contribution to
survival and reproduction. This difference does not matter here, however. Thus, for ease of
exposition, we treat Wakefield's view as if it were identical to Boorse's view but for the addition of a harm condition.

However, there is a special problem for sufficientarian accounts: The role of environmental and social factors in impeding the achievement of valuable goals makes it difficult to set and apply a uniform threshold of physical and mental functioning for different societies. A sufficientarian adopting a goal-oriented account of health would have two unsatisfactory options for threshold-setting. She could adopt a single threshold for both societies, with reference to which the first blind individual but not the second would be "healthy enough." However, this raises a significant practical problem. We might have thought that once a health threshold had been set through the political process, the question of whether a particular person meets it would be a strictly medical determination. However, on the single-threshold view, this will not be the case—an ophthalmologist could not make this determination without extensive knowledge of the Braille resources and other print alternatives available in his society.

Alternatively, the two societies could set different thresholds, both of which could be readily applied by an ophthalmologist. In the Braille-poor society, a blind individual would fall below the threshold; in the Braille-rich society, he would not. However, this would not only undermine any universalist ambitions of health-sufficiency justice but also raise practical problems. A threshold that took account of the totality of a society's social and economic conditions would have to change to reflect changing conditions. The opening of a large Braille production facility in the Braille-poor society might place blind people above its health-sufficiency threshold, whereas a sharp increase in the price of specialized paper in the Braille-rich society might push blind people below its threshold. This is much more troubling than the prosaic observation that what counts as "healthy enough" for justice may change as medical science marches on; this more radical variability would place a severe strain on the agencies responsible for health justice. They would have to monitor the entire society to ensure that people's bodies continued to work "well enough" to pursue their purposes in their changing social context. Although proponents of goal-oriented approaches such as Venkatapuram might endorse this holistic "social" conception of health, we believe that it would be unwieldy at best—and thus that there is, at the very least, good reason to search for a more narrowly "medical" approach to sufficiency thresholds.

4. A Non-instrumental Normative Account: Health as the Absence of Harmful Disease Entities

In the remainder of this chapter, we outline a normative approach to health that is more appropriate for a workable health sufficiency standard. Such an approach must meet two challenges raised by our examination of other accounts: (1) It must identify physical and psychological conditions that are either harmful in themselves or cause harm in ways not primarily mediated by prejudice, exclusion, neglect, or other independently identifiable social responses (including inappropriate and damaging medical procedures); and (2) the classification of a condition or effect as harmful cannot be based on the specific goals, history, or circumstances of the affected individual.

In ignoring harm, naturalistic accounts such as that of Boorse fail to provide any basis for assigning priority to disease conditions for purposes of setting a health sufficiency standard and assessing when it is reached. In requiring only that Boorsian atypicalities cause harm, a hybrid account such as that of Wakefield fails to distinguish harms that are matters of health from those that are matters of social attitudes or practices. Nordenfeldt's fully normative account likewise fails to distinguish harms that fall into the domain of health from other harms, and it makes the individual's health depend on his or her personal goals. Venkatapuram's more general goal-orientated approach avoids the latter problem, but it makes the domain of health coextensive with the domain of well-being. Those seeking a basis for a health-sufficiency standard will find little guidance in any of these accounts. Ram-Tiktin's account, discussed previously, does narrow the range of health-relevant capabilities. However, in ignoring the role of social factors in disadvantage, it fails to provide a domain-specific understanding of health or health care.

We propose an account of health for health justice tailored to avoid the previously mentioned difficulties—one that defines health in terms of the absence of harmful or harm-causing disease entities, excludes harms mediated by social factors, and understands harm independently of individual goals or circumstances.

Ron Amundson was perhaps the first to suggest a conception of health as the absence of disease, with disease narrowly defined as biological processes that lead to pain, loss or disruption of physical or mental function, or premature death.[27] Amundson noted that although disabilities were often consequences of diseases, they were not diseases themselves—they were not harmful processes, even if they were caused by such processes. This is not merely an academic distinction: Many people are born without sight, hearing, or limited mobility but also without active disease processes that threaten further loss of function, pain, or premature death. It is these individuals who, we have argued, can be disabled but healthy, or at least healthy enough for justice.

An account building on that of Amundson would define disease in terms of harm-causing biological processes, thereby distinguishing disability, which is, per the social model, often caused by social practices rather than biology. An understanding of disease as a harm-causing process should, we suggest, adopt a

---

27. Amundson, "Disability, Handicap, and the Environment," 105ff.

"noncomparative" account of harm of the kind offered by Seana Shiffrin.[28] Shiffrin identifies a class of states and events that can be regarded as bad or harmful for the individual regardless of how she would otherwise have fared; their badness is not understood in terms of how she was doing before experiencing them or how she would have done if she had not experienced them. These harms include pain, mental distress, discomfort, disruption, disability, death (at least premature death), and other losses—of cherished functions, people, activities, environments, and so on.

Shiffrin's account can be adapted to health by limiting the harms to those directly involving bodily conditions: the loss of a spouse would not make one less healthy, although the major depression it triggered would. Enslavement would not make one less healthy, although the material conditions of one's servitude likely would. Her account can also be adapted to a social model by removing disability from the list—the disruptive loss of a physical or psychological function through disease or injury would make one less healthy, but its mere absence (as in stable congenital conditions) need not. Treating the loss but not the absence of sensorimotor functions as presumptively harmful accords with a perspective that emphasizes the prospects for flourishing with less than a species-typical complement of human functions.[29] People with disabilities will, of course, often be unhealthy, but not simply by virtue of having a disability. Because we all must experience some or many noncomparative harms, no one can be perfectly healthy (at least for very long).

Shiffrin's account of noncomparative harm is not developed for health; still, the basic idea that health is to be defined in terms of certain kinds of harm is not unfamiliar. As discussed previously, Wakefield develops a broadly Boorsean notion of health that adds a "harm condition"; a disease is a departure from species-normal functioning that causes harm. This sort of account is more plausible if we restrict the harms in question to the distinctively health-related ones we have been discussing. Suppose that extreme shortness resulting from insensitivity to human growth hormone undermines lifetime earning power. If this were the only harm this abnormality caused, we would not want to say it was unhealthy. However, suppose also that this shortness led to reduced life expectancy, but solely because

---

28. Seana Valentine Shiffrin, "Wrongful Life, Procreative Responsibility, and the Significance of Harm," *Legal Theory* 5, no. 2 (1999): 117–148.

29. We recognize, of course, that the absence of certain species-typical functions, such as reasoning or moving any part of one's body, can be plausibly claimed to reduce the prospects for flourishing. We do not want to draw a line or suggest how one could be drawn. We merely insist that some common conditions classified as major disabilities, such as blindness, deafness, and paraplegia, need not preclude full flourishing.

of reduced earning power. Even a modified Wakefield-style account would have to state that shortness, as a harmful bodily abnormality, is a health problem because that view still puts no restrictions on causal pathways. However, this seems wrong as an account of the kind of health that matters to health justice—the problem here is not short stature but, rather, a society that does not provide fair opportunity to short people.

It is not enough, then, for a biological abnormality to cause harm; rather, this abnormality must do so directly, biologically, and in its own right (what these modifiers can mean is discussed later), not merely because social or environment conditions are inhospitable. The Boorsean element of Wakefield's account again renders it incapable of drawing this distinction.

Peter Hucklenbroich has proposed (what we would call) a harm-based account of health that does better on this score.[30] Health, Hucklenbroich states, is the absence of a "disease entity"; it is a biological process that is *pathological* in the sense that

1. It is immediately lethal or definitely life-shortening, [or]
2. It is a condition of pain, suffering, or other specific complaints, [or]
3. It is a condition of infertility (incapability of biological reproduction), [or]
4. It is a condition of inability or impairment for living together in human symbiotic communities, [or]
5. It is a non-universal disposition of the organism to develop a condition that is pathological according to one or more of these criteria.[31]

Hucklenbroich's account is congenial to our concerns for two reasons. First, it defines health in terms of a list of reasonably health-specific harms—albeit not necessarily the exact same list we would specify.[32] Second, more important, it has the resources, unlike Wakefield's account, to exclude harms due to social aspects of disability. It restricts health to the absence of biological conditions that either (1) directly *involve* harm or (2) *dispose* one to suffer harm.

This appeal to the notion of a "disposition," we believe, is the key to distinguishing health-relevant causal pathways from a bodily condition to a harm from health-irrelevant pathways (Hucklenbroich devotes little attention to this issue). The problem with Wakefield's definition of health, as it stands, is that

30. Hucklenbroich, " 'Disease Entity' as the Key Theoretical Concept of Medicine."

31. Hucklenbroich, ibid., 12. Note that "disease entity" in this sense includes some states we would not ordinarily call "diseases," such as internal bleeding as a result of traumatic injury. We use the term "disease process" to emphasize loss and disruption.

32. We are not sure, for instance, whether or when infertility generates claims in health justice, nor what precisely it takes to live in "human symbiotic communities."

any biologically abnormal bodily condition that makes harm more likely entails ill health. This makes health dependent on the state of a body's (actual or typical) environment, whereas it should be dependent only on the state of the body itself.[33] The idea of a *disposition* to produce certain harms, as opposed to a mere *likelihood*, can help solve this problem. Extreme short stature does not *dispose* one to a shorter life expectancy, even if it makes a shorter life expectancy more likely (only) via its effect on income. Disposition, unlike likelihood, must be *intrinsic*.[34] To illustrate, suppose I place a large glass statue of George Washington next to a similarly sized glass statue of Barack Obama in a public park in rural Texas. Unfortunately, Obama's statue is more likely to be broken. However, it is not any more fragile, or disposed to break, than Washington's statue. It is the same size and material; their difference in appearance does not affect intrinsic properties that determine their fragility. Similarly, we propose, a bodily condition—such as short stature—that reduced life expectancy in one social setting but not another would not be unhealthy in one social setting but healthy in the other. It is *biologically, intrinsically*, the same condition (in a bioscientific sense that Hucklenbroich spells out in detail); thus, it cannot be any different with regard to health. Short people who suffer adverse health consequences from discrimination do not have a claim of *health justice* against the harms their bodily condition produces in them; if their society stops discriminating against them, it does not make them healthier.

Defining health in terms of bodily dispositions therefore helps to explain why extrinsic factors, such as those cited by social models of disability, are irrelevant to health. Admittedly, there are problems yet to be solved here. Consider, for instance, sickle cell trait, a hematological condition that is advantageous in malarial environments, neutral in nonmalarial environments, and allegedly disadvantageous at high elevation.[35] Should we say that it is not a disease process in the (malarial) jungle but that it is a disease process in the (nonmalarial) mountains? Pressing as this sort of question may be for the analysis of health, it is less important for the purposes of health justice. Someone with sickle cell trait who lives at a high elevation might be disposed to develop (other) disease processes. He or she will certainly have a claim in health justice to the treatment of those, if they are sufficiently severe.[36]

---

33. This is not to say that health does not have "social determinants" but, rather, that the determinants in question are *causal* rather than *constitutive*: Social conditions affect our health, but only by affecting the state of our body.

34. David Lewis, "Finkish Dispositions," *Philosophical Quarterly* 47, no. 187 (1997): 147.

35. Boorse, "A Rebuttal on Health," 86ff.

36. Moreover, health justice will often generate claims to purely *preventive* medicine: When a nondisease bodily condition threatens to become disease, in the future, given the environment we will likely inhabit and that medical intervention is the best means to prevent this,

Our restriction of health justice to the prevention and treatment of harmful disease processes also has some controversial implications. It would regard a condition that disposed an individual to lose vision after age 65 years as a disease process with some claim to medical treatment. However, no such claim would apparently arise from a genetic microdeletion that resulted solely in congenital blindness, even if fetal gene replacement were available. Most people would surely judge it worse to be born (untreatably) blind than to be disposed to lose sight at age 65 years.[37] One way to accommodate this judgment would be to treat the microdeletion as a disease process leading to a loss of function. However, because the loss is sustained prenatally, we doubt it should count as a health harm because there is no (experienced) loss or disruption. Rather, we believe that if avoiding the congenital loss of sight has priority as a matter of justice over preventing the possible loss of sight at age 65 years, it is not because congenital blindness is a more serious health condition. It is because a life without sight could reasonably be expected to be more difficult overall, if only because our society does not do nearly enough to accommodate blindness.

It appears, then, that a Hucklenbroich-style approach to health has all the right features for developing the sort of "health" standard we need for a health-sufficientarian approach to justice. Unlike purely non-normative accounts, it only finds a health decrement where something bad comes from the state of the body. Unlike more capaciously normative accounts, it defines these "bads" in terms of a general and health-specific harm; one is not made unhealthy by any body-based limitation on the pursuit of any (potentially idiosyncratic) goal. Finally, unlike other harm-based accounts, it can distinguish harms that come from social responses to the body from harms that come from the body itself, thereby distinguishing between harms that generate claims on health care from harms that generate claims against social injustice.

5. Conclusion

Our account of health offers a way of assessing the health burden of disease that does not depend on personal or social factors. We therefore believe that it offers a clear, satisfactory response to the question with which we began about the boundaries of health. John Broome states the concern as follows:

> Pain is bad in itself, and it also reduces your ability to enjoy music. Is the latter an instrumental effect? It depends on whether we regard your ability

---

we may have a claim in health justice to such intervention, despite not now being sick. If sickle cell trait were sufficiently dangerous at high elevations, then whether it is in itself a disease there or not, it might still generate claims of this preventive kind.

37. We thank an anonymous reviewer for challenging us with an example similar to this one.

to enjoy music as a health or non-health factor in your well-being. I am not sure where to draw the boundaries of health.[38]

Although we are not sure how to measure the intensity or severity of pain, its effect on health would not, on our account, depend on the specific activities it affected for an individual or how much he or she valued those activities. In assessing pain, interference with musical appreciation would not count as a health burden.

Questions remain, of course, about how free of Hucklenbroichian "disease processes" we must be to count as "healthy enough" for purposes of justice. Our goal here is not to answer these difficult empirical and political questions but, rather, to provide some reason to think that these are the questions about health we should care about if we care about justice. We reach this conclusion by inference to the best explanation: This sort of account explains our considered judgments about which disadvantages ground claims to health care and which do not. In particular, as we have shown, it explains two important convictions concerning the relevance of disability to justice:

1. That some people disadvantaged due to disability have claims in justice that are primarily or exclusively claims to respect and inclusion rather than claims on health care (although health care claims may be a "second-best" response if respect and inclusion claims are ignored).
2. That when people with disabilities have claims of health justice, this is not because they are disabled per se but, rather, because their disabilities involve medical conditions that are harmful *in themselves*—that is, not harmful only because of the social environment or the disabled individual's particular goals or interests.

As we have argued, extant accounts of health and of health sufficiency fail to capture these convictions. They therefore have us asking the wrong question when we ask how "healthy" someone must be to be healthy enough for justice. This question should not be construed as one about whether the individual has a "normal complement of human capabilities" (per Venkatapuram and Ram-Tiktin) or a "normal complement of typically functioning parts" (per Boorse). Nor should we understand it as a question about whether a person's body is well-suited to help her achieve her goals (per Nordenfelt) or to avoid harm in general (per Wakefield). Rather, it should be understood as a question about our freedom from certain specific sorts of harmful processes: bodily processes that involve, or dispose us to suffer, certain specifically bodily harms.

---

38. John Broome, "Measuring the Burden of Disease," 26, accessed March 3, 2015, http://users.ox.ac.uk/~sfop0060/pdf/measuring%20the%20burden%20of%20disease.pdf.

Therefore, a just world is not a world in which everyone's body is sufficiently close to some statistical norm or in which everyone's body suits each person sufficiently well to pursue his or her valued goals. Rather, it is a world in which bodily differences do not cause too much pain, suffering, disruption, or premature death.

Acknowledgments

We thank the editors, Carina Fourie and Annette Rid, for extensive and extremely helpful comments on several drafts of this chapter. We also thank the participants of the First-Year Fellows Seminar at NIH Bioethics and Luke Gelinas and Holly Kantin for extended discussion of these and related issues. The views presented in this chapter are our own; they do not represent the Department of Bioethics, the National Institutes of Health, or the United States Federal Government.

10

Sufficiency of Capabilities, Social Equality, and Two-Tiered Health Care Systems

Carina Fourie

A TWO-TIERED HEALTH care system can be described as "a system that allows patients to buy access to medical services that others with the same needs cannot obtain."[1] Whether or not tiered care is morally acceptable, or which kinds of tiered care may be acceptable, has caused debate for many decades.[2] Critics could claim, for example, that medical services are special social goods, access to which should be distributed equally, unlike goods such as income. On the other hand, defenders could claim, for example, that individuals should be as free to buy medical services as they are to buy smartphones or cars, even if others are not able to afford them or choose not to spend money on them.

There are two theories in political philosophy—a sufficiency of capabilities approach and social-relational egalitarianism (for short, social egalitarianism)—that have not yet been applied to the ethics of tiered health care systems but that could contribute to helping to assess them. At a quick glance, it seems that sufficientarians would argue that if we take care of everyone's medical needs up to an adequate threshold (the sufficiency threshold), then it may be acceptable to allow individuals to buy further medical services if they so choose. On the other hand,

---

1. Benjamin J. Krohmal and Ezekiel J. Emanuel, "Access and Ability to Pay: The Ethics of a Tiered Health Care System," *Archives of Internal Medicine* 167, no. 5 (2007): 433.

2. For a summary of a number of the arguments for and against tiered care, see Krohmal and Emanuel, "Access and Ability to Pay."

social egalitarians could be seen to object to two-tiered systems because of the status hierarchies that they instantiate or reinforce.

In this chapter, I investigate how these two theories assess the ethics of two-tiered health care systems. I argue that a plausible specification of a particular kind of sufficientarian approach, a sufficiency of capabilities approach (CA), can help us to reconcile sufficientarianism with a social egalitarian critique of two-tiered systems. Using this approach as a basis for health care justice will allow for only limited and specific kinds of two-tiered systems.

The structure of the chapter is as follows. In the first section, I provide more detail about two-tiered health care systems. In the second section, I provide a sketch of a sufficiency of CA, which I will apply, in the third section, to tiered health care. In the fourth section, I formulate the social egalitarian objection, and in the last section, I indicate how a sufficiency of CA can respond to this objection.

The upshot of the chapter is both practical and theoretical. In addition to considering what practical application this analysis has for the ethics of two-tiered health care systems, on a theoretical level, I show how two-tiered care provides us with an illustrative example for pointing to significant ways in which we need to specify a sufficientarian CA in order to make it more plausible in application to health care justice. Two-tiered care also provides a catalyst for explaining how best we can reconcile what may appear to be two conflicting theories, egalitarianism and sufficientarianism.[3] Particularly, highlighting the (potential for the) different kinds of pluralism of Martha Nussbaum's CA—a theory with a sufficientarian commitment but a lack of detail about that commitment—will help show how these approaches can be reconciled.

1. Two-Tiered Health Care

Let's elaborate on the description of two-tiered care with which we started. We can distinguish a "first tier" of this system that usually relies on a statutory public health care insurance or delivery system, providing guaranteed access to what is often referred to as essential or basic medical care where needed. Individuals are said to belong to a second tier when they choose to contribute to voluntary insurance schemes. There are two primary kinds of voluntary insurance—gap and parallel insurance.

---

3. Although sufficientarianism is often considered incompatible with distributive egalitarianism, social egalitarianism has been used as a basis for defending sufficientarian principles. See, for example, Elizabeth Anderson, "What Is the Point of Equality?" *Ethics* 109, no. 2 (1999): 287–337. Much more work needs to be done to elaborate on the relationship between sufficientarianism and social-relational egalitarianism. This chapter helps to start filling in the gap in the literature.

Gap insurance covers " 'services excluded or not fully covered' by the statutory system."[4] Parallel insurance includes supplementary insurance and substitutive insurance. Supplementary insurance occurs when individuals opt in to paying for additional coverage on a separate voluntary track, but they must also continue to pay fees to support the coverage offered as part of the first tier. In contrast, substitutive insurance is said to hold when individuals receive care on a separate insurance track and opt out of or are excluded from paying for statutory insurance[5]—in this case, being part of the second tier excludes one from the first. It is not always clear in the literature which of these kinds of insurance should be included as part of two-tiered care, and indeed there seem to be many different ways of understanding two-tiered care. I prefer using a relatively broad description, which would include two-tiered systems with gap insurance or parallel insurance or both. We can then consider whether the type of insurance makes a moral difference.

In reality, it would be difficult to find a country that did not fall into the two-tiered system classification if we use this broad description, but the details can differ considerably (even Canada, which is often described as not having a two-tier system, indeed has one under this description).[6] For example, in some countries, the first tier is seriously underfunded or not universally accessible, such as in the United States. In contrast, in countries such as Sweden, the first tier is universal, mandatory, and extensive; few individuals have voluntary health insurance and thus few belong to a second tier of care.[7]

Although the ethics of two-tiered systems have been debated for many decades within public and political discourse, it remains a topical aspect of health justice as debate and controversy are ongoing. For example, as part of the arduous

---

4. Joseph White, "Gap and Parallel Insurance in Health Care Systems with Mandatory Contributions to a Single Funding Pool for Core Medical and Hospital Benefits for All Citizens in Any Given Geographic Area," *Journal of Health Politics, Policy and Law* 34, no. 4 (2009): 543–583, at 547.

5. Joseph White, "Gap and Parallel Insurance in Health Care Systems," 456–457.

6. What we can say is that Canada does not have a *parallel* two-tiered system but has a gap coverage two-tiered system. Goran Ridic, Suzanne Gleason, and Ognjen Ridic, "Comparisons of Health Care Systems in the United States, Germany and Canada," *Materia Socio-Medica* 24, no. 2 (2012): 112–120, at 113.

7. For the United States, consider Ezekiel Emanuel, *Reinventing American Health Care: How the Affordable Care Act Will Improve Our Terribly Complex, Blatantly Unjust, Outrageously Expensive, Grossly Inefficient, Error Prone System* (New York: Public Affairs, 2014). For Sweden, see Anders Anell, Anna H Glenngård, and Sherry Merkur, *Sweden: Health System Review 2012*, Health Systems in Transition, vol. 14, no. 5 (Brussels, Belgium: European Observatory on Health Systems and Policies, 2012), http://www.euro.who.int/en/about-us/partners/observatory/publications/health-system-reviews-hits/countries-and-subregions/sweden-hit-2012.

process of attempting to reform its health care system, questions have been asked as to whether it is fair for the United States to continue with its tiered system;[8] in Canada, there are ongoing arguments and legal conflict over attempts at increased privatization that would encourage a two-tiered system with parallel substitutive insurance.[9]

On a theoretical level, we also require an update—the potential of certain kinds of political philosophical theories to contribute to the debate still need to be explored. As mentioned previously, at least at first glance, a sufficiency view may seem to support two-tiered systems, whereas social egalitarianism would seem to object to them. My starting point for why I believe that these two theories should be assessed in application to tiered care is that something like sufficientarianism and like social egalitarianism are already reflected in the public and political discourse on tiered health care, but they need to be explored in greater theoretical detail.

It seems like a fairly well-trodden idea, corresponding to sufficientarianism, that there should be universal access to social goods up to a certain level but that it is less urgent for these goods to be provided once individuals have enough care to achieve an adequate level of health. In line with social egalitarianism, it is similarly a rather well-rehearsed idea that such systems cause divisions in society by reinforcing class structures. Indeed, the label "two-tier" seems to imply precisely what the social egalitarian is concerned about, and the term itself already seems to be ethically loaded (I use it, however, because it is a well-known term in public discourse, and it is often even used by its advocates). It remains to be seen, however, whether sufficientarianism does indeed support two-tiered care and whether social egalitarianism does indeed provide a critique once we delve into the details of particular theories. I now turn to examining a particular sufficientarian theory to understand what it might have to say about tiered systems.

2. Sufficiency of Capabilities

A good starting point is to examine a sufficiency of capabilities approach. A number of CAs, partially based on or at least motivated by aspects of Martha Nussbaum's CA, have been developed to apply to health justice.[10] For the purposes

---

8. Benjamin J. Krohmal and Ezekiel J. Emanuel, "Tiers Without Tears: The Ethics of a Two-Tiered Health Care System," in *The Oxford Handbook of Bioethics*, ed. Bonnie Steinbock (Oxford: Oxford University Press, 2009).

9. Lauren Vogel, "Medicare on Trial," *Canadian Medical Association Journal* 186, no. 12 (2014): 901.

10. See, for example, Madison Powers and Ruth Faden, *Social Justice: The Moral Foundations of Public Health and Health Policy* (New York: Oxford University Press, 2006); Jennifer Prah

of this chapter, I examine how the sufficientarianism of Nussbaum's CA can be specified in brief and, in the next section, applied to health care justice and two-tiered health care systems rather than focusing on one of these specific theories of health justice. I think it is important to start with Nussbaum because there is very little direct discussion of the sufficientarianism of her view or of how it relates to social egalitarianism, so it would be significant to articulate this. Once we have established these aspects of Nussbaum's theory, we can then consider, in a step beyond the scope of this chapter, how the CAs that focus on health justice would compare.

Let me provide a few comments on CAs as an introduction. If our aim is to design just social institutions, such as health care systems, then one of the ways of determining whether these are indeed just is to focus on their implications for the distribution of a morally relevant "currency" of justice. This is often said to imply the following two central questions: What is the pattern of distribution for which we are aiming—for example, equality or sufficiency? What is the currency of that pattern—for example, resources, opportunities for welfare, or capabilities? According to CAs, the currency of justice should be capabilities for functionings.[11] Functionings refer to what people are or what they do (their "beings and doings")—these could be as specific as swimming or walking or the more general functionings of being mobile or being healthy.[12] Capabilities can be understood as the real opportunities an individual has to achieve functionings.[13]

Certain functionings can be seen to be particularly central to a human life. Nussbaum identifies 10 of these: life; bodily health; bodily integrity; senses, imagination, and thought; emotions; practical reason; affiliation; relationships with other species; play; and control over one's environment.[14] For Nussbaum's

---

Ruger, *Health and Social Justice* (New York: Oxford University Press, 2009); Efrat Ram-Tiktin, "A Decent Minimum for Everyone as a Sufficiency of Basic Human Functional Capabilities," *American Journal of Bioethics* 11, no. 7 (2011): 24–25; Efrat Ram-Tiktin, "The Right to Health Care as a Right to Basic Human Functional Capabilities," *Ethical Theory and Moral Practice* 15, no. 3 (2012): 337–351; Sridhar Venkatapuram, *Health Justice: An Argument from the Capabilities Approach* (Cambridge, UK: Polity, 2011). Powers and Faden's account is probably not strictly a CA because it focuses on well-being rather than capabilities, but it is similar enough to be included as part of a loose category of CA.

11. For example, see Amartya Sen, *Development as Freedom* (Oxford: Oxford University Press, 1999); Amartya Sen, *Inequality Reexamined* (Oxford: Oxford University Press, 1995); Martha Nussbaum, *Women and Human Development: The Capabilities Approach* (New York: Cambridge University Press, 2000); Martha Nussbaum, *Frontiers of Justice: Disability, Nationality, Species Membership* (Cambridge, MA: Harvard University Press, 2007).

12. Sen, *Inequality Reexamined*, 39.

13. Sen, *Inequality Reexamined*, 40.

14. Nussbaum, *Women and Human Development*, 78–80.

CA, these are central because they are required in order to live a truly human life, which means a life of human dignity. A minimum requirement for justice, according to Nussbaum, is for each person to have the capabilities to achieve a threshold level of each of the central functionings (sometimes I shorten this to "sufficiency in the central capabilities").[15] The state aims at helping people achieve the capabilities—in other words, the opportunities for functionings and not the functionings themselves—in order to uphold the capability of practical reason and to satisfy a political notion of justice.[16]

Although much of what I have described is furiously debated—for example, whether capabilities should really be the currency of justice, or whether these are indeed the central capabilities, and so on—I take it for granted in this chapter that these claims can be justified or revised to make them more plausible in order to make progress with the sufficientarian and health-related aspects.[17]

We can identify the Nussbaumian approach as sufficientarian. As I understand it, to be sufficientarian one must be committed, at least, to the idea that it is a priority for individuals to reach a certain morally significant threshold (or thresholds) and that this threshold(s) should be understood as having non-instrumental moral value. It is non-instrumental in the sense that it is not (merely) the means to achieving another distributive pattern but, rather, should be seen to be an end in itself. This means it has, at least, final or ultimate value.[18] Sufficiency of capabilities, then, cannot simply be the means to another distributive pattern that in itself has final value; it is not the claim that achieving sufficiency of capabilities is good because it helps us to achieve, for example, equality of capabilities.

---

15. Nussbaum tends to refer to threshold levels of *capabilities*, whereas I have referred to capabilities for threshold levels of functionings. I am inclined to think that what should ultimately matter is that people are able to achieve the central functionings and thus it is threshold levels of these, rather than threshold levels of capabilities, that are at play. However, a full consideration of this is not possible here.

16. Nussbaum, *Women and Human Development*, 86–96; Nussbaum, *Frontiers of Justice*, 79–80.

17. An example of an influential critic of the CA (and sufficiency views) is Richard Arneson. For example, see "Distributive Justice and Basic Capability Equality," in *Capabilities Equality: Basic Issues and Problems*, ed. Alexander Kaufman (New York: Routledge, 2006), 17–43.

18. The form that morally significant value takes is much debated—for example, whether or not what is of genuinely final value must also have intrinsic value—and I refer to this debate here only cursorily. See, for example, Christine M. Korsgaard, "Two Distinctions in Goodness," *Philosophical Review* 92, no. 2 (1983): 169–195. For the purposes of this chapter, what is important is only that the way in which sufficientarians value sufficiency could correspond to the way in which egalitarians value equality—whatever this precise value may be. Taking my cue from Korsgaard, I use the term "final value" to describe how sufficientarians value sufficiency, but I make no claims about its relationship to *intrinsic* value.

However, Nussbaum says very little about the sufficientarian aspect of her approach and does not engage with the growing body of literature on sufficientarianism. Her theory requires further specification of the sufficientarian elements. An element that seems necessary to specify here—if we are also going to consider two-tiered systems in the light of an egalitarian critique—is its potential relationship with equality. In trying to understand this relationship, I provide some basic details of Nussbaum's sufficientarianism, particularly highlighting the different kinds of pluralism to which the theory could be committed. As discussed later, particularly in the last section, highlighting the different kinds of pluralism of the theory also provides more specific answers as to how the CA is able to respond to the social egalitarian objection.

Sufficientarian theories are often said to have a positive and a negative thesis—I refer to these rather as a positive and a positioning claim.[19] We can call the commitment to sufficientarian thresholds of capabilities as a final value part of the positive thesis of Nussbaum's sufficientarianism. The positive claim is that justice demands that it is a priority for individuals to achieve sufficiency in each of the 10 central capabilities. That sufficiency in each of the 10 central capabilities has independent value can be called a kind of pluralism. It is a pluralism related to the currency of justice, or what I refer to as dimension pluralism—that is, pluralism in the dimensions of well-being that the theory identifies.[20] Compare Nussbaum's dimension pluralist view to a sufficientarian view that insisted that we should "add up" the various capabilities to give us an overall capability and it is sufficiency in this overall capability for which we should be aiming.

The positioning claim of sufficientarianism can be seen to specify the relationship of sufficientarianism to other distributive patterns or other moral goals. Some sufficientarian theories could claim to be sufficientarian alone—this means that only sufficientarian thresholds are of moral value. Many versions of sufficiency are not this extreme and can rather be called pluralist in a different sense to dimension pluralism. According to this form of pluralism, although a sufficientarian threshold is of final value, there are other goals that are also of final value. I refer to this kind of pluralism as value pluralism in order to distinguish it from dimension pluralism. Value pluralism can be further broken down into what I call pattern and external pluralism.

Pattern pluralism recognizes that even other patterns of distribution could have final value, and thus we should not only care about achieving sufficiency but

---

19. For more detail, see Chapter 1 of this volume (Fourie, "The Sufficiency View: A Primer").

20. Consider also Axelsen and Nielsen's discussion of the aspect-pluralism of a sufficientarian approach in this volume (Chapter 6).

also we could care, for example, about achieving the best position for the worst-off below or above the threshold. According to external pluralism, moral goals outside of those represented by distributive patterns could be valuable. For example, a theory could claim that there are two final values: procedural justice, which is not a commitment to a specific distributive pattern, as well as sufficiency of capabilities, which is a distributive pattern. Such a theory might claim, for example, that we should care about what happens above a sufficientarian threshold, but not because *patterns* above the threshold have real moral significance; rather, inequalities above the threshold are morally problematic if and only if they are caused by violations of procedural justice.

The two forms of value pluralism I have identified are not exclusive—one can be both a pattern and an external pluralist (furthermore, value pluralism can also, but need not, be combined with dimension pluralism). Being a value pluralist does not mean that you accept that equality has final value, but you need to be a value pluralist in order to claim that both sufficiency and equality do have such value.

Some defenses of sufficientarianism root at least part of the appeal of their accounts in anti-egalitarianism.[21] Nussbaum's sufficientarianism, however, is not justified by anti-egalitarianism. There are a number of reasons why I make this claim. First, and directly, she does not indicate that we should support sufficientarianism because of problems with egalitarianism. Furthermore, she claims that sufficiency of capabilities is only a partial theory of justice, and that justice probably requires more than merely these threshold levels.[22] In addition, she indicates that various forms of egalitarianism could be morally significant and compatible with her CA.[23]

Although she does not provide detail on these claims, it seems that it would be consistent with her theory to identify it as value pluralist, possibly both external and pattern pluralist, and to maintain that it has the potential to recognize the non-instrumental value of equality. This merely indicates a certain *structure* to the CA without giving it specific content; much more needs to be specified and developed in terms of the CA's sufficientarianism (which is beyond the scope of this chapter). However, merely highlighting that the CA is dimension pluralist and that it has the potential to be value pluralist is helpful in that either or both of these forms of pluralism could help to accommodate egalitarianism, at least in certain forms. This is examined further in Section 5. First, let us consider whether this version of sufficiency of CA can indeed be used to defend two-tiered care.

---

21. See, for example, Harry Frankfurt, "Equality as a Moral Ideal," *Ethics* 98, no. 1 (1987): 21–43.

22. Nussbaum, *Women and Human Development*, 211–212; Nussbaum, *Frontiers of Justice*, 71.

23. See, for example, Nussbaum, *Women and Human Development*, 86.

3. Sufficiency of Capabilities Applied to Two-Tiered Health Care Systems

I understand "health justice" here as one part of overall social justice, and which is particularly concerned with the functionings and the social goods associated with health, often overlapping with the kinds of concerns and policies that are dealt with by government departments of health, and clinical medicine. Considering the CA, we could say that here the functioning that Nussbaum refers to as "bodily health" would be of particular concern. If justice requires the capability for a threshold level of each of the central functionings, (part of) what health justice requires is that individuals have the capability for achieving threshold levels of bodily health. I will use a stopgap description of this capability based on an ordinary language notion of health with some help from Madison Powers and Ruth Faden.[24] This capability would include the physical and mental health associated with a common-sense understanding of the biological functioning of the body, and in its absence one would find disease, pain, malnutrition, or a combination of these. For the purposes of this chapter, this understanding of the capability of "bodily health" should serve. For a full theory of the CA and how it applies to health, we would need to wade into the complex debate about the definitions of health, disease, and biological functioning, but I set that aside for now.[25]

The public provision of medical care (including primary medical care and hospital care), a central example of what health care systems deliver, could be justified on the basis that it helps to contribute to sufficiency in the capability of bodily health. However, considering the dimension pluralism of Nussbaum's approach, we cannot assess the distribution of the goods associated with medical care from the perspective of the capability of health alone. If medical interventions can be used to help establish thresholds in other central functionings besides health, or the way in which they are distributed would interfere with other central capabilities, we would need to take this into account. Consider nontherapeutic contraception and abortion, for example: Even if these interventions are not required for a woman's health per se, they can be justified as requirements for achieving sufficiency in a number of other capabilities (control over one's environment and bodily integrity seem, at least intuitively, to be relevant here). Medical care institutions and the provision of basic medical care should be understood according to their contribution to any one of the central capabilities, where it is indeed clear that they do

---

24. Powers and Faden, *Social Justice*, 16–17.

25. For an analysis of an appropriate sufficientarian understanding of health, consider Aas and Wasserman's chapter in this volume (Chapter 9).

have an influence on these capabilities, and not merely on health (indeed, there need be no relationship between medical care and health to justify the need for medical care as long as it contributes to other capabilities). It is for this reason that it is important not to limit concerns of health justice merely to the capability of bodily health because we might then erroneously believe that certain "health" care benefits or services are unnecessary because they do not contribute to sufficiency in this particular capability of health. This point about the importance of other capabilities will become especially important when we consider responses to the social egalitarian objection.

From here, we can consider one particular aspect of health justice—the ethics of two-tiered health care systems—in relation to the CA. In practice, a line is often drawn between the benefits of basic care and the benefits of additional care. Universal access to basic care is part of what one could call the first tier of a health care system, whereas additional care, provided via a second tier, includes treatments that are only provided to individuals when they opt in to additional insurance.[26] Dental care and prescription drugs are examples of treatments that are often not included in the first tier of many health care systems.[27] The difference between a second and a first tier, however, may not necessarily be in terms of the *benefits* themselves but, rather, in how they are delivered or how much choice is involved in their delivery. For example, the same benefit, such as a hip replacement operation, may be provided as part of basic care, but it could be delivered more quickly or with a choice of which specialist will perform the surgery when individuals pay for supplementary insurance; thus, this kind of service would fall under what is offered as part of a second tier.[28] To take account of this difference, I refer in what follows to "benefits," on the one hand, and "services," on the other hand, where "services" has to do with the way in which benefits might be delivered or how much choice one has regarding how they are delivered.

I cannot provide a comprehensive picture of what the CA would say about all the different aspects of two-tiered systems, but I point out four significant features. First, this approach can provide a *normative* justification for the overall structure of two-tiered systems. The CA would claim that it is morally necessary, and morally

26. For an in-depth discussion of basic care packages, see Panteli and van Ginnekin's chapter in this volume (Chapter 13).

27. For example, in Canada: Ridic, Gleason, and Ridic, "Comparisons of Health Care Systems in the United States, Germany and Canada," 113.

28. For example, in the United Kingdom: Thomas Foubister et al., *Private Medical Insurance in the United Kingdom* (Geneva: World Health Organization Regional Office for Europe, and European Observatory on Health Systems and Policies, 2006), http://apps.who.int//iris/handle/10665/107741, e.g., xi.

most urgent, for individuals to achieve sufficiency in the central capabilities. Everyone in a society should have access to the medical care they require so that they are able to achieve a threshold level of the capabilities, or to maintain a threshold level, as much as this is socially possible. Which benefits and which services should be included as part of basic medical care should be judged according to their potential role for contributing to the sufficiency of the central capabilities for those in need. As a matter of justice, these medical care benefits and services should be funded, at least partially, via a public health care insurance or delivery system. If they are not, individuals will be at high risk of falling below sufficiency thresholds considering the potential of exposure to the extremely high costs of medical care.

However, the CA would distinguish between benefits and services that are a priority to provide individuals and those that are not (as much of) a priority because they would only improve the capabilities above a threshold. This moral distinction could provide a justifiable line for claiming that benefits and services above the threshold do not need to be provided publicly or are less of a priority to provide. Using this distinction as a basis, the CA could stipulate that individuals could be allowed to buy voluntary health insurance as part of a second tier as a concession to acknowledging that gains in capabilities above the threshold are also of value but are not as morally urgent for society to provide. In this way, the general outlines of a two-tiered system seem to be justifiable.

Second, the first tier of the system as understood by the CA would be quite comprehensive in terms of which benefits should be provided normatively. It is difficult to think of kinds of treatments that would not under some circumstances help to provide sufficiency in capabilities. More analysis is needed here, but it seems to make sense to claim that according to the CA, excluding entire types of services—for example, dental care and prescription drugs—is impermissible because the grounds to exclude them on the basis of this theory could only be that they cannot contribute to sufficiency of capabilities, and this does not seem plausible. This may imply that although a second tier of such a system is justifiable, it will be quite limited in terms of the actual benefits that should be covered exclusively in such a tier.

In contrast, there are probably a wide range of different ways in which benefits could be delivered—for the sake of convenience and efficiency, for example—that would not be related to sufficiency, and thus there may be much more scope for services to differ between tiers. As emphasized previously, both benefits and services can influence sufficiency, and what must be included in the first tier in terms of benefits and their delivery must be judged according to this influence. Thus, where services do influence sufficiency—for example, if the choice of the surgeon or hospital makes a substantial difference to whether an operation is likely to succeed—then the relevant service should be part of the basic package. However, there could be a number of services that will not make a substantial difference to health, such as receiving comfort, privacy, and quality of food similar to those offered by a five-star hotel (in Section 5, we consider whether this can be said to make a difference to sufficiency in capabilities other than health).

Third, under real-life practical conditions, it is likely that certain specific treatments that would be judged to be a necessary part of basic care according to their contribution to sufficiency of capabilities would not in reality be included in basic care under the first tier because of their costs. In an ideal world, all benefits that could contribute to sufficiency should be so covered as part of the first tier, but I do not believe that this could be practically implemented, especially because the CA would demand such comprehensive basic care. This concern with costs is not merely a practical consideration. The CA would demand that resources are distributed in such a way that over time, sufficiency of capabilities will be sustained. Thus, if benefits contribute to sufficiency but providing these benefits as part of the first tier would threaten the whole system, then they could be justifiably excluded.

It seems that the benefits that would need to be excluded, but that should have been included ideally, must have some sort of special moral status in the second tier. What I mean by this is that there is a further moral distinction to be drawn between benefits besides those that contribute to sufficiency and those that do not. We can also distinguish then between those benefits that could contribute to sufficiency of capabilities but that are excluded from the first tier because of costs and those benefits that do not contribute to sufficiency at all. There is greater moral urgency for the former to be provided than the latter.

How exactly this would be cashed out practically is not entirely clear, and under certain circumstances, especially depending on exactly how expensive these treatments may be, we may not be able to make anything practical out of this moral distinction. However, there are a couple of ways in which we could understand the potential implications. First, it seems that under these circumstances, a second tier that functions as a gap insurance system (in which individuals can opt in to receiving benefits that are not covered by the first tier) is not merely permissible but may well be obligatory because it seems essential for individuals to have some sort of access to these benefits as they contribute to sufficiency (if it is feasible for insurers to cover these expensive treatments even on a second tier). Second, it seems that trying to make these interventions less expensive—for example, via research and development and patenting regulations—would be a priority.

The fourth and last point I make is that under specific empirical, non-ideal conditions, the CA would rule out certain kinds of two-tiered systems entirely. Concerns have been raised that the second tier can undermine the first tier of basic care.[29] As an example of how this might occur, we can compare gap insurance with parallel substitutive insurance. Gap systems allow individuals to "top-up" health care, but everyone is still obliged to pay into the system of basic care. In contrast, a parallel substitutive system will exclude the individuals who opt in to private insurance from funding the first tier or allow them to opt out of it, and this could threaten the funding for the first tier. The CA would rule out any cases in which the first tier is undermined by the second tier because the sufficiency of those who are only part of the first tier would be threatened.

To conclude this section, we could state that the CA provides a limited justification for certain kinds of two-tiered systems. It would also insist on quite comprehensive basic care benefits and would (morally) prioritize benefits in the second tier according to whether or not they contribute to sufficiency. It may allow for a range of services to be offered on the second tier, as long as these services are not requirements for achieving sufficiency. It may also promote a gap system particularly where benefits that should be covered cannot be covered on the first tier due to costs but would rule out systems in which the first tier is undermined by the second tier.

4. Two-Tiered Health Care and Morally Significant Inequalities: An Objection from Social Egalitarianism

I examine one particularly significant objection to two-tiered health care systems, which is that they violate social equality. What is particularly interesting about this objection, as I have mentioned, is that something like it is often raised in the public and political discourse. Two-tiered systems—of health care or wages, for example—are often disparaged for creating or reinforcing a class system, and they are said to create or reinforce "second-class" citizenship. As of yet, little or no direct reference has been made to the burgeoning recent theory on social equality that arguably could be said to provide a basis for this kind of claim.[30]

Although social equality has been characterized in different ways, I take it to indicate, in part, that the ways in which major social institutions are set up and the way in which social goods, such as medical care benefits, are distributed should

---

29. See Krohmal and Emanuel, "Tiers Without Tears."

30. Philosophers and bioethicists have only very recently started exploring the potential of social-relational egalitarianism for health and health care policy. See J. Paul Kelleher, "Health Inequalities and Relational Egalitarianism" (n.d.); Kristin Voigt and Gry Wester, "Relational Equality and Health," *Social Philosophy and Policy* 31, no. 2 (2015): 204–229.

not create or reinforce (even unintentionally) certain kinds of unequal relationships, especially relationships that imply that some people have lower social status than others. The concern then with two-tiered systems would be that they create these unequal relationships.

A preliminary attempt to claim that two-tiered systems do create such problematic differences in status might focus on the links between social status and health. Research on the social determinants of health indicates that inferior social status has a negative impact on health; at the least, one's relative position in many kinds of social hierarchies is correlated to health.[31] Consequently, it may be tempting to claim that two-tiered systems imply that those who can only afford to be part of the first tier suffer inferior status, which in turn could negatively affect their health. However, the CA could respond that if two-tiered care were set up according to the demands of the CA, it seems much less likely that it would lead to any serious health discrepancies between those on the first and those on the second tier because it requires such comprehensive care. Also, even if the health of those on the first tier were negatively impacted due to their inferior social status, the CA would claim that as long as this did not threaten sufficiency of health, then it is not an urgent moral problem. In this case, even if the CA conceded the point, it could claim that the concerns about equality here are only instrumental—the inequality of status is only a problem if it leads to insufficiency. I think as a criticism of the CA's understanding of two-tiered care, we need to develop our objection beyond this preliminary attempt.

So let us add a little more detail to our notion of social equality, especially in terms of trying to understand where the moral problem with tiered care may lie. Social equality tends to be focused foremost on what it means for people to *be* social equals. I take it that in order for people to be social equals, they should, first, be *treated* as equals, and, second, *feel* that they are equals (and they should feel this reasonably so, meaning we can rule out, for example, feelings of inferiority that stem primarily from personality traits and that do not stem from a social hierarchy).[32] Constitutive of treating people as equals would be treating them with respect-for-persons. Part of fulfilling the demands of respect-for-persons would be upholding individuals' claims to both procedural and distributive justice. In

---

31. See, for example, Michael Marmot, *The Status Syndrome: How Social Standing Affects Our Health and Longevity* (New York: Holt, 2005).

32. T. M. Scanlon, "The Diversity of Objections to Inequality," in *The Ideal of Equality*, ed. Matthew Clayton and Andrew Williams (Basingstoke, UK: Palgrave Macmillan, 2002), 41–59. These are developments of previous claims I have made, for example, in Carina Fourie, "What Is Social Equality? An Analysis of Status Equality as a Strongly Egalitarian Ideal," *Res Publica* 18, no. 2 (2012): 107–126.

terms of the second aspect, people might reasonably feel as if they are not equals, for example, even without them necessarily being treated as inferior. For example, if someone frequently found herself at the bottom end of social hierarchies even where there was no violation of respect-for-persons, she could be made to feel inferior.[33]

The following are the direct moral wrongs that we can refer to in relation to social equality:

1. In the case of people not being treated as equals, respect-for-persons is violated.
2. In terms of violations of both conditions—that is, when people are not treated as equals as well as when they do not feel that they are equals—a sense of self-worth can be damaged.
3. Also in terms of violations of both conditions, civic friendship (or what is often called fraternity) is violated; another way to put this is that social cohesion and social trust are damaged.[34]

Social egalitarians tend to understand social equality as having final value—that is, it is not purely of derivative value. Thus, the claim is not that treating people as equals is instrumental to achieving respect-for-persons, for example, or even vice versa. Rather, part of what constitutes treating people as equals is achieving respect-for-persons.

Let us apply this description of social equality to the CA's understanding of the permissibility of two-tiered care. I think that for most of what we have discussed about two-tiered health care systems under the version of the CA proposed previously, it would not make sense to claim that people are actually being *treated* as inferior; thus, there is no violation of respect-for-persons. That someone is receiving fewer services and benefits does not seem to imply that she is being treated as inferior. Furthermore, under ideal conditions, considering only the benefits of basic care and the fact that they would be quite comprehensive, it also seems unlikely that people could be said to be made to feel inferior or that the social bonds between people will be damaged by a two-tiered system that, in the end, allows for very few benefits to be excluded.

---

33. Carina Fourie, "To Praise and to Scorn: The Problem of Inequalities of Esteem for Social Egalitarians," in *Social Equality: On What It Means to Be Equals*, ed. Carina Fourie, Fabian Schuppert, and Ivo Wallimann-Helmer (New York: Oxford University Press, 2015), 87–106.

34. See Andrew Mason, "Justice, Respect, and Treating People as Equals," in *Social Equality: On What It Means to Be Equals*, ed. Carina Fourie, Fabian Schuppert, and Ivo Wallimann-Helmer (New York: Oxford University Press, 2015), 129–145; Scanlon, "The Diversity of Objections to Inequality."

However, I think the objection from social equality would hold, first, if there were very many *services* that were available to people on the second tier and not on the first tier. The CA would appear to find permissible an extensive range of services on the second tier. These might make care much more efficient or comfortable, as well as provide a greater choice in terms of how benefits are delivered. A major difference between what was offered on the first tier and what was offered as part of the second tier would seem to contribute to a large division between social groups that threatens civic friendship. This would be exacerbated if, due to costs, there were also a large range of *benefits* that were only available on the second tier. This would be even further exacerbated if society generally, thus looking beyond health care, were highly hierarchical, and the same people or groups of people were frequently at the bottom of a variety of social hierarchies. Although the main threat that I am describing here seems to be to civic friendship, the more extensive the divisions, the more plausible it may be for an egalitarian to claim that these systems might make those receiving coverage only via the first tier feel inferior, damaging their self-worth.

Skeptics may deny that these kinds of instances that I have described can indeed be said to make people feel inferior or interfere with civic friendship, but it seems to me that the stronger the divide between those on the first tier and those on the second tier, the more convincing these claims become. Furthermore, denying that these are examples of social inequality may seem to be conceding the social egalitarian's overall point—that is, that where these kinds of social inequalities are prevalent, they are problematic, and it is a question of interpretation or further analysis as to whether particular cases do actually constitute morally problematic inequalities.

Second, parallel substitutive insurance systems would most likely be ruled out by social equality, and not merely for the reasons the CA might rule them out. As discussed previously, the CA would worry about these systems if they threatened the sufficiency of capabilities of those receiving coverage only via the first tier. For social egalitarians, these systems would be problematic even if they did not threaten sufficiency, however; substitutive systems seem strongly to threaten morally significant forms of equality because individuals in society are no longer "in the same boat" so to speak—those with more money live in a separate world of social goods and privilege. This particularly would seem to break the bonds between community members and threaten civic friendship.

Although the CA provides only a limited defense of certain forms of two-tiered care and this blunts a social egalitarian critique somewhat, overall social equality still seems to have some plausible objections. We would still need to be concerned about the kinds of two-tiered system the CA finds permissible. The problem for the CA, then, is that it does not seem to have the theoretical resources to respond to these social inequalities and would not be able to recognize that there are moral problems with systems that it can justify—at least that is how it seems according to the discussion thus far.

5. The CA's Potential Responses to the Social Egalitarian Objection

I think there are at least three possible responses that the proposed version of the CA can make to these objections: the independent value response, the foundational social egalitarian response, and the internal response. I briefly outline them here; they will require further elaboration, however.[35] The first two responses are related mainly to how we understand the pattern of justice of the capabilities approach (i.e., its sufficientarianism), and the third response primarily has to do with its dimensional pluralism (that we are aiming for sufficiency in all 10 central capabilities).

A first attempt at forging a response from the capabilities approach's external pluralism (the claim that we can endorse sufficiency of capabilities as well as other values that do not constitute distributive patterns) could be the following: According to the CA, one could value social equality as a final end and value sufficiency of capabilities in the same way. If these were considered to be two independent ends, then we would need to evaluate public policy from the perspective of its influence on sufficiency in the central capabilities as well as from a socially egalitarian perspective. In terms of judging the moral permissibility of two-tiered systems, we would then need to weigh social equality against achieving sufficiency of capabilities. We could call this first response *the independent value response*.

In contrast, it is possible to understand the relationship between sufficiency and equality as interdependent rather than as independent, and this leads us to a second response: *the foundational social egalitarian response*. Consider, for example, Elizabeth Anderson's claim that a sufficiency of capabilities approach is what follows from an egalitarian starting point.[36] Sufficiency of capabilities is in this sense an interpretation and requirement of what it means for people to be equals. Let's try to understand how this might work for my proposed version of the CA. We can say that the social and political ideal of social equality flows from the idea that

---

35. Two-tiered care is only one example of how the CA could run afoul of social egalitarianism. I think that social egalitarianism also has potential, for example, to be concerned about how a sufficientarian approach would assess other aspects of health justice, such as the social gradients in health, and thus it would be particularly significant to explore the response the CA can make in more detail.

36. Anderson, "What Is the Point of Equality?"; Elizabeth Anderson, "Justifying the Capabilities Approach to Justice," in *Measuring Justice Primary Goods and Capabilities,* ed. Harry Brighouse and Ingrid Robeyns (New York: Cambridge University Press, 2010).

everyone has equal moral worth, or what Nussbaum refers to as everyone having dignity. As we have seen, social equality is fulfilled when individuals are treated as equals and they feel that they are equals. As part of the requirement of treating people as equals, we need to provide them with respect-for-persons. This will include adhering to their claims of distributive justice, and can be fulfilled, at least partially, by achieving sufficiency of capabilities. Thus, in this sense, rather than social equality and sufficiency of capabilities being two independent final values, sufficiency of capabilities is constitutive of justice and, in turn, of social equality.[37]

This second response is incomplete, however. The point of the previous discussion was to highlight that the CA does not seem to be able to register the problems with two-tiered care that social egalitarianism identifies. The CA cannot state in its defense that because the claims to sufficiency of capabilities are founded on social equality, it is immune to those egalitarian criticisms, if on an applied level, we are still left with the problem that a sufficiency of CA does not show us, at least as we have seen thus far, that two-tiered care may well be impermissible under certain circumstances and in certain forms. If we did want to go down the route of viewing a sufficiency of CA as partially constitutive of social equality, we would need to find a way to add something to the theory to accommodate social egalitarian concerns with these systems. This may simply require further elaboration— we need sufficiency of capabilities and "something else," some separate standard of social equality, which we could use to judge two-tiered care.

I call the third response *the internal response*. I have said that health care justice needs to be judged not merely according to the capability of health but also according to the other central capabilities; this is the dimension pluralism of the CA. What Nussbaum refers to as the capability of affiliation overlaps significantly with social equality. According to this capability, first, one is "able to live with and toward others, to recognize and show concern for other human beings, to engage in various forms of social interaction" and, second, to have "the social basis of self-respect and non-humiliation; being able to be treated as a dignified human being whose worth is equal to that of others."[38] Social equality then could be seen to be expressed and fulfilled, at least partially, through both of these components of affiliation that demand civic friendship and respect-for-persons.[39] Social equality

---

37. Would such a response still allow the CA to be a *sufficientarian* theory? I think so. Consider that sufficiency is not instrumental to achieving equality; it is constitutive of it. Sufficiency of capabilities remains the morally urgent final goal of *distribution*.

38. Nussbaum, *Frontiers of Justice*, 77.

39. Wolff and De-Shalit have emphasized the overlap between social equality and affiliation. They emphasize that other capabilities, such as emotional well-being, may also overlap with aspects of social equality: Jonathan Wolff and Avner de-Shalit, *Disadvantage* (Oxford: Oxford University Press, 2007), especially 6, 167–180.

and its critique of two-tiered care might thus be accommodated internally in the CA by being understood as part of the capability of affiliation.

What would this mean in terms of two-tiered systems? It would mean that within the CA we would be able to recognize the justification for two-tiered systems via sufficiency of capabilities (according to whichever capabilities require medical care to achieve sufficiency) and we would also be able to acknowledge the problems we have identified with these systems via the capability of affiliation. In terms of assessing tiered systems, we would then need to weigh the significance of the capability of affiliation against the significance of distributing resources according to sufficiency in the other capabilities. In some sense, this response would be similar to the first response except that instead of claiming that sufficiency and equality are two separate values, it would understand the importance of social equality as covered by the capabilities, and the weighting between values would be between two forms of sufficiency (of independent capabilities).

Although we do not have enough information from this chapter to make any kinds of overall claims about how this weighting between capabilities could be done, preliminarily, we might be able to state that we have reasons, generated by the CA alone, to reject two-tiered systems in which they seem to violate social equality and thus sufficiency in the capability of affiliation. As a reminder, based on our discussion in Section 4, two-tiered systems would be impermissible:

- if there were major discrepancies between the benefits or services, or both, made available in the first tier in comparison to the second tier; and
- if parallel substitutive insurance systems were instituted.

As I have already mentioned, the three responses from the CA I have discussed here would require further elaboration. However, I think they are promising, and the third implies that the CA may well be able to accommodate a social egalitarian critique using only its internal resources. Also, the second and third responses need not be viewed as exclusive, and perhaps they could be combined.

Let me end this chapter with a brief summary. I analyzed how a CA can be consistently expanded to generate the basis for a sufficientarianism, which is pluralist in nature. This sufficientarian CA can be usefully applied to health justice, determining, for example, the normative basis for a limited version of two-tiered health care. At the same time, it may be able to respond to objections from social egalitarianism, which would question the permissibility of two-tiered systems, under certain circumstances. It is an advantage of this theory, I believe, that it seems to have the structure to accommodate both the normative commitments that underlie why we might think that two-tiered systems are indeed acceptable and those that accommodate the concern, often expressed within the public and political discourse, that these systems create or reinforce class divisions.

Acknowledgments

I am particularly grateful to Agomoni Ganguli Mitra, Jan-Christoph Heilinger, Sabine Hohl, Sebastian Muders, Annette Rid, Fabian Schuppert, Liam Shields, and Verina Wild for their feedback on draft versions of this chapter, which was very useful in helping me to revise it. I also thank participants of the Ethics Research Institute's colloquium on Applied Ethics at the University of Zurich and faculty and students at the Department of Philosophy of the University of Washington, Seattle, whose questions and feedback were also extremely beneficial for improving the chapter. I am grateful for the generous financial support of the Swiss National Science Foundation.

11

Determining a Basic Minimum of Accessible Health Care

A COMPARATIVE ASSESSMENT OF THE WELL-BEING
SUFFICIENCY APPROACH

Paul T. Menzel

1. Introduction

Access to a basic minimum of health care is a matter of justice and a moral right.[1]
Delineating the minimum that forms the content of this right can be difficult. The
right's importance will vary significantly, depending on whether the basic minimum is lean or extensive.

In the larger debate about whether access to a basic minimum is a moral right,
one might proceed by being fairly definite about the content at the beginning and
then proceed to determine whether access to this minimum is a matter of justice
and a right. On what basis, however, would one select this initial content? And
what if the answer from the ensuing debate is "No, access to this minimum is
not a right and not required as a matter of justice"? Other possible minima might
generate "Yes" answers. To which other minimum should one turn next?

---

1. I assume that it is for purposes of this chapter. I have argued it is in Paul T. Menzel,
"Justice and Fairness: A Critical Element in U.S. Health System Reform," *Journal of Law,
Medicine, and Ethics* 40, no. 3 (2012): 582–597; and Paul T. Menzel, "A Cultural Moral Right
to a Basic Minimum of Accessible Health Care," *Kennedy Institute of Ethics Journal* 21, no.
1 (2011): 79–120. The principle of distributive justice I employ is equal opportunity for welfare, and the principle of fairness is prevention of free-riding (see Section 2). I argue that,
as embedded in a wide range of political views, these principles amount to cultural "moral
facts." Combined with several legal and economic facts, they generate a realistic, "existing"
moral right to health care.

An alternate course reverses this order.[2] First, leave the minimum's content provisionally ambiguous. Second, be clear what the claim at issue, "access to (a basic minimum of) care is a person's right," means: that people have a justified claim that access should not be left to vagaries of the market, where because of financial means and health status some will have access and others will not, and that society is obligated to restrain or sidestep the market to ensure everyone's access. Third, getting such a right actually recognized and the obligations associated with it met will inevitably involve the collective power of the state, but then the task of discerning a basic minimum takes the following form: What amount and scope of health care may and should a society use its collective power to make universally accessible? If society has chosen to realize the right through multipayer insurance with an insurance mandate (e.g., as in Germany or Switzerland), the right's content will be the level of care for which the society can justify requiring people to purchase insurance. If society has chosen a single-payer or national health service system (e.g., as in Canada or the United Kingdom), the content will be the level and scope of care for which the requisite taxation is justified. Finally, in either case, we return to the moral principles and social facts central in constructing the case for universal access to determine what they imply about the content of the minimum. Those implications will concern not only what the basic minimum should include but also what it need not.

In this chapter, I

- review several closely allied arguments for the right to an accessible basic minimum with this "reversed" order—arguments that initially leave the minimum unspecified but that, upon further analysis, can be seen to imply certain elements of and limits to the minimum. These arguments involve widely shared principles of justice and fairness not found in sufficiency theory;
- articulate a prominent sufficiency theory of justice, the essential dimensions of well-being view of Madison Powers and Ruth Faden, and compare the broad outlines of the content of the basic minimum this theory generates with the minimum generated by the previous nonsufficiency arguments;
- pursue in detail the implications of this sufficiency theory for one particular controversy about how to configure the basic minimum, prioritizing care by age of recipient ("age-related prioritizing"),[3] and compare those with the implications from the earlier arguments for the right to a basic minimum; and
- conclude with observations about the degree to which sufficiency theory can assist in delineating the health care to which people have a moral right.

---

2. Such a reversed order is explicitly provided in Menzel, "A Cultural Moral Right," at 83–90.

3. I typically speak of age-related or age-based "prioritizing," not "rationing." My reasons are explained in Paul T. Menzel, "Statistical and Identified Lives: Why Not to Use the 'R' Word," in *Fair Resource Allocation and Rationing at the Bedside*, ed. Marion Danis et al. (New York: Oxford University Press, 2015), 238–252.

2. A Realistic Moral Right Based on Principles of Justice and Fairness

A moral right of access to a basic minimum of health care can be a "realistic" moral right, resting on certain actual facts and existing moral principles in a given society. [4] For a moral principle to "exist" in this sense is for it to be widely acknowledged in the society in which it is being employed. Politically, it would be shared by most people on both left and right. Connecting the dots between several such principles and key social facts can reveal the existence of a moral right.[5]

One pattern of connected dots begins with a central fact in the economics of health insurance, *market failure*. A voluntary market for insurance offered by unrestrained insurers to unrestrained subscribers will not make insurance accessible to the people who most need it, the most likely ill. For the market to serve them, insurers must be barred from using the preexisting condition exclusions and "experience-rated" premiums that render insurance often unaffordable. If insurers are not so barred, they will keep lowering premiums to the youngest and healthiest to a level that is still profitable but much lower than premiums for the less healthy. Without young and healthy in a common pool, premiums for many of the less healthy will become unaffordable. Those people, however, are most in need of insurance for protection against devastating expenses, producing a "failed market." Premiums for policies that exclude care for preexisting conditions or preserve the insurer's right to rescind insurance when a subscriber gets too expensive may remain affordable, but those policies leave subscribers exposed to the very risks insurance is designed to blunt—still a failed market.[6]

Simply prohibiting insurers from segmenting premiums, rescinding insurance, and excluding preexisting conditions does not solve the problem. Such restrictions—requiring "guaranteed issue" for a "community-rated" premium—can be self-defeating. By themselves, they will increase, not decrease, the ranks of the uninsured. Guaranteeing common-premium rates inevitably raises premiums for the healthy and young, who are then even less likely to insure. In turn, premiums for those who still do insure rise still further. A "death spiral" for insurance ensues.

---

4. More detailed versions of the argument in this section and the next are in Menzel, "A Cultural Moral Right"; and Menzel, "Justice and Fairness."

5. I intend the claim to hold even for a society such as the United States that does not have universal access to health care (which it does not, even under Obamacare). In the rest of this section, I sometimes cite particular facts from the United States. Because of the basic nature of insurance markets, most of the moral argument will apply in other economically advanced countries with more universal access.

6. Left unrestrained, subscribers as well as insurers contribute to this failure. If subscribers were barred from dropping insurance or from switching to much leaner insurance when they considered themselves to need less care, insurers' behavior might need less restraint.

The obvious solution is mandatory insurance: Do not allow people to postpone or revoke their purchase of insurance merely because they think it is a poor bargain given their current health. People need to pay in all along. Not only must insurers be barred from using preexisting condition exclusions, waiting periods, and widely varying risk-rated premiums but also everyone must have insurance.

The language of this argument, focused on "market failure," is the language of economic *fact*: Unfettered competitive markets in health insurance are bound to fail. No one should be misled, however, into thinking that the argument requires no moral premise. Suppose someone says, "Yes, market failure characterizes unfettered markets for insurance, but we should just let this failure lie where it falls. After all, many things in how a market plays out may be unfortunate or inequitable, including lack of affordable insurance for the likely ill. *So what?*"

The argument cannot proceed here without some moral principle that condemns the segregation of financial burdens between well and ill. Fortunately, a widely shared principle is available—what I refer to as the *just sharing* of financial burdens of illness:

> *Principle of just sharing:* The financial burdens of medical misfortunes should be shared equally by well and ill alike, unless people can be reasonably expected to control those misfortunes by their own choices.

The just sharing principle does not tolerate preexisting condition exclusions, premium variation by subscriber risk, rescission of insurance when subscribers become high cost, and other market segmentation devices that inevitably arise in unfettered markets and leave the likely ill high and dry. To avoid that, insurance must be made mandatory. Why shouldn't we leave the likely ill high and dry? The reason expressed by the just sharing principle is that the likely well should contribute more to insurance than their own individual risk situation by itself warrants.

The just sharing principle also bolsters another crucial element in universal access. For a mandate to be fair and care to be truly accessible, premiums must be affordable. For some, affordability comes with narrowing the permissible range of premiums between well and ill, a direct consequence of the just sharing principle. For others, with lower incomes, affordability requires publicly funded premium subsidies as well. Such subsidies that alleviate the unfairness of mandating insurance that people cannot afford are also a consequence of the just sharing principle.

The principle does not come out of nowhere or stand alone in its specific realm of health care. It manifests a general principle of relational justice that is much more widely shared than debates about universal access might indicate. To see this, we need only to probe briefly what the proper degree of equality should be in the distribution of life's goods (e.g., wealth, education, health, and—to the extent that it preserves and promotes health—health care).

We find two extremes in people's beliefs. On the arch-egalitarian end stand those who would strive for equal well-being or equal resources for all. Their position may have some intuitive attraction, but it encounters pointed objections concerning incentives and differences in merit and desert related to varying investments of talent and effort.

On the other end stand arch-libertarians, who argue that short of contract, individuals have no obligations of justice to others; obligations never arise out of fate alone. Their position has some intuitive attraction, conveyed by a question that they presume to be rhetorical: If through no act or oversight or inaction of yours, I am struck, for example, by lightning, why should you be obligated to help me?

It is not difficult to remove the rhetorical power this question is presumed to have. Even in the United States, few people think about overall burdens and advantages in life along such strictly "separatist" lines. The burden of proof implied in the question when heard as rhetorical can be flipped: If there is no relevant difference between people (e.g., one person is no more deserving than another), *why shouldn't* we be obligated to share in another's most unfortunate, life-agenda-setting burdens? Being alive at all is a gratuitous fortune for each of us. On what basis, therefore, may any of us legitimately complain if truly undeserved burdens are pooled to help equalize life chances and overall opportunities for well-being? Obligations of justice are simply not grounded only in contract by actual individuals from their existing natural situations.

The vast middle ground in a moral culture such as that of the United States echoes this. In a middle-ground sense of justice, some (but not all) burdens should be pooled, and some inequalities of well-being (but not all) should be accepted, preserving a limited role for liberty and choice, merit and talent, and incentives to produce helpful goods and services. The following is one articulation of such a view:

Principle of equal opportunity for welfare (EOW): People should not be worse off than others through no fault or voluntary choice of their own. Situations in which people are worse off because of their own sufficiently blameworthy actions or choices are not unjust, as painful or compassion-eliciting as those situations may be.[7]

---

7. EOW is Richard Arneson's label: Richard Arneson, "Equality and Equal Opportunity for Welfare," *Philosophical Studies* 56 (1989): 77–93; and Richard Arneson, "Liberalism, Distributive Subjectivism, and Equal Opportunity for Welfare," *Philosophy and Public Affairs* 19 (1990): 158–193. G. A. Cohen articulates a similar view: G. A. Cohen, "On the Currency of Egalitarian Justice," *Ethics* 99 (1989): 906–944. EOW resides in a family of views known as "luck egalitarian" justice. Shlomi Segall in *Health, Luck and Justice* (Princeton, NJ: Princeton University Press, 2010) provides an admirable summary: "It is unjust for individuals to be worse off than others due to outcomes that it would have been unreasonable to expect them to avoid" (p. 13). The views are "luck egalitarian" because they consider justice not as *generally* equalizing whatever is the proper object of equalization (e.g., welfare) but equalizing it only in order to compensate for bad "brute luck" (e.g., being hit by a falling tree

In this notion of justice, equal *opportunity* for welfare differs from equality of welfare. Focusing on opportunity, not welfare per se, EOW preserves a considerable role for individual choice. Applied to health care, EOW implies something like the just sharing principle. Both point toward rectifying inequality when the factors that create it are beyond people's control, just as both tolerate inequalities that result from sufficiently blameworthy choices within people's control.

There is considerable evidence within US health policy history that a view of justice that includes the just sharing principle is widely held:

- The existence of Medicare reflects the need for the likely well to share in the expenses of the elderly who are more likely ill.
- The Emergency Medical Treatment and Active Labor Act, first passed in 1985 and reaffirmed since,[8] recognizes that the costs of treating one portion of those who are particularly ill, nonpaying patients who present at emergency rooms, need to be shared.[9]
- Within the fractious debates in the United States about health insurance reform, one of the few elements on which liberals and most conservatives agree is that people should not be prevented by their health status from obtaining or maintaining insurance.

Thus, even though the argument for mandatory universal insurance for basic care goes beyond facts to rely also on principles of justice, it is still realistically powerful. The foundation of its central moral premise is a view of justice that is not only philosophically defensible but also widely shared.

This case for universal access is bolstered by a similar argument from a different fact and related principle of fairness. Not even in the United States are people willing to see those who are uninsured go without emergency care. Reflecting a rescue ethic, legislation gets passed that obligates hospital emergency rooms to provide care regardless of patients' insurance and ability to pay.[10] However, that creates a temptation for people not to insure; after all, one will still get emergency

---

one had no reason to suspect would fall), not for bad "option luck" that occurs in a chain of events in which one's own voluntary choices play a role. See Chapter 3 of Segall for extensive discussion.

8. The Emergency Medical Treatment and Active Labor Act (1998), Pub. L. No. 99–272, 100 Stat. 164, codified as amended at 42 U.S.C. 1395dd (hereafter EMTALA). Notably, no suggestions to repeal this law have emerged from conservative voices even in the vigorous US debates about health care reform.

9. Funding of EMTALA is largely accomplished through cost shifting to paying patients who are insured, which in turn raises premiums for everyone who buys insurance. Most of those who are insured are less ill than those needing the emergency care.

10. EMTALA (1998).

care. Most of the cost of the resultant "free" emergency room care then gets shifted to people who have insured, raising their premiums. In some cases, this will constitute unfair free-riding by those who chose not to insure on those who have insured. In any case, the resulting overreliance on emergency care to substitute for primary and preventive care is inefficient. A principle of fairness about free-riding then comes into play:

> *Principle of prevention of free-riding*: People should pay their share of the costs of a collective enterprise that produces benefits from which they cannot be or are not excluded, unless they would actually prefer to lose all the benefits of the enterprise rather than pay their fair share of its costs.[11]

With the free-riding and inefficiency that occur when universal emergency care is decreed without other insurance, the remedy is either mandatory insurance for health care more generally or a single-payer arrangement.

The gist of these two arguments, illustrated by the United States as a case study, is that as a matter of consistency, in any society characterized by certain preexisting factual realities and widely shared moral principles, everyone has a moral right of access to a basic minimum of health care, to be realized by either subsidized mandatory private insurance or single-payer insurance.

3. Implications for the Content of the Basic Minimum

The facts and principles on which the previous two arguments rely—market failure, the already obligatory access to emergency care, the principle of just sharing based on equal opportunity for welfare, and prevention of free-riding—point to several essential elements in the basic minimum for which everyone should be insured:[12]

- Emergency care, primary care (including preventive care), and post-emergency acute care must be included. These are the first ingredients needed to remedy the unfairness and waste in a situation in which the only universal access is to emergency care.

---

11. For greater detail in the argument for universal insurance based on preventing free-riding, see Menzel, "Justice and Fairness," at 586–591; and Paul T. Menzel, "Justice, Liberty, and the Choice of Health System Structure," in *Medicine and Social Justice* ed. Rosamond Rhodes, Margaret Battin, and Anita Silvers, 2nd ed. (New York: Oxford University Press, 2012), 35–46, at 37–41.

12. Here I provide only a brief summary. For further explanation, see Menzel, "A Cultural Moral Right," at 92–105; and Paul T. Menzel, "Setting Priorities for a Basic Minimum of Accessible Health Care," in *Medicine and Social Justice*, ed. Rosamond Rhodes, Margaret Battin, and Anita Silvers, 2nd ed. (New York: Oxford University Press, 2012), 131–141.

- There should be no lifetime cap on the benefits an individual can receive from insurance. Equality of opportunity for welfare is distinctly compromised by lifetime health benefit caps that disadvantage precisely those facing the most serious challenges from illness.
- Patient cost-sharing may be employed to discipline the use of insured care, but it should be carefully limited and graduated with income so as not to discourage care needed to preserve equality of opportunity for welfare.
- Comparative effectiveness assessments should be used to exclude treatments that are less effective than alternatives, even if they are no more costly, and treatments that are more expensive even when they are no more effective. Ignoring such assessments is wasteful and benefits largely only the special interests behind comparatively ineffective or unnecessarily expensive care.

Further moral principles involved in the same sense of justice and fairness employed in these arguments generate additional capacity to discipline the basic minimum. The chain of reasoning here begins with a factually pervasive phenomenon in insurance:

> *The insurance effect*: Insurance distorts patients' and providers' sense of relationship between cost and value. In the context of insurance, their preferences no longer restrain care to keep it worth its cost. Neither patient nor provider will need to reckon with whether the resources required by an item of care (its "cost") are warranted by its benefits.

Yet in a situation in which much care is insured, are any perspectives other than those of the patient and provider available?

There is one. In a context of fair, just, person-respecting insurance that is the concern of the previous arguments for a right to a basic minimum, there is another, more logical perspective. Because the cost-fueling culprit is embedded in the very situation of insurance itself, why not use the initial point associated with insurance, the act of insuring, to delineate some discipline on the use of care? The approach this suggests is the perspective of the "prudent insurer" or "reflective subscriber":

> *Principle of the prudent insurer*: Care that is sufficiently effective and resource-efficient to be worth its expense is care for which subscribers who are knowledgeable and imaginative about what is at stake in their current insurance decisions for coverage of their later care, and who are cognizant of the resource trade-offs involved, would choose to insure.[13]

---

13. "Prudent insurer" is the term used by Ronald Dworkin, "Justice and the High Cost of Health," in *Sovereign Virtue: The Theory and Practice of Equality* (Cambridge, MA: Harvard

Using such a prudent insurer perspective will reveal limits on the basic minimum:[14]

- Last-chance care at the end of life that has a very low probability of benefit, or a somewhat higher probability but only of a very small benefit, especially if it is relatively expensive, should not be included.[15]
- Life-extending care for patients in a persistent vegetative state or with end-stage dementia need not be included, especially when it incurs significant expense. The benefit of extended survival is very small, and for many people it is zero or even negative.[16]
- Preventive screening with a very low statistical chance of benefit for a particular patient, and where the measures used to follow up on false positives pose risks, should not be included. This is especially the case when costs are considerable.

In addition to such limits on the minimum that the prudent insurer perspective generates, it combines with the previously employed EOW principle to suggest additional limits. One of the most plausible is lower priority for life-extending care after one has reached a "complete life" age. Prudent insurers, looking ahead (or back, too) over their life spans, may very well want to see more resources invested in life-extending care at younger ages when more life-years are at stake and relatively fewer resources invested at much older ages when the gains of successful treatment for one's whole life are smaller.[17] Not just from such a prudential perspective but also from a societal perspective of relational justice, age-related

---

University Press, 2000), 307–319. Mark Hall, in *Making Medical Spending Decisions: The Law, Ethics, and Economics of Rationing Mechanisms* (New York: Oxford University Press, 1997), uses "bundled consent." An argument that this, by whatever label, is the appropriate conceptual perspective to use for disciplining costs is provided by Menzel, "Setting Priorities," at 134–135.

14. For arguments for and explanations of these conclusions, see Menzel, "Setting Priorities," at 137–138; and Menzel, "A Cultural Moral Right," at 97–103.

15. A complex example is glioblastoma. See the sensitive discussion of age-prioritizing treatment for this particular disease by Michael K. Gusmano, "Is It Reasonable to Deny Older Patients Treatment for Glioblastoma?" *Journal of Law, Medicine, and Ethics* 42, no. 2 (2014): 183–189.

16. For the justification of this judgment in the case of PVS, see Paul T. Menzel, "Determining the Value of Life: Discrimination, Advance Directives, and the Right to Die with Dignity," *Free Inquiry* 25, no. 5 (2005): 39–41. For justification in the case of end-stage dementia, see Paul T. Menzel and Bonnie Steinbock, "Advance Directives, Dementia, and Physician-Assisted Death," *Journal of Law, Medicine, and Ethics* 41 (2013): 484–500, at 492–493.

17. This is essentially the "prudential life span" account for placing a lower priority on life-extending care in older age articulated by Norman Daniels in *Am I My Parents' Keeper? An Essay on Justice Between the Young and the Old* (New York: Oxford University Press, 1988), 40–65.

priorities may plausibly emerge: The well-known "fair innings" argument[18] for greater priority on life extension at younger ages is fundamentally a claim about equal opportunity for well-being over people's whole lives. Much more will be said about this in Section 5.

To be sure, not all of the content of the basic minimum can be determined as an implication from the primary facts and principles that generate the argument for universal access in the first place. For some kinds of care, the principles and facts that generate the right of access to a basic minimum will point to neither inclusion nor exclusion. In these cases, there can be no substitute for a collective process of debate and discussion that brings the voices of citizens, subscribers, and taxpayers into play, not merely the voices of patients and providers.

Throughout the consideration of what should be included in the basic minimum, one must keep in mind that it amounts to the following question: What care may a society use its collective coercive power to make universally accessible? Consideration of what the basic minimum does *not* need to include, not only what it should include, is morally important. Setting the basic minimum unduly high will constitute exploitation. Insurance itself already greatly diminishes the likelihood that providers and patients will weigh value relative to cost. With insurance made legally mandatory, the ordinary leverage of insurers and providers gets expanded by the power of the state. This is a perfect recipe for exploitation of those who must provide the necessary premiums and taxes. In such a setting, the task of discerning a defensible basic minimum must not be handed primarily to providers and insurers. To be fair, decisions about the basic minimum must consider the perspective of citizens required to purchase insurance and pay taxes as well as the perspectives of providers with expertise and patients needing care. It is never appropriate simply to presume that because some medical treatment is designed to contribute to health, it should be included in the basic minimum to which everyone is guaranteed access.

4. Justice as Sufficiency of Well-Being

If a sufficiency theory of justice is to ground the right to a basic minimum of health care, we expect it to enlighten the content of the basic minimum. One naturally supposes such a theory will do this directly, for just sufficiency is already the argument for the right. I argue that this picture of the role of sufficiency in defining the basic minimum in a sufficiency theory is only partially accurate.

The claim I make is narrow and does not necessarily address sufficiency theories generally. It is about one theory: the multidimensional theory of justice for health

---

18. Alan Williams, "Intergenerational Equity: An Exploration of the 'Fair Innings' Argument," *Health Economics* 6 (1997): 117–132.

care by Madison Powers and Ruth Faden.[19] In their view of justice (as in the views of many others), people are "entitled" to what is just,[20] so their sufficiency view of justice is a view about rights. Reflecting their "sufficiency" theory, the right to health care they assert is automatically going to be to some sort of basic minimum.

Their view has major elements in common with the previously developed arguments for the right to health care not grounded in sufficiency theory. First, just as EOW takes well-being ("welfare") as one of its objects, the object of justice in Powers and Faden's theory is also well-being (though sufficient well-being). Powers and Faden prefer an Aristotelian notion of well-being as human flourishing rather than one of the contemporary notions focused on desire/preference satisfaction,[21] but their theory's focus is still human welfare. Second, Powers and Faden's notion of well-being that focuses on flourishing, capabilities, and functionings is expansive relative to a narrower preference-satisfaction notion of welfare, just as EOW is expansive relative to equal welfare.

On other scores, there are significant differences. Powers and Faden's claim of justice is to a sufficient level of actual health, not merely *access* to health or the *opportunity* for it. Health needs occur when a level of health is insufficient for human flourishing, and injustice occurs when those needs are not met. Moreover, health is fundamentally valuable for its own sake as a component of human flourishing; it is not just instrumentally valuable by contributing to equality of opportunity. In asserting the right to health care, we care about the sufficiency of human health itself.

Powers and Faden's view, however, is not exclusively focused on health. Social justice is the achievement of sufficiency in five additional essential dimensions of well-being (EDsWB) as well: personal security, reasoning capacity, respect, self-determination, and bonds of attachment. Each must be satisfied to achieve justice. Thus, Powers and Faden are able to take agency, responsibility, and self-determination seriously right within justice, as parts of it, just as does the previously employed middle-ground view of relational justice, EOW. Powers and Faden do not build elements of choice and self-determination into the very object of health justice, as *access* to health care and *opportunity* for welfare do, but self-determination

---

19. Madison Powers and Ruth Faden, *Social Justice: The Moral Foundations of Public Health and Health Policy* (New York: Oxford University Press, 2006). The ambiguities in "sufficiency" that emerge from my analysis of how their view could help construct the basic minimum may apply to sufficiency theories more generally, but I will not make such a claim. My focus here is narrowly comparative: how one derives some conclusions about the basic minimum within a view about the right to health care like the one I have articulated previously, which uses certain principles of justice and fairness not found in sufficiency views, compared with how Powers and Faden derive conclusions about the basic minimum in their theory.

20. Ruth Faden and Madison Powers, "Sufficiency, Relational Egalitarianism, and Health," unpublished manuscript (May 8, 2012), at 23–24.

21. Ibid., 11–14.

is as essential a dimension of the just distribution of well-being as is health. Because social justice concerns the sufficiency of each and all of the six, justice in health policy cannot be focused solely on the achievement of sufficient levels of health. Health is not a separate, much less a privileged, sphere of justice.

What, though, is a level of health sufficient for human flourishing? For Powers and Faden, there needs to be "enough health for a decent human life ... enough health to live a full life course without preventable, significant functional disability or ... treatable pain or suffering."[22] To what resources for realizing such a sufficient level do people have a right? To "the resources necessary to achieve health sufficiency, understood as sufficient health for a decent life."[23]

Although this initial assertion of theirs is unqualified, it would seem to mean *all* the resources necessary to achieve such sufficiency. Add to this the fact that although it may not be difficult to get unanimous agreement that many treatments and services are critical to preserving or restoring the health necessary for a "decent life," people will vary greatly in some of their perceptions of what qualifies as a "decent life." Then sufficiency defined by reference to a "decent life" would seem to be so elastic as to provide little, if any, discipline on resource expenditure—little, that is, beyond the requirement that the care to which one has a right should be effective in actually achieving health.

Faden and Powers, however, do not leave resource matters this elastic. They add two cautions: To constitute justice, health sufficiency will often be dependent on sufficiency in other EDsWB. Moreover, health has social determinants that range far beyond health care.[24] Insofar as high expenditures on health care make it difficult or impossible to achieve sufficiency in any other EDWB, or to the extent that the lengths to which we might go in health care exacerbate negative social determinants of health, then *as a matter of justice and rights and the sufficient basic minimum*, investments in health care may need to be restrained.

These restraints, however, suffer from a "does too much, yet does too little" difficulty. On the one hand, negative effects on another EDWB can be plausibly alleged for almost any health care expenditure except the most clearly cost-effective ones. On the other hand, the negative effects on the other EDsWB and on the larger social determinants of health from an expenditure on health care are usually so ambiguous or opaque that any restraint that should flow from carefully considering these effects tends to evaporate.[25]

---

22. Ibid., 22.

23. Ibid., 23.

24. Ibid., 24.

25. For example, it may be thought that a given extra investment in health care would do more good if it were invested in improved education—both by getting closer to sufficiency in reasoning (another EDWB) and by perhaps improving health through having a better educated populace (one of the social determinants of health).

We can summarize these capacities of Powers and Faden's sufficiency view to define a basic minimum. First, the care included must be effective in promoting, preserving, or restoring sufficient levels of health. It is not health care per se or the intentions in providing it that constitute its connection with justice; it is care's real effect on health. Second, some elements of a sufficient level of health are readily agreed to be necessary for a "decent life": prevention of serious disability, avoidance of early death, and freedom from pain and suffering that significantly interfere with appreciating the common, everyday goods of life. Care that is clearly known to accomplish any of these is included in the basic minimum. Third, potentially negative effects of excessive health care spending on the social determinants of health and on the other EDsWB constitute an ever-present source of concern to keep the basic minimum within bounds. Such effects are usually so difficult to pin down, however, that as a matter of realistic practice, few discrete limitations are likely to be put on the basic minimum because of these negative effects.

To discern other aspects of the capacity of Powers and Faden's sufficiency theory to enlighten the basic minimum, one will need to get beyond typical treatments and services and take up specific controversies at the margins.[26] One such area is age-related prioritizing. Because Powers and Faden have spoken to it explicitly and because treatments at the end of life and in old age take up a major portion of health care spending, I pursue it here.

5. Age-Related Prioritizing

"Age-related prioritizing" refers to any prioritizing of care on the basis of a recipient's age; it can include comparisons between recipients of any age. Here, I ignore major parts of the full spectrum of age comparison—for example, between young children and young adults—to pursue only one segment, arguably the most plausible: reduced priority in "old age," when someone is past the life span commonly viewed as constituting a "full life." I refer to this age as "complete-life age."

Any remotely plausible lower priority for health care for persons older than this age will not remove all of their care from the basic minimum. Quality-of-life improving care should retain the same priority. At any age, pain and suffering can turn the time one lives into something less than "decent," acceptable life. In the case of pain-relieving, quality-improvement care, the patient is going to live regardless. Pain or deficient quality of life from going without

---

26. Consideration of such controversies is important in evaluating any foundational argument for the right to a basic minimum. How much "core" content of the minimum a foundation provides is one aspect of that evaluation; how much it enlightens and defines the minimum at the margins is another.

care is as harmful to someone past a complete-life age as it is in earlier years. Plausible age-related prioritizing will concern only *life-sustaining, life-extending* care. Moreover, plausible prioritizing for complete-age persons will not exclude all life-extending care. Any lower priority can be graduated by the degree and probability of the care's effectiveness, as well as by how much older a person is past a complete-life age.

Consider a plausible candidate for complete-life age—for example, 85 years.[27] Within age-related prioritizing, treatment that is *clearly life-saving* for an 85-year-old—treatment that will almost certainly prevent death and whose omission virtually ensures death—could have the same priority as similar life-saving care for someone younger. Age prioritizing can still operate if a lower priority is given for treatments with less chance of success, or "success" only for a short time for an 85-year-old, in comparison to that same sort of treatment for a younger person. If diminished priority is not a blunt cutoff, it is presumably more acceptable because the value of a person's life to herself does not simply drop away when she reaches complete-life age. *Graduated* priorities that decline with age still constitute prioritizing directly by age. They do not merely use age as a surrogate for something else (e.g., years of life potentially remaining).

Even if understood in this moderate, graduated way, however, should we exclude a significant portion of life-extending care from the basic minimum for those who have reached complete-life age? No, say Powers and Faden.[28] They admit it could be fair to give lower priority to life-saving care after the age that constitutes a person's "fair innings,"[29] a conception similar to my notion of complete-life age. Even within their own theory, they could regard reaching such an age as "sufficient health" if they thought that life, for purposes of justice and sufficiency, should be viewed in whole life spans. But they do not view it that way, or not only in that way: "Any plausible account of sufficiency in health must be concerned not only with ... health over a lifetime but also with ... levels of people's health at

---

27. There are numerous ways of discerning the age that is a "full life." Ordinary language within a culture is one—what ordinary people, when someone dies, typically refer to as a full life. Statistical average is another—national, multinational regional, or multinational by similarity of economic demographic. For her notion of "shortfall inequality," for instance, Jennifer Prah Ruger uses the highest national average life span—that of Japan, 83 years. See Jennifer Prah Ruger, *Health and Social Justice* (New York: Oxford University Press, 2010), at 200–201.

28. Powers and Faden, *Social Justice*, at 162–166. Previously (at 159–162), Powers and Faden discuss the different age-prioritizing effects of cost–utility analysis (QALYs in particular) and a "fair innings" approach, and they explain why they reject both. One reason for rejecting a fair innings approach is its bluntness (162). The graduated age-related prioritizing I have described avoids this criticism.

29. Williams, "Intergenerational Equity."

any point in time."[30] Even if they viewed sufficiency in health in life span terms, however, they make it clear that they would still oppose age-related prioritizing. Justice requires sufficient levels of all six DsWB, and two non-health dimensions, they argue—respect and bonds of attachment—are threatened by any age-related prioritizing. Sufficiency of *health alone*, if focused on whole life spans, would grant that an 85-year-old has already had a sufficient level of health, but life-extending care still makes claims on justice because its denial threatens sufficiency of respect and bonds of attachment.

This move has its own difficulties. If having already had 85 years can be viewed as fair and sufficient health in regard to life itself, why should people react to any failure to provide life-extending care after age 85 years as a failure to respect them? Sufficiency of *respect* must have its own standard, and it certainly cannot be that people are accorded insufficient respect simply by being denied something they very much want (i.e., continued life).

Perhaps, though, the disrespect is not that people are denied something they very much want but, rather, that the basis for doing so is group membership—an age group. However, treatment of persons as members of a class or group is not, by itself, disrespect. To categorize someone as a member of a class in order to *discriminate* against the individual, of course, is unacceptable (and disrespectful). However, the whole weight of the objection then comes down to showing that there has been (illegitimate) discrimination, not merely categorization. Any plausible argument for age-related prioritization of life-extending care is precisely an argument that categorization by age for this limited purpose is not (objectionable) discrimination. But then to claim that it is discriminatory begs the very question at issue: Is such prioritizing discrimination?

These more complex dimensions of respect may be revealed by certain non-sufficiency theories of justice, such as the view of Norman Daniels that focuses on fair equality of opportunity.[31] The broad category of equal opportunity theories includes the EOW view employed in my previous arguments for a right to health care. Within those theories, and for life-extending care in a context in which the cost fueling insurance effect needs constraint, enlightened insurance subscribers may take a prudential life span view. Especially if some element of prior consent thus undergirds the age prioritization of life-saving care, age-related limitations need not disrespect patients as persons.

---

30. Powers and Faden, *Social Justice*, at 166. The reasons they give focus on the continuing importance, at any age, of quality of life. However, those matters have already been set aside in my treatment here. The age-related prioritizing with which I am concerned—the only plausible form, I would argue—focuses exclusively on life-extending care.

31. Daniels details his view in Norman Daniels, *Just Health: Meeting Health Needs Fairly* (New York: Cambridge University Press, 2008). Justice will require basic levels of long-term

There are similar problems in Powers and Faden's claim that sufficiency in bonds of attachment requires providing life-extending care in old age. We form attachments in the face of our mortality all the time. Their disruption by it, unless the mortality is "premature," is hardly grounds for viewing death past a complete-life age as a rupture of the bonds of attachment that puts this dimension of a person's life below sufficiency. An example illustrates the point. People marry or remarry at age 90 years, and soon after marriage, one of the spouses develops a life-threatening illness. They can hardly complain that the bonds of attachment in their lives have not had a chance to grow to a level of sufficiency. The death and broken bonds are very sad, but why should they be viewed as *unjust*?

Viewed in one way, these discussions illustrate how vague and undefined the central notion of "sufficiency" ends up being in Powers and Faden's theory. Sufficiency of health, by itself, would seem to tolerate diminished priority for life-saving for those who have reached a complete-life age. At that point, the laudable nuance and sensitivity of Powers and Faden's multidimensional notion of sufficiency comes into play, and sufficiency levels of respect and bonds of attachment are alleged to be violated.[32] But are they? Respect for people as they attempt to prioritize some things over their whole life spans, as well as bonds of attachment for people who have learned to adjust to all sorts of things in their old age, may well still tolerate age prioritizing.

We could see this discussion as pointing to the conclusion that in a sufficiency view, life-saving care past a complete-life age can justly be omitted from the basic minimum. Having lived to age 85 years, one has already lived a reasonably

---

care in order to provide the opportunity for normal quality of life in old age, but life-extending care would not appear to be required. In earlier work—*Am I My Parents' Keeper?* (1988)—Daniels thought that self-interested, prudential life span thinking justified such prioritizing. In the more recent *Just Health*, Daniels has his doubts that such reasoning can get him this far: When the use of age to prioritize different cases of life extension has been put through a fair process of discussion with accountability for reasonableness, it has been rejected (*Just Health*, at 180–181). Neither an intuitive "fair innings" defense of age prioritizing nor his own prudential life span defense seem to survive an open public process to be socially sustainable.

Why, though, should Daniels give up the argument he previously made *if it was correct* in claiming that frontloading lifesaving efforts within their life-spans really *is* in each person's overall self-interest? If the problem is that people find themselves *unable to live by their own prudential judgments*, age-prioritizing does not thereby become *unjust*. The inability could be "weakness of will" in achieving moral justice, not a sign that age-prioritizing is unjust.

32. The whole package of Powers and Faden's view on age-related prioritizing, with its distinctions between life span health, respect, and attachment, is explicated and assessed in detail by Carina Fourie, "What Do Theories of Social Justice Have to Say About Health Care Rationing? Well-Being, Sufficiency, and Explicit Age-Rationing," in *Rationing Health Care. Hard Choices and Unavoidable Trade-Offs*, ed. Andre den Exter and Martin Buijsen (Antwerp: Maklu, 2012), 65–86.

complete, long, and healthy life; no disrespect is shown in the denial of life-extending care if that is paired with priorities for life-saving for those who are younger (which all of us who are old once were). Bonds of attachment, too, are somewhat different in old age; losses, even very sad ones, may not constitute insufficiency. If this is the view taken within a sufficiency theory, the basic minimum may be bounded by age-related lower priorities for life-extending treatments.

Instead of emphasizing its ambiguity as a weakness, perhaps it is a merit of sufficiency theory that it harbors argumentative resources for both excluding age-related life-saving care from the basic minimum and including it. However, this discussion does reveal that discerning what constitutes a defensible basic minimum is not made any clearer by having a sufficiency theory for the health care to which one has a right as a matter of justice. The sufficiency element may seem to give sufficiency theory a built-in advantage in defining the basic minimum because "sufficient" and "minimum" are conceptually so close. However, at least in one sophisticated, attractive version of the theory—that of Powers and Faden—it does not.

6. Conclusion

Any moral theory or set of principles that provides the foundation for a universal right of access to a basic minimum of health care will face a host of challenges in delineating that minimum. Among other things, it will need to provide a strong basis for excluding care that is not effective in achieving health. Even on this most evident of scores, potential controversies abound—allegedly effective, yes, but how much evidence, for example, should be needed to back that up?[33] Equally, if not more, difficult controversies surround cost-effectiveness generally and end-of-life care and assisted reproduction specifically. And the list goes on.

Powers and Faden's sufficiency theory is intuitively attractive as a theory of human rights (universal moral rights that presumably should be legal rights): Isn't a basically "decent" life—reasonably long, safe, and secure, with respect accorded one when one develops and uses reasoning, feeling, and attachment capacities—the thing that we believe most strongly every person who lives at all should have? Yet when one parses out their theory's implications for a basic minimum of health care, which one expects that a sufficiency theory would be particularly good at, the

---

33. How reluctant should we be to include unproven but promising therapies in the basic minimum? The "next big thing" in health care has not always held up; cardiovascular stents are the rage one decade but in the next the big failure where we barked up the wrong tree. For the problem under these labels, see Eduardo Porter, "Acceleration Is Forecast for Spending on Health," *New York Times*, April 23, 2014, B1–B2.

theory does not get as far as one would hope. If the previous discussion of age-related prioritizing is any indication, sufficiency theories per se may provide no greater assistance in delineating boundaries for the basic minimum than other foundations for a right to health care. Another set of foundations yields a rich variety of suggestions[34] even though it begins with no preconceptions from "sufficiency" for the minimum's content. Nonsufficiency foundations do not have to fare worse in discerning the substantive content of the basic minimum that collective resources and power should be used to provide, and some may fare better.

Whether with sufficiency or nonsufficiency theories for the right to health care, there will also likely be considerably different implications for the basic minimum as cultural, political, and practical surroundings vary. Different theories may have different implications, but the variation with cultural context in plausible implications from any given theory may be at least as great. Perhaps it is the right to health care as socially embedded in a historical context that supplies the most content of the basic minimum, not whether its moral foundation is a sufficiency theory.

Acknowledgments

I am grateful to Bonnie Steinbock, Annette Rid, and Carina Fourie for their numerous critical and constructive suggestions.

---

34. Note the many bulleted points in Section 3.

12

Just Caring

THE INSUFFICIENCY OF THE SUFFICIENCY PRINCIPLE IN HEALTH CARE

Leonard M. Fleck

1. Introduction: Why Sufficiency?

No society can devote unlimited resources to meeting health care needs, no matter how morally demanding those needs might be. If health care costs are going to be contained, then some health care *needs* will not be met. This is the problem of health care rationing. This view represents a rejection of the pseudo-moral belief that human life is priceless.[1] Some health care needs might be characterized as being life-prolonging, but the cost of an intervention to meet that need might be so great and the likely degree of medical success so small or remote that it would be unreasonable and unjust to try to meet that need. Such a denial of life-prolonging care is a matter of justice because, strictly speaking, our patient will die "prematurely."

Every advanced country is faced with the problem of escalating health care costs. In 1960, health expenditures in the United States, for example, totaled $26 billion, or 5.2% of the gross domestic product (GDP). In 2014, the comparable expenditure figure was $3.1 trillion, or 17.5% of GDP.[2] European nations are currently

---

1. For an extended critique of the claim that human life is priceless, see Peter Ubel, *Pricing Life: Why It's Time for Health Care Rationing* (Cambridge, MA: MIT Press, 2000). See also Leonard Fleck, *Just Caring: Health Care Rationing and Democratic Deliberation* (New York: Oxford University Press, 2009), 71–99.

2. S. Keehan et al., "National Health Expenditure Projections, 2014–2024: Spending Growth Faster Than Recent Trends," *Health Affairs* 34, no. 8 (2015): 1407–1417.

in the 8–11% range of GDP for health expenditures. The primary drivers of escalating health care costs are emerging health care technologies. In the 1960s, patients with end-stage renal disease died relatively quickly from their disease. However, renal dialysis was perfected at that time, which meant that these patients could have their lives sustained for many years on dialysis. The US government created a program in 1972 to pay for kidney dialysis for these patients. The result is that more than 615,000 US citizens currently have their lives sustained by this technology at a cost to the federal government in 2011 of approximately $34 billion.[3]

Daniel Callahan notes that there was no *need* for renal dialysis until dialysis was invented. Prior to the invention of dialysis, no one had a just claim to dialysis. Since then, thousands of costly new medical technologies (transplant surgeries, artificial hearts, targeted cancer drugs, prosthetic limbs, etc.) have been introduced into our health care system, thereby expanding the domain of health care needs and concerns about health care justice.[4] Given this historical background, if a just society does not owe anyone, as a matter of justice, *unlimited* access to needed health care, then what are the limits of what a just society owes all its citizens? I explore the answer proponents of various sufficientarian conceptions of justice will give to this question.

2. Sufficientarianism: What Is Enough?

Early versions of sufficientarianism tended to be abstract and theoretical. Its proponents asked: What does a just, relatively wealthy society owe each of its citizens in the way of resources so that each can live a decent enough life? No special attention was given to health care. Rather, the goal was to articulate a conception of distributive justice that was an alternative to egalitarian, prioritarian, and utilitarian conceptions of justice. However, it seems clear that access to needed and effective health care is fundamental to protecting access to many other social goods (i.e., careers open to talents, financial sufficiency, and caring for children) viewed as key elements of a satisfying human life. Furthermore, the complexity and heterogeneity of health care needs, as well as their cost, generate distinctive issues of justice for the sufficientarian (as well as all other advocates for other conceptions of justice). I articulate and critically assess those issues in Section 3. More recent sufficientarians have returned to a broader, more explicitly complex

---

3. US Renal Data System, "2013 Atlas of End-Stage Renal Disease," accessed June 11, 2014, http://www.usrds.org/2013/pdf/v2_00_intro_13.pdf. See especially 158–159.

4. Daniel Callahan, *What Kind of Life: The Limits of Medical Progress* (New York: Simon & Schuster, 1990), 31–68.

conception of sufficiency wherein health is given special attention as a critical component among multiple components. These are "well-being" and "capabilities" conceptions of sufficiency, which I critically assess in Section 4. I conclude that even these more nuanced conceptions are still too indeterminate for purposes of providing ethical guidance to complex problems of health care justice in the real world. In the final section, I argue that some form of rational democratic deliberation must supplement any conception of health care justice in order to provide specific and "just enough" guidance for more complex allocation problems of health care justice.

Harry Frankfurt, an early proponent of a sufficientarian perspective, wrote,

> What is important from the point of view of morality is not that everyone should have the *same* but that each should have *enough*. If everyone had enough, then it would be of no moral consequence whether some had more than others.[5]

He then noted that the apt response to scarcity "is to distribute the available resources in such a way that as many people as possible have enough, or, in other words, to maximize the incidence of sufficiency."[6] Roger Crisp is another prominent sufficientarian. His key claim is that the sufficiency principle best captures our collective sense of just compassion "for those who are badly off."[7] Furthermore, absolute priority is to be given to providing nontrivial benefits to those below some threshold of sufficiency.

Sufficientarianism may be thought of as a version of a weak egalitarianism because a just society will see to it that everyone has enough. That is, equality is only required up to a point to satisfy the concerns of justice. Hence, society can be morally indifferent to how justice-relevant goods are distributed beyond that sufficiency boundary, at least for the "upper limit" version of sufficientarianism.[8] Sufficientarianism may also be thought of as a species of prioritarianism because its advocates are especially attentive to the needs of those who are *less well-off*. However, sufficientarians are not prioritarians. If the majority of individuals in a

---

5. Harry Frankfurt, "Equality as a Moral Ideal," *Ethics* 98 (1987): 21–43, at 21.

6. Frankfurt, "Equality as a Moral Ideal," at 31.

7. Roger Crisp, "Equality, Priority, and Compassion," *Ethics* 113, no. 4 (2003): 745–763, at 745.

8. To be clear, most sufficientarians would view themselves as critics of egalitarianism. Crisp and Frankfurt would be such critics, as would Efrat Ram-Tiktin and Yitzak Benbaji. See Efrat Ram-Tiktin, "The Right to Health Care as a Right to Basic Human Functional Capabilities," *Ethical Theory and Moral Practice* 15, no. 3 (2012): 337–351; and Yitzak Benbaji, "Sufficiency or Priority?" *European Journal of Philosophy* 14, no. 3 (2006): 327–348.

society have annual incomes of $1 million, but a reasonably decent life is possible on an income of $50,000 per year, then that society would have done all that justice required from an "upper limit" sufficientarian perspective if that income level were assured. Prioritarians, on the other hand, would require social policies that maximized the income potential of the least well-off; it would not be just enough to only bring them up to some minimally decent income level.[9] Thus, sufficientarianism represents a distinct conception of justice.

The following is our critical question: How much health care is *enough* to satisfy a sufficientarian conception of justice? A generic definition of sufficientarianism includes two theses. First, justice has no or only secondary concern with inequalities of health or wealth above a threshold of sufficiency. Second, the focus of justice needs to be on those individuals whose health or wealth is below some threshold of sufficiency. Furthermore, the goal of justice is to bring as many people as possible up to that sufficiency threshold.[10]

Next, we can distinguish "absolutist" and "non-absolutist" versions of sufficientarianism. Crisp is an advocate of the absolutist view, according to which it is unjust to give up a small benefit for someone just below the threshold of sufficiency in order to provide a very large benefit for many already above the sufficiency threshold, even if just slightly above the threshold.[11] For the non-absolutist, such as Ram-Tiktin, if individuals very far below the threshold cannot benefit more than a little from a large provision of social resources, then those resources may be distributed to other individuals capable of deriving large benefits, whether they are above or below the threshold. As she states, "Priority will not be given to the worst-off if the predicted benefit to her is trivial."[12] It is also part of Ram-Tiktin's non-absolutist view that if individuals above a specified health threshold are in danger of falling far below that threshold, perhaps from an untreated cancer, such individuals will have strong just claims to the care that they need to prevent their falling below that threshold. In some cases, their just claims will supersede the claims of those very far below that health threshold. What will determine for Ram-Tiktin how such trade-offs are made will be the severity of the condition for certain types of patients, the potential size of the benefit for such patients, and the number of beneficiaries in each case.

---

9. For Rawls' discussion of the difference principle, see John Rawls, *A Theory of Justice* (Cambridge, MA: Harvard University Press, 1971), 75–83, 100–105.

10. Paula Casal, "Why Sufficiency Is Not Enough," *Ethics* 117, no. 2 (2007): 306–310.

11. Crisp, "Equality, Priority, and Compassion."

12. Ram-Tiktin, "The Right to Health Care," Section 4.

Ram-Tiktin's non-absolutist version of sufficientarianism is clearly more sophisticated, and less open to obvious criticism, than any absolutist version. However, I argue that this more refined version of sufficientarianism cannot provide a reasonable or adequate answer to the question of where that sufficiency threshold is, in part because of the complexity, heterogeneity, and uncertainty associated with most health care needs and their corresponding possible interventions. Sufficientarian considerations may well be a part of a much more complex and pluralistic conception of health care justice, but as the dominant or primary source for reasonable judgments of health care justice, sufficientarianism will be inadequate, especially in relation to individual patients or individual types of patients.

The core sufficientarian principle (just claims are about having "enough" of various social goods) has plausible application with regard to distributional concerns for some range of social goods. A just society is not required to provide filet mignon to those with refined tastes.[13] However, health care is very different in this respect. Some individuals will have excellent health for 100 years. Other individuals, such as 500-g premature infants, may require $1 million in health care just to achieve the first year of life. Still other individuals may have enormous and costly health needs relatively late in life. What does the sufficiency principle tell us is *enough* with regard to meeting such health care needs justly?

Norman Daniels notes that health care needs tend to be "lumpy" rather than being describable as a smooth continuous function.[14] No one can have half a heart transplant or even half the dose of an expensive antibiotic. Imagine, then, a 60-year-old patient with end-stage heart failure and a 6-month life expectancy. His heart failure is a product of a poor genetic endowment and a 40-year, two-pack per day cigarette habit. Does the sufficiency principle require that we provide him with a $300,000 heart transplant? The supply of transplantable hearts is extremely limited (roughly 2500 per year in the United States). However, we are currently clinically testing a totally implantable artificial heart, which can be manufactured in unlimited quantities. Roughly 800,000 Americans die of heart disease annually, and 350,000 of them could be candidates for this device, which would add $100 billion to annual health costs in the United States.

---

13. On the problem of expensive tastes in relation to a conception of justice, see Ronald Dworkin, *Sovereign Virtue: The Theory and Practice of Equality* (Cambridge, MA: Harvard University Press, 2000), 65–119.

14. Norman Daniels, "Justice, Health, and Health Care," in *Medicine and Social Justice: Essays on the Distribution of Health Care*, ed. Rosamond Rhodes et al., 2nd edition (New York: Oxford University Press, 2012), 17–33.

Does the sufficiency principle require funding all 350,000 of these artificial hearts as a matter of justice? Let us assume all 350,000 of these individuals are above the threshold of sufficient health. However, if they are denied the artificial heart, they will fall very far below that threshold—that is, they will die prematurely (2–10 extra years of life lost without the artificial heart). Ram-Tiktin tells us that what should matter in this situation, as far as justice is concerned, is the severity of the patients' condition, the potential size of the benefit, and the number of beneficiaries. These considerations would seem to justify providing the artificial heart to all these individuals. However, if we glibly accept that conclusion, we are not taking seriously the health care rationing problem. We stipulated that all these heart failure patients were currently above the health-related sufficiency threshold. However, there will still be considerable heterogeneity and uncertainty regarding health status among these patients. The age range will be 45–85 years. Should the sufficientarian make any justice-relevant distinctions in that regard? Many patients will exhibit a complex mix of comorbidities. Some will have a metastatic cancer that will kill them in 2 years, although their heart failure will kill them in 6 months. Should sufficientarians make any justice-relevant distinctions in this regard? There is a vagueness in many sufficientarian accounts, such as that of Ram-Tiktin, that undermines the need for practical guidance in making just allocation decisions.

3. What Should Be the Goals and Currency of Sufficiency?

Two major problems must be addressed with respect to the sufficiency principle. First, at what level should sufficiency in health care be set, and for what purpose? Should the goal of health care for a sufficientarian be a dignified enough life, perhaps defined as a life of adequate self-sufficiency? Or should the goal be a satisfying enough quality of life, a life in which ill health is minimized? Or should the goal be an adequate length of life with whatever degree of quality an individual finds acceptable? Or should the goal be access to enough effective health care that one can develop enough capabilities to have a satisfying enough life? All these goals involve some mix of objective and subjective considerations that require access to limited social resources. Given the vagueness of these goals and the essential heterogeneity of health needs and costly health care options, how can a society judge non-arbitrarily anyone's just claims to health care? If that level of sufficiency is set too low, many compelling health needs could be unjustly ignored (from the perspective of other reasonable conceptions of health care justice). If the level is set too high, then the problem of health care rationing (setting limits) is not being taken seriously. That brings us to our second question.

What precisely is the currency of sufficiency supposed to be in health care? Should it be sufficiency of resources, or health outcomes, or health needs satisfied, or health needs satisfied cost-effectively, or health-related capabilities, or well-being (broadly conceived)? We consider several concrete health care allocation scenarios. At an abstract level, appeals to these different sufficiency considerations seem useful and adequate. However, when concrete allocation scenarios must be addressed, these considerations are too vague to provide the specific direction needed to yield well-justified allocation judgments. Later, we consider more nuanced versions of sufficientarianism.

3.1. Sufficiency of Resources

Is the currency of sufficiency supposed to be about sufficiency of *resources*? For example, would entitling everyone to a million dollars' worth of health care over a lifetime be sufficient? Individuals must take responsibility for using limited resources wisely. But then there is the story of Mr. Dawson, as reported in *The Wall Street Journal* in 2007.[15] He had a lifetime cap on his insurance of $1.5 million. However, at age 61 years, he developed a staph infection, possibly related to a pacemaker implant. He required 5 months in three different hospitals to address the multiple complications associated with that infection at an overall cost of $2.7 million. Did he receive "more than enough" health care, at least from the perspective of a sufficientarian conception of health care justice?

The vast majority of us will never use a million dollars' worth of health care during our lifetime. If the sufficiency level is set too high, then many individuals would demand very costly and very marginally beneficial health care, especially in terminal circumstances, thereby worsening problems of health care justice. However, if the sufficiency level is set too low, then hundreds of thousands of patients each year would be denied very costly but very effective health care. In the United States, for example, 5% of the population in any given year accounts for 49% of total health expenditures.[16] Something similar is likely to be true in most of Europe as well. To illustrate, approximately 4% of cystic fibrosis patients with the most severe form of the disease and a distinct genotype, the G551D mutation, can benefit enormously from a drug, ivacaftor, which currently costs approximately

15. Joe Mantone, "Even with Insurance, Hospital Stay Can Cost a Million," *Wall Street Journal* (November 29, 2007), accessed June 11, 2014, http://blogs.wsj.com/health/2007/11/29/even-with-insurance-hospital-stay-can-cost-a-million.

16. Mark Stanton, "The High Concentration of U.S. Health Care Expenditures," Agency for Health Care Research and Quality (2006), accessed June 11, 2014, http://www.ahrq.gov/research/findings/factsheets/costs/expriach/index.html#diff1.

$300,000 per year.[17] Instead of a 20-year life expectancy, these patients could achieve age 50 years, but at lifetime medical costs of approximately $15 million. Should a sufficientarian endorse reimbursement for this drug as a matter of justice? From one perspective (limited resources), this seems hugely excessive, but from another perspective (30 extra years of life) it seems "just enough." Defining sufficiency in terms of *monetary* resources, whether equalized for all or individualized, does not seem to be either an ethically or an economically viable position. Health needs, and corresponding possible health care interventions, are too variable to permit some economic formula to yield consistently just ethical allocations.

An alternative form of resources would be a "basic," "minimally decent," "adequate," or "medically necessary" package of health care benefits guaranteed to everyone in our society. These terms are all inherently vague. We could say that for defining the content of an *adequate* health care benefit package, "basic" will be defined as everything physicians would judge to be "medically necessary" for achieving a specific therapeutic objective for an individual patient. That, however, yields an incredibly high standard of sufficiency or adequacy. Targeted cancer therapies that yielded only extra weeks or months of life for $100,000, as well as artificial hearts for nonagenarians in heart failure, would be just as "medically necessary" as infliximab for rheumatoid arthritis or surgery for an inflamed appendix. Virtually nothing in the current medical armamentarium would be excluded, which means the problem of escalating health care costs would be ignored.[18]

3.2. Sufficiency of Outcomes

If sufficiency of resources is not viable, should we be talking about sufficiency of *outcomes*? If so, what outcomes are most important from the perspective of health care justice? Is everyone entitled to whatever effective health care that might be needed to achieve age 70 or 75 years, independent of the associated costs? Or must quality of life be given some moral weight as well? If so, who would have the authority for determining the balance of those two objectives? Is this a matter of respect for individual autonomy, even though social resources are at stake?

---

17. Jocelyn Kaiser, "New Cystic Fibrosis Drug Offers Hope, at a Price," *Science* 335 (2012, February 10): 645. It is fair to ask whether the justice issues would be greatly diminished if the prices of these drugs and other interventions were much lower. Sometimes this will be true. I argued for that point in a recent essay titled "The Ethical Challenges Raised by Hepatitis C Drugs," accessed November 23, 2014, http://msubioethics.com/2014/10/23/hepatitis-c/?utm_source=Center+Newsletters&utm_campaign=6db5c63009-Bioethics_in_the_News10_2014&utm_medium=email&utm_term=0_ebda7a82a0-6db5c63009-158359345.

18. I have discussed these issues in a much longer essay; Leonard Fleck, "Just Caring: Defining a Basic Benefit Package," *Journal of Medicine and Philosophy* 36 (2011): 589–611.

In the early days of the AIDS epidemic, infection with HIV was a death sentence. Last-year-of-life costs were approximately $127,000.[19] If some sufficientarians at the time were asked whether their sufficiency principle required providing such care, they would likely have answered in the affirmative. This might be because these individuals were among the medically least well-off and were generally relatively young—that is, not having had enough of life. Then nucleoside reverse transcriptase inhibitors were introduced, followed by protease inhibitors, integrase inhibitors, and fusion inhibitors. The result of current four-drug combinations is likely 30 or more years of life for HIV-positive individuals at a cost per person per year of $35,000, or a lifetime cost of approximately $1 million. Again, I imagine that at least some sufficientarians would approve this expenditure as just because of the relative excellence of the outcome (both a reasonable quality of life and length of life).

Another difficult question remains for these sufficientarians. If these patients achieve 30 extra years of life for $1 million, would they also have a just claim to $127,000 worth of last-year-of-life costs because they were now among the medically least well-off? Or would that be "more than enough" because they had already achieved a normal life expectancy? Would these patients have a just claim only to necessary comfort care because aggressive life-sustaining care would yield only marginal benefits and a greatly diminished quality of life? Clearly, outcomes matter as far as health care justice is concerned. However, outcomes will not matter equally because multiple considerations (including cost-effectiveness, aggregate costs, seriousness or urgency of need, and personal responsibility) will often be relevant to assessing outcomes. This requires a complex pluralist conception of health care justice that will include sufficiency considerations as one relevant component.

3.3. Sufficiency as Satisfaction of Serious Health Needs

Is sufficiency to be judged by the quantity or seriousness of health *needs* satisfied? Consider someone with a late-stage cancer or late-stage heart failure. He *needs* a $100,000 targeted cancer drug, such as bevacizumab or ipilimumab, for an extra year or two of life or else a left ventricular assist device (LVAD) for $200,000 that might yield an extra year or two of life. Does the sufficiency principle require that such serious and urgent needs be met as a matter of justice? If an individual has an inflamed appendix with a high likelihood of bursting, is her *need* for an

---

19. Lawrence Altman, "Cost of Treating AIDS Patients Is Soaring," *New York Times* (July 23, 1992), accessed June 11, 2014, http://www.nytimes.com/1992/07/23/us/cost-of-treating-aids-patients-is-soaring.html.

appendectomy just as serious and urgent from a sufficientarian perspective as the previously mentioned person's need for an LVAD or targeted cancer drug? These questions deserve a compelling and well-justified response from sufficientarians. Can a more robust version of sufficientarianism meet this challenge?

As Callahan has argued, health care needs are endless because of the constant stream of emerging medical technologies. [20] Hence, health care needs must be prioritized. What does the sufficientarian principle tell us about how health care needs should be prioritized in order to be "enough"? Patients in the early stages of heart failure are given multiple drugs that effectively manage heart failure. Is that "enough"? Are the LVAD and the artificial heart beyond the limits of sufficientarian justice? If so, will that conclusion be equally true whether we are considering a 25-year-old patient with heart failure due to a bacterial infection of the heart muscle or a 72-year-old patient with bacterial infection of the heart muscle? Furthermore, should it make a difference for the sufficientarian that with access to an artificial heart the 72-year-old patient would be restored to a somewhat vigorous state of health, as opposed to a 72-year-old with several chronic degenerative conditions? Or should a sufficientarian state that these health differences do not make a difference as far as justice is concerned—that both individuals have had "enough" of life because both would have achieved a normal life expectancy? What if our patient were a vigorous 92-year-old prior to his bacterial endocarditis? Would he have a just claim to an artificial heart? His needs are also *serious* and *urgent*. Again, serious and urgent health needs are presumptively matters of health care justice. However, the circumstances and costs and likely outcomes associated with those needs are extremely diverse and require equally diverse and complex judgments of health care justice. Straightforward versions of egalitarianism, prioritarianism, utilitarianism, or sufficientarianism will not by themselves yield adequately nuanced judgments of health care justice in relation to the previously discussed scenarios.

3.4. Sufficiency as Only Satisfying Health Needs Cost-Effectively

If a sufficientarian were to endorse providing an artificial heart to the 92-year-old discussed previously, that would be too high a bar for societally affordable sufficiency. Consequently, sufficiency must be judged with cost-effectiveness in mind, not just needs. There is much argument in the relevant literature about how judgments and calculations regarding cost-effectiveness should be made. [21] We cannot

---

20. Daniel Callahan, *What Kind of Life*, 31–68.

21. Dan Brock, "Ethical Issues in the Use of Cost-Effectiveness Analysis for the Prioritization of Health Care Resources," in *Public Health, Ethics, and Equity*, ed. Sudhir Anand, Fabienne Peter, and Amartya Sen (New York: Oxford University Press, 2006), 201–224.

explore those arguments here. One reasonable reference point might be the cost of facility-based dialysis for 1 year, which was approximately $88,000 in the United States in 2013.[22] This is publicly funded. In essence, the moral and political argument would be that if society is willing to spend at that level through a public program for an intervention that yields many extra years of life of reasonable quality, then other comparable interventions with similar costs and effectiveness should be funded as well. No one has a just claim to interventions that are likely to yield only small benefits at a very high cost. Call this the *insufficiency* perspective. Then the problem a sufficientarian (and all other proponents of a principled approach to health care justice) must be prepared to address is the "ragged edge" problem.[23]

In brief, we have a "ragged edge" problem when we have a therapeutic intervention that sometimes yields a substantial health benefit at significant cost, at other times yields a very marginal benefit at substantial cost, and most of the time yields varying degrees of benefit with varying cost-effectiveness ratios all along a continuum. No bright moral line distinguishes all these costworthy interventions from the non-costworthy interventions. Consider the following cases.

Researchers recently found that women with metastatic breast cancer and various vascular endothelial growth factor (VEGF) genotypes received very different degrees of benefit from the drug bevacizumab combined with paclitaxel compared to paclitaxel alone.[24] Paclitaxel alone yielded a median gain in life expectancy of 26 months. For the 7% of women with the most responsive genotype, bevacizumab and paclitaxel yielded a median gain in life expectancy of more than 50 months, or a cost per quality-adjusted life-year (QALY) gained of $50,000. For the 11% of women with the next most responsive genotype, the median gain in life expectancy was 31 months, or a cost per QALY gained (5 extra months) of approximately $240,000. The following is our critical question: Would a cost-effectiveness-based variant of the sufficiency principle endorse as "just enough" providing bevacizumab only to the 7% group, given that it falls below the cost of $88,000 per year for dialysis? And would this still hold even though, keeping in mind what a median represents, the weakest responders of the 7% group might overlap slightly with the best responders in the 11% group?

---

22. US Renal Data System, "2013 Atlas of End-Stage Renal Disease," at 159.

23. Daniel Callahan, *What Kind of Life*, 31–68.

24. Bryan Schneider et al., "Association of Vascular Endothelial Growth Factor and Vascular Endothelial Growth Factor Receptor-2 Genetic Polymorphisms with Outcome in a Trial of Paclitaxel Compared with Paclitaxel Plus Bevacizumab in Advanced Breast Cancer ECOG 2100," *Journal of Clinical Oncology* 26 (2008): 4672–4678. See also Ransdell Pierson, "Looking for Lessons in Cancer's 'Miracle' Responders," *Reuters* (September 15, 2013), accessed June 12, 2014, http://www.reuters.com/article/2013/09/15/us-cancer-superresponders-idUSBRE98E07420130915.

Granted, sufficientarians reject a strict egalitarian standard of health care justice, so they could be morally comfortable with providing the drug only to the 7% group. But then many of the women in the 11% group will be relatively young (some years from achieving a normal life expectancy). They may be among the medically least well-off and regard those extra 5 months of life as a not-insignificant benefit. If this were an isolated issue (just breast cancer and bevacizumab), we could likely justify regarding this as an exception. However, recent medical literature suggests that the connections between these ultra-expensive targeted cancer therapies and genetic features of an individual or his or her cancer that are predictive of responsiveness may be ubiquitous.[25] If future medical research generates consistently reliable predictions of such degrees of response to these ultra-expensive drugs, then are there considerations of health care justice that would allow us to fairly distinguish cancer patients who would have a just claim to these drugs from those who would not? I am arguing that all accounts of health care justice, including sufficientarian accounts, are too abstract and too vague to provide those answers. A procedural response is needed, such as the account of rational democratic deliberation for which I advocate.[26]

Another area of cancer research that will generate even more complex health care justice issues is related to cancer drug resistance and the emerging understanding of intratumor genetic heterogeneity. In brief, most of these $100,000 targeted cancer drugs yield gains in life expectancy measurable in weeks or months because these drugs target the primary genetic driver in a tumor. Defeating that primary driver permits another genetic driver in the tumor to emerge as the primary driver, for which a different targeted cancer drug can be given. These drugs can be given sequentially, but researchers believe the "AIDS strategy" is to be preferred—that is, giving these drugs in combination and switching combinations as the primary genetic driver of the tumor changes, resulting in progression.[27] This strategy might yield 5 extra years of life expectancy for these cancer patients with reasonable quality. In one report on non-small cell lung cancer, first-line treatment with erlotinib yielded 9.7 months of progression-free survival at a cost of $6,300 per month. Adding bevacizumab

---

25. The literature on this topic is vast. The following is a representative citation: Thomas Urban and David Goldstein, "Pharmacogenetics at 50: Genomic Personalization Comes of Age," *Science and Translational Medicine* 6, no. 220 (2014), 220ps1.

26. Fleck, *Just Caring: Health Care Rationing and Democratic Deliberation.*

27. Some of the relevant literature about cancer drug resistance and tumor heterogeneity is discussed in Leonard Fleck, "Just Caring: Can We Afford the Ethical and Economic Costs of Circumventing Cancer Drug Resistance?" *Journal of Personalized Medicine* 3, no. 3 (2013): 124–143.

yielded 16.0 months of progression-free survival at a cost of $16,700 per month or $200,000 per year.[28] If we imagine this strategy being successful for 5 years by switching in and out various targeted drugs, the cost of saving those 5 years would be $1 million per person. How should sufficientarians think about the question of whether or not cancer patients have a just claim to this therapeutic option? The cost per QALY clearly exceeds the norm we discussed. However, the aggregated benefit would be quite significant for patients who would seem aptly characterized as being among the medically least well-off who were still capable of significant benefit.[29]

At this point, we have "rough justice or non-ideal justice" issues emerging. We are paying for ivacaftor at $300,000 per year for those cystic fibrosis patients with a distinctive genetic characterization. That seems to justify our paying for this combination cancer strategy. Likewise, HIV patients who survive 30 years with the help of these four-drug combinations would seem to provide another justificatory reference point. Their cost per QALY is $35,000, but they too incur lifetime costs for their drugs of approximately $1 million. Should those aggregated lifetime costs for a particular therapy have justice-relevant significance for sufficientarians? But then we are taken back to our 11% breast cancer group that gains 5 extra months of life with a bevacizumab–paclitaxel combination at a cost of $240,000 per QALY. Members of this group now contend they are within the cost-effectiveness parameters of these other patients and, consequently, they have a just claim to these drugs at social expense. Furthermore, they note that in the case of all the metastatic breast cancer patients who get this drug combination, whatever the survival gain, it is *the same real* $100,000 that is spent, not this abstract theoretical cost-effectiveness number. By way of contrast, it is a real $200,000 that must be spent to buy 1 year of life for our non-small cell lung cancer patients, the implication being that sufficiency considerations should not justify their having their life-prolonging needs met before these breast cancer patients.

Our conclusion is that cost-effectiveness is a justice-relevant consideration in making fair rationing/allocation decisions, but a number of other considerations will be justice-relevant as well in making "all things considered" judgments. We turn now to more complex versions of sufficientarianism.

28. Crystal Phend, "ASCO: Targeted Tx Combo Stalls NSCLC," *MedPage Today* (June 3, 2014), accessed June 11, 2014, http://www.medpagetoday.com/MeetingCoverage/ASCO/46127.

29. The category of patients who are among the "medically least well off" is very complex, morally speaking. See Leonard Fleck, "Just Caring: Health Care Rationing, Terminal Illness, and the Medically Least Well Off," *Journal of Law, Medicine, and Ethics* 39 (2011): 156–171.

4. Sufficiency of Well-Being: Still Insufficient?

We next consider the views developed by Madison Powers and Ruth Faden in addition to Efrat Ram Tiktin.[30] We critically assess those views in relation to the problem cases introduced previously, specifically the "ragged edge" and "rough justice" cases. Our conclusion will be that significant inadequacies remain with their views as applied to these challenging scenarios.

Powers and Faden defend what they describe as a *sufficiency of well-being* view that includes six dimensions of well-being. Ram-Tiktin defends a view that defines sufficiency in relation to basic human functional capabilities. For Powers and Faden, those six dimensions are health, personal security, reasoning, respect, attachment, and self-determination. Each of these dimensions is believed by Powers and Faden to capture "a morally salient aspect of human flourishing that is not reducible to the others."[31] Their conception of social justice requires that a just society will put in place social policies and social practices such that all its citizens might achieve a sufficient level of well-being in each of these six dimensions. Individuals will be free to make trade-offs among these dimensions of well-being in their own lives (risk their health for great fame and respect), but a society may not make trade-offs that put at risk sufficiency in one dimension of well-being in order to maximize well-being in another. A society may not severely constrain individual liberty (outlaw all salty snacks and sugar-laden desserts) in order to maximize the health of the population as a whole.

For Ram-Tiktin, the basic functional capabilities are all health-related physiological capabilities. She names nine of them, including thinking and emotions, senses, circulation, respiration, digestion, metabolism, and immunity. Her view is that a just society will guarantee everyone a right to whatever is medically available and necessary to protect or restore each of those functional capabilities to an age-relativized normal status. This will permit individuals to live dignified lives and carry out their life plans. Following Frankfurt, she adds that normal status defines the requirements of sufficiency. Above that level is beyond the domain of justice. Unlike Frankfurt, she adds another threshold below the sufficiency threshold that she refers to as the "personhood" threshold. At that level, *all* capabilities are lost or can be lost—that is, when patients are in a persistent vegetative state or at risk of dying. The risk of dying has immense moral urgency for her, and it will have very high priority for health care resources below the sufficiency threshold. She

---

30. Madison Powers and Ruth Faden, *Social Justice: The Moral Foundations of Public Health and Health Policy* (New York: Oxford University Press, 2006); Efrat Ram-Tiktin, "The Right to Health Care," 337–351.

31. Powers and Faden, *Social Justice*, 21.

adds, however, that in setting priorities below the sufficiency threshold, what will matter will be how badly off people are, how many there are, and the size of the expected benefit for those people. She illustrates her point by stating that if we have a limited amount of money and can either fund growth hormones for very short children or a drug that will yield 5 extra years of life for lung cancer patients, the latter choice should have priority because those individuals are saved from a premature death—that is, the loss of all capabilities.

Powers and Faden list six dimensions of well-being, each of which can influence the other dimensions, and this may be especially true with regard to health. They write, "Inequalities of one kind beget and reinforce other inequalities."[32] Health will be in that position. Individuals afflicted with poor health will generally have less ability to learn valuable skills, less ability to hold anything but a marginal job, and less effective liberty to function in society and earn the respect of others. This suggests that a just society will provide secure access to needed health care up to a sufficient level of health.

At the same time, however, a just society with only limited resources to meet unlimited health care needs will not have unlimited obligations of justice for meeting health needs, especially when those needs require extraordinarily expensive interventions that yield only minimal benefits. If that were a matter of justice, other essential dimensions of well-being would be underfunded and potentially massive numbers of individuals would be condemned to insufficiency in those other dimensions. To illustrate, patients who are in either a persistent vegetative state or a late stage of various dementing illnesses will have only very minimal just claims to needed health care because contemporary medicine has little to offer of benefit. That is, neither employment opportunities nor bonds of attachment or any capabilities that might yield increased respect will be improved. These patients are very far from any threshold of health sufficiency. However, if patients in either of these categories were to be identified with a serious life-threatening cardiac condition, Powers and Faden would not argue that these patients would have a just claim to an artificial heart, an LVAD, or any costly form of cardiac surgery. This seems to be a just and reasonable conclusion, especially if meeting such costly needs meant resources were diverted from meeting the less costly and more medically amenable needs of those below the threshold of health sufficiency. This is because there are no meaningful functional gains for patients who are so severely disabled. Powers and Faden are in agreement with Ram-Tiktin on this point.

It was noted previously that sufficientarians tend to be indifferent about matters of justice above a sufficiency threshold. However, Powers and Faden argue

32. Powers and Faden, *Social Justice*, 31.

that attention to inequalities above the threshold in various dimensions is necessary because those inequalities may have adverse health consequences for others
below the threshold.[33] This becomes a reason on their view for not being indifferent to such inequalities. Individuals far above the threshold in terms of wealth
may not use their wealth to buy a heart transplant (or any other absolutely scarce
medical good) to the disadvantage of those below the threshold in terms of both
health and wealth.

Powers and Faden claim that one of the virtues of their conception of sufficiency compared to resource-based conceptions of sufficiency is that they have an
objective reference point for judging what level of resources will be sufficient.[34] If
individuals are burdened by preventable disease or an ameliorable disability and a
shortened life span, then those individuals have a just claim to effective resources
needed to address those deficiencies. Their view is that "each of us [should] have
enough health over a long enough life span to have a decent life."[35] They add that
the appropriate understanding and application of this abstract principle will be
context sensitive. That is, as they state, "sufficiency can be pegged to what is technologically feasible with regard to both length and health-related quality of life."[36]
The example they give pertains to death from AIDS in the early 1990s. Such a
premature loss of life then could be viewed as tragic but not unjust. However, the
development of the protease inhibitors and all the other HIV-/AIDS-managing,
life-prolonging drugs since 1996 creates a very different moral background.
Denying HIV-positive patients effective access to these drugs today with a subsequent premature death would be clearly unjust for Powers and Faden.

Many of these HIV/AIDS drugs cause cardiac problems over a period of years.
These individuals will be in their sixties, short of a normal life expectancy. Their
cardiac problems should be treated. I am confident Powers and Faden would agree
with that judgment. However, then we get to those last-year-of-life costs for these
patients. They may be faced with opportunistic infections, which are costly to treat
and not ultimately defeatable. Would Powers and Faden then conclude that their
version of sufficientarianism did not require very costly medical efforts to gain
that last year of life? Would justice require that such patients be provided with
comfort care only?

We need to keep in mind that it is often not possible to predict with a high
degree of medical confidence that *this patient* has only a small chance of surviving

33. Ibid., 58–59.

34. Ibid., 59.

35. Ibid., 61.

36. Ibid., 61.

another year. Some comments by Powers and Faden quoted previously would suggest that there was a presumptive obligation of justice to use these technologies. It is not clear what their conception of sufficiency would require in these circumstances. The same will be true for Ram-Tiktin. Is the benefit too marginal, period? Or too marginal relative to cost? These are not patients with end-stage dementia; these are patients who might very much like to live that last year of life even if the quality of that life is somewhat diminished.

Powers and Faden could argue that these last-year-of-life costs for these AIDS patients are excessive and that these same resources could be saved and redeployed to meet other more basic needs for patients who are far below health sufficiency and could be brought closer to health sufficiency with those resources. This is a reasonable option, not obviously unjust. However, what would justify restricting this rationing/reallocation protocol to AIDS patients? Prima facie this looks discriminatory. To correct for that, we would need to articulate a much broader rationing/reallocation protocol, perhaps stating, in effect, that if there is a confident medical judgment that a patient with end-stage heart disease or end-stage liver disease or end-stage cancer (and so on) has less than a 20% chance of surviving another year, then he or she would no longer have a just claim to very expensive life-prolonging care. Instead, the patient would be provided with high-quality palliative care. Again, this seems reasonable enough and just enough, given limited resources and unlimited health care needs.

This last conclusion, however, does not seem incongruent with either Ram-Tiktin's or Powers and Faden's sufficientarian perspective. One implication of this view would be that metastatic cancer patients would not have a just claim to these $100,000 targeted cancer drugs that yielded only months of additional life. But then we would be left with that 7% cluster of breast cancer patients who might gain 2 or more years of extra life. This appears to be significant from Ram-Tiktin's capabilities perspective. What would Powers and Faden judge is the just response to the needs of these patients? Recall that Powers and Faden place much emphasis on the justice-relevant implications of a changing medical technology landscape. This is why AIDS patients had a just claim to the protease inhibitors. Why would not the same logic apply to the fortunate 7% of our breast cancer patients as well as whatever other cancer patients turn out to be genetically favored by other of these targeted cancer drugs? The problem is the "ragged edge" and "rough justice" issues. All these cancer patients are among the medically least well-off. However, as John Harris, a strict egalitarian, would argue, those are very meaningful months for these patients during which they hope to fully exercise their remaining human capabilities.[37] The challenge to sufficientarians is to justify

---

37. John Harris, *The Value of Life* (Oxford: Routledge & Kegan Paul, 1985), 110.

from within their framework setting the bar in this case at 1-year survival rather than 5-month survival or 2-year survival.

Currently, at least 50 of these very expensive targeted therapies ($50,000 to more than $150,000 for a course of treatment) are approved in the United States. Furthermore, although the median gain in life expectancy from any one of these drugs is very marginal, thousands of patients experience gains in life expectancy measurable in a small number of years, not months. Researchers do not know why these individuals are so fortunate. From the sufficientarian perspective of Powers and Faden, what is the most just response to the needs of these patients? If we cannot segregate the strong from the weak responders (although all are terminally ill in a broad sense because none of these drugs are curative), are we morally obligated to provide these expensive drugs to all no matter what the degree of their effectiveness? Alternatively, should all be denied these drugs if the savings would be redeployed to meet effectively the health care needs of patients who were even less well off?

Recall current proposals from cancer researchers to follow the "AIDS strategy" and attack cancers with combinations of these targeted cancer drugs as a way of addressing the problem of genetic heterogeneity. The hope would be to gain 5 extra years of life for these patients, although the cost per patient for those 5 years could be in excess of $500,000 each. Again, given 600,000 cancer deaths in the United States each year, the cost of a 5-year cohort of 3 million patients at "only" $100,000 each would be $300 billion in additional annual cancer costs. It seems something like this must be beyond the moral demands of the sufficiency principle. However, the analogy with AIDS and the protease inhibitors is compelling. Of course, AIDS patients would tend to be much younger than either heart failure or cancer patients. However, many younger individuals are faced with a very premature death from either heart failure or cancer. Does the sufficiency principle, as understood by either Powers and Faden or Ram-Tiktin, make an exception for them? If so, where would the cutoff be? Would there be an objective basis for such a cutoff in the sufficiency principle as understood by Powers and Faden or Ram-Tiktin? The problem is that 5 extra years of life expectancy would be a very substantial gain in well-being or capabilities by any measure, although these would be mostly older patients.[38] However, the aggregate costs threaten other important health care needs. Some trade-offs would be required. Appeals to considerations of well-being or capabilities will not yield the justified discriminating judgments

---

38. Carina Fourie would have concerns, as a sufficientarian, that unjust age rationing would be at issue here. See Carina Fourie, "What Do Theories of Social Justice Have to Say About Health Care Rationing? Well-Being, Sufficiency, and Explicit Age Rationing," in *Rationing Health Care: Hard Choices and Unavoidable Trade-Offs*, ed. Andre den Exter and Martin Buijsen (Antwerp: Maklu, 2012), 65–86.

called for, especially if we consider all the other terminally ill or nearly terminally ill noncancer patients who will have significant health needs as well.

Again, a 5-year gain in life expectancy is a significant health benefit. At age 80 or 85 years, these individuals would have lived a complete life. However, if they are otherwise vigorous, either because of excellent health habits or because of an excellent genetic endowment, what would justify a just and compassionate society not providing an effective medical intervention likely to yield 5 extra years of life? Alternatively, what if otherwise vigorous 85-year-olds in heart failure were also exhibiting some early indications of dementia? In a span of 5 years, the dementia might not progress beyond the moderate stage. However, if these individuals were given the artificial heart, that would facilitate their progressing to late-stage dementia (and substantial social costs). Should Powers and Faden conclude that these individuals would not have a just claim to the artificial heart for that reason? What if the story were the same as mentioned previously except these individuals were only 65 years old? Would Powers and Faden deny these individuals an artificial heart as well? If so, what would be the sufficientarian justification for that judgment? Again, the challenge has to do with trade-offs, ragged edges, and rough justice. Sufficiency, whether a matter of well-being or capabilities, is relevant in addressing practical problems of health care justice. But so are equality, utility, cost-effectiveness, quality of life, resource limits, protecting fair equality of opportunity, and personal responsibility for health. This is why, in my view, a pluralist conception of health care justice is required.

5. Conclusion

Powers and Faden, as well as Ram-Tiktin, offer sophisticated versions of sufficientarianism.[39] However, their versions are still unable to yield clear and unambiguous moral guidance regarding the most contentious problems of health care justice generated by contemporary medicine. In that respect, their views are inadequate. They might well ask what other conception of health care justice would do better.

I offer three brief responses. First, no other principled conception of health care justice will do much better. Norman Daniels has also offered a more sophisticated principled account of health care justice based on protecting fair equality

---

39. To be clear, what makes their accounts more sophisticated is their recognition that protecting health adequately is about much more than access to everything the contemporary medical armamentarium has to offer. There are social determinants of health that require the attention of policymakers as a matter of justice. I have not been able to address those complexities.

of opportunity for accessing the normal opportunity range of a society. However, he concedes that his account cannot adequately address the most difficult and challenging problems of health care rationing, such as those I discussed previously, because his theory is too abstract and indeterminate.[40] In my view, this is a limitation of every principled account of health care justice. Daniels speaks comprehensively to this issue in his more recent theory of "accountability for reasonableness."[41] Second, I would be inclined to defend a pluralistic conception of health care justice. That is, given the complexity and heterogeneity of the problems of justice in health care, no single conception of health care justice will yield "just enough" judgments of justice consistently for the full range of problems related to emerging medical technologies. Sometimes considerations of utility in relation to a specific health care allocation issue will yield a "just enough" response. Other times, considerations of equality, priority, fair equality of opportunity, liberty, or sufficiency will yield a "just enough" response. Moral argument will sometimes make clear which consideration should be determinative. However, other times, rational democratic deliberation will need to settle the matter because moral argument will not generate a clearly superior judgment. Third, John Rawls calls attention to the "burdens of judgment"; that is, no theory of justice can have all the theoretical resources necessary to address adequately the complexity of ethical issues in the real world.[42] This creates space for another kind of moral deliberation.

Often, multiple considered judgments of health care justice with regard to a specific rationing problem, such as access to the $100,000 targeted cancer drugs, might all be "just enough," although the justifications might be very different (sometimes egalitarian, sometimes utilitarian, etc.). In such cases, it might not be morally possible to offer a rationally compelling argument for saying one judgment was clearly morally superior to the other. However, consistency is needed to protect fairness. In such circumstances, I have argued that we then need to appeal to processes of rational democratic deliberation to identify what we, citizens in a just and caring society, would judge to be a just enough policy.[43] This is a form of constrained, imperfect procedural justice that supplements a more principled pluralist account of health care justice.

40. Norman Daniels, *Just Health Care* (Cambridge, UK: Cambridge University Press, 1985). Daniels concedes the limitations of his account in Norman Daniels, "Rationing Fairly: Programmatic Considerations," *Bioethics* 7 (1993): 224–233.

41. Norman Daniels, *Just Health: Meeting Health Needs Fairly* (Cambridge, UK: Cambridge University Press, 2008).

42. John Rawls, *Political Liberalism* (New York: Columbia University Press, 1993), 54–58.

43. Leonard Fleck, *Just Caring: Health Care Rationing and Democratic Deliberation*, especially Chapter 5 for a fuller account of rational democratic deliberation.

To return to the breast cancer example, we could choose to fund bevacizumab exclusively for the 7% of breast cancer patients who were strong responders, or we could choose not to fund bevacizumab with social resources for any of these patients. Morally reasonable arguments exist for both choices. For purposes of democratic deliberation, virtually all of us will be behind a health care "veil of ignorance." We might be vulnerable to breast cancer (or care about someone with that vulnerability), or we might not. We might be in the genetically favored group, or we might not. We are aware of an enormous range of disease vulnerabilities that we, or those we care about, might have reason to fear. We are also aware of how costly some of those medical interventions might be, their limited degree of effectiveness, and the limits of our willingness to spend for health needs. So we are capable in these circumstances of making thoughtful impartial judgments of health care justice that should be a product of a deliberative democracy. That impartiality is part of what ensures that the outcome of the deliberations is "just enough."

In addition, the conversation is constrained by what I refer to metaphorically as "constitutional principles of health care justice." Allocation or rationing proposals that violated any of these constitutional constraints would be ethically illegitimate. My pluralistic conception of health care is the source of these constitutional principles. They also help ensure that the outcomes of these deliberations are "just enough." Then there are many "considered judgments of health care justice" that are widely endorsed with which outcomes of these democratic deliberations must be congruent. This is what is typically referred to in the ethics literature as wide reflective equilibrium. Finally, mutual respect is essential to fair and successful democratic deliberations. This is a kind of moral sufficiency to which we should aspire.

Acknowledgments

I thank Annette Rid and Carina Fourie for numerous helpful critical comments that have certainly improved the quality of the chapter. I also thank Jean Edmunds for outstanding research support.

PART IV

Implementing Sufficiency in Health Care Policy and Economics

Chapter 13

Defining Health Care Benefit Packages

HOW SUFFICIENTARIAN IS CURRENT PRACTICE?

Dimitra Panteli and Ewout van Ginneken

1. Introduction

In May 2005, countries at the 58th World Health Assembly committed to re-structuring health financing mechanisms in order to achieve universal health coverage.[1] The World Health Organization (WHO) followed up with two reports providing guidance both for policymaking and for research priorities,[2,3] reflecting the increasing momentum of the universal coverage notion in many countries. Whereas most high-income countries have established mechanisms that ensure their populations have access to quality services that meet their needs without risking financial hardship due to their acquisition (cf. definition of universal health coverage given by WHO in *The World Health Report: Research for Universal Health Coverage*), many low- and middle-income countries are still in the process of introducing the necessary changes to make this possible.

1. World Health Organization, "World Health Assembly 58, Resolution 33. Sustainable Health Financing, Universal Coverage and Social Health Insurance," WHA58.33, presented at the 58th World Health Assembly, Geneva, May 16–25, 2005, accessed April 4, 2015, http://apps.who.int/medicinedocs/documents/s21475en/s21475en.pdf.

2. World Health Organization, *The World Health Report: Health Systems Financing: The Way to Universal Coverage* (Geneva: World Health Organization, 2010).

3. World Health Organization, *The World Health Report: Research for Universal Health Coverage* (Geneva: World Health Organization, 2013).

Traditionally, low-income countries have placed greater emphasis on the personal finance of health care, usually by means of out-of-pocket (OOP) payments, because public funding for health care is limited. Nevertheless, whereas a low-income country may be faced with low health spending, limited capacity to raise revenue, a rapidly growing population, and lack of access to care of good quality, a typical high-income country may be struggling with unsustainable growth in health spending, a rapidly aging population, the challenge of costly technology, and increasing OOP spending. However, both have a similar challenge: how to best utilize scarce resources given the financial constraints. An important aspect in this challenge is the definition of coverage—that is, the question of which services to include in a country's benefit package, to what extent, and for whom.

In the context of finite resources in any health care system, it is impossible for everyone's health needs to be met exhaustively, even under universal coverage aspirations. In practice, most high-income countries that have achieved universal coverage seem to have adopted models that approximate the two-tiered conception suggested by Beauchamp and Childress, which entails "enforced social coverage for basic and catastrophic health needs (tier 1), together with voluntary private coverage for other health needs and desires (tier 2)."[4] Mandatory ("enforced") social coverage represents a country's statutory health system. Voluntary private coverage can take the form of complementary policies that cover services excluded from, or only partially covered by, the mandatory package. It can also take the form of supplementary policies, which include services already covered in the mandatory package but offer additional advantages, such as better facilities or immediate access.

Beauchamp and Childress posit that the two-tiered model presents a compromise between different theories of justice because it offers equal treatment for a given range of services (egalitarian approach), an opportunity for free-market production (libertarian approach), a maximization of social good and decision-making based on cost-utility (utilitarian approaches), and an opportunity for many to achieve better health through quality health care (capabilities/well-being theories). Beauchamp and Childress do not specifically mention sufficientarianism as one of those theories. However, if one adopts an "ordinary language" understanding of sufficiency (i.e., "having enough"), one could argue that the model in itself is sufficientarian because some services or part of services are included in statutory coverage in order to guarantee that "basic" care is available for all, whereas the excluded services become an individual responsibility. The concept of "basic and catastrophic health needs," which are meant to be addressed by the statutory

---

4. Tom L. Beauchamp and James F. Childress, *Principles of Biomedical Ethics*, 7th edition (New York: Oxford University Press, 2013), 272–274.

system, is reminiscent of two aspects of sufficiency. On the one hand, it is important to ensure that individuals can "live a life that is sufficiently good"[5]—that is, necessitating a basic level of coverage. On the other, "what matters is whether individuals have enough not to fall below some crucial threshold of advantage"[6]—that is, also meaning that they are protected against catastrophic health expenditure. According to Crisp, "no priority is to be given" beyond the sufficiency threshold,[7] and this is also embodied in Beauchamp and Childress' conception of two-tiered health coverage because individuals can choose to insure themselves additionally to statutory coverage if they are prepared to bear the financial burden. In fact, the pervasiveness of the two-tiered coverage model may indicate that the concept of sufficiency has largely informed coverage decisions in high-income countries with universal coverage. However, the model itself does not prescribe thresholds of sufficiency, neither in the volume or types of health care one aims to cover nor in the amount of health this volume should achieve.

Other chapters in this volume discuss the notions of a "decent" or "adequate" minimum of health and "basic" or "essential" services that society should grant its citizens under constrained resources.[8] Although a general definition of health (and thus its boundaries) may form the background against which coverage decisions are taken, in practice these decisions deal with sufficiency of health *care*. Both the understanding of "what is enough" and the mechanisms for determining which services are considered "basic" (and should therefore be covered or prioritized in the statutory system) are bound to vary with system objectives and organization, which in turn relate to a country's economic, political, and cultural context. Indeed, although similarities exist in the way statutory benefit packages are determined in different countries, each system has a unique combination of substantive principles, according to which services are considered for the statutory benefit package, and relevant decision-making processes.[9]

As a general rule, a broad definition of the statutory benefit package can be found at a higher legislative level, mostly delineating the areas of care to be covered. Packages are then determined more concretely by a variety of actors at

---

5. Roger Crisp, "Equality, Priority, and Compassion," *Ethics* 113, no. 4 (2003): 745–763.

6. Paula Casal, "Why Sufficiency Is Not Enough," *Ethics* 117, no. 2 (2007): 296–326.

7. Crisp, "Equality, Priority, and Compassion"

8. In this volume, see chapters by Leonard M. Fleck (Chapter 12), Efrat Ram-Tiktin (Chapter 8), Paul T. Menzel (Chapter 11), and Carina Fourie (Chapter 10).

9. Jonas Schreyögg et al., "Defining the Health Benefit Basket in Nine European Countries: Evidence from the European Union Health BASKET project," *European Journal of Health Economics* 6, Suppl. 1 (2005): 2–10.

the regulatory level, centrally or regionally, and usually within each area of care. This results in more or less explicit benefit catalogs, which can consist of recommendations and/or the inclusion or exclusion of specific services. How these catalogs are set up is often related to how countries pay for services in different areas of care.[10]

In health systems that are financed mainly through social security, coverage decisions are taken by public institutions. By contrast, in mixed systems, such as in the United States, such decisions befall both public authorities and private insurers. A number of approaches have been adopted thus far to guide decisions on coverage priorities and thus the composition of benefit packages. They range from ranked lists based on cost–benefit ratios and spanning all areas of care (e.g., the Oregon Medicaid program) to the establishment of new institutions tasked with identifying necessary, appropriate, and cost-effective care (e.g., NICE in England).[11] Tools supporting evidence-based decision-making, such as health technology assessment (HTA), are increasingly incorporated in formal decision-making structures. HTA essentially encompasses the evaluation of a given technology (e.g., pharmaceuticals, medical devices, procedures, or interventions) across a number of domains, usually including clinical effectiveness, safety, and costs, using scientific methods.

Aiming to facilitate the understanding of how much health care is considered "enough," this chapter examines a number of country case studies with two main questions in mind: (1) Do the principles underlying the definition of benefit packages correspond to notions of sufficiency? and (2) Assuming that two-tiered systems of health coverage fundamentally embody the idea of sufficiency, is this idea implemented in practice?

It is beyond the scope of this chapter to give a normative interpretation on whether the countries under review provide sufficient coverage. However, it could be considered a first step toward systematically analyzing the extent to which the definition of essential benefit baskets is consistent with a sufficientarian approach. To date, no studies have examined sufficiency of coverage in an international comparative context with a universally agreed definition of what can be deemed sufficient or not. The analytical framework presented here could serve as a basis for future research that will aim to determine, from a normative perspective, to what extent essential health care packages are "sufficient."

10. Schreyögg et al., "Defining the Health Benefit Basket in Nine European Countries."

11. Lindsay Sabik and Reidar Lie, "Priority Setting in Health Care: Lessons from the Experiences of Eight Countries," *International Journal for Equity in Health* 7, no. 4 (2008): accessed March 5, 2015, doi: 10.1186/1475-9276-7-4.

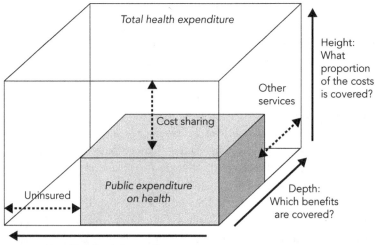

FIGURE 13.1 Dimensions of health coverage

Source: Reinhard Busse and Sophia Schlette, *Health Policy Developments 7/8 Focus on Prevention, Health and Ageing and Human Resources* (Gütersloh, Germany: Verlag Bertelsmann Stiftung, 2007).

2. Analytical Framework

Coverage in a statutory system encompasses three distinct dimensions: *breadth*, depicting the extent to which the population is covered; *depth*, describing the type and number of services covered; and *height*, accounting for the extent to which included services are covered and not subject to cost-sharing.[12,13] As is evident from Figure 13.1, coverage may take different shapes. For example, universal systems in terms of population coverage can include a limited amount of services that are fully covered, or they can have a comprehensive services package but with more cost-sharing per service.

To understand the extent to which current practice seems to overlap with important aspects of sufficiency along these three dimensions, substantive criteria

12. Schreyögg et al., "Defining the Health Benefit Basket in Nine European Countries," 2–3; Reinhard Busse and Sophia Schlette, *Health Policy Developments 7/8 Focus on Prevention, Health and Ageing and Human Resources* (Gütersloh, Germany: Verlag Bertelsmann Stiftung, 2007), 96; World Health Organization, *The World Health Report: Primary Health Care Now More Than Ever* (Geneva: World Health Organization, 2008), 26.

13. Rechel, Thomson, and van Ginneken introduce a slightly different terminology, still using breadth to denote how much of the population is covered but describing which services are covered as the "scope" of coverage and the proportion of the benefit cost covered as the "depth." Essentially, the three-dimensional model is applied identically; Bernd Rechel, Sarah Thomson, and Ewout van Ginneken, *Health Systems in Transition: Template for Authors* (Copenhagen: World Health Organization, 2010), 37.

and procedural mechanisms used for (partially) including or excluding services are explored with the help of relevant examples from a number of countries. Subsequently, notable (past) approaches toward priority-setting relevant to the sufficiency approach are briefly illustrated. The countries were chosen to cover different types of health systems (predominantly tax-funded, predominantly insurance-based, and mixed; centrally administered and decentralized) that adopt some form of a two-tiered system of coverage.[14]

Table 13.1 provides a brief overview of the coverage schemes in the reviewed countries. It presents level of application (central vs. decentralized), specifications along the three dimensions of coverage illustrated in the analytical model, existing measures for financial protection (e.g., cost-sharing caps or exemptions), types of voluntary health insurance available and the level of use of such packages,[15] the proportion of total health expenditure attributed to OOP payments, and experienced access barriers due to cost among respondents to an international survey.[16] Unless otherwise indicated, country information both in the table and in the text is from the The Commonwealth Fund.[17]

3. How Sufficientarian Is Current Health Coverage Decision-Making?

3.1. Regulation Underpinning Coverage Decisions and Sufficiency

As previously mentioned, a country's general approach toward coverage and the areas of care to be covered in the benefit package are determined at a higher

---

14. Schreyögg et al., "Defining the Health Benefit Basket in Nine European Countries"; Sabik and Lie, "Priority Setting in Health Care"; Christine Hoffmann and Reinhard Busse, "Priorisierung in Anderen Gesundheitssystemen; Was Kann Deutschland Lernen?" *Bundesgesundheitsblatt* 53 (2010): 882–889.

15. Primary insurance policies replace statutory coverage and cover people not eligible for or opting out of the statutory system. As mentioned previously, complementary policies may cover services not included in the statutory system or copayments necessary for included services, whereas supplementary policies provide additional advantages for services covered in the statutory system, such as shorter waiting times and enhanced choice of provider or amenities; Rechel et al., *Health Systems in Transition*, 50. Note that the Organization for Economic Co-operation and Development (OECD) uses a slightly different nomenclature; Organisation for Economic Co-operation and Development, *OECD Study on Private Health Insurance* (Paris: OECD, 2004).

16. The Commonwealth Fund, *Commonwealth Fund International Health Policy Survey 2014* (New York: The Commonwealth Fund, 2014).

17. Elias Mossialos et al., *International Profiles of Health Care Systems 2014* (New York: The Commonwealth Fund, 2015).

(legislative) level.[18] Given the variety of organizational structures and financing mechanisms across health care systems, one can expect the content and terminology of relevant provisions to differ substantially, along with the legal or regulatory documents in which they are anchored (Table 13.2). If, once again, one adopts an ordinary-language understanding of sufficiency to explore the stated goal of statutory provision (e.g., understands terms such as "adequate," "basic," and "essential," as indicating "having enough") and which types of services would thus be covered, as reflected in countries' relevant regulation, this hypothesis is confirmed (see the terms in italics in Table 13.2).

For example, the Canada Health Act refers to "*reasonable* health access without financial or other barriers" (italics added) as its goal for all residents. Responsibility for organizing and delivering health services in Canada is decentralized and befalls provinces and territories. The federal government subsidizes these health insurance programs through the Canada Health Transfer as long as they adhere to the criteria of the Canada Health Act (public administration, comprehensiveness, universality, portability, and accessibility). Thus, whereas comprehensiveness and universality are prerequisites for regional insurance plans, the "reasonableness" element suggests that there is a certain limit to what the system is prepared to offer.

Similarly, in New Zealand's devolved model, the government determines health policy goals, health service requirements, and the annual budget for publicly funded health care, but it is the district health boards (DHBs) that are responsible for meeting these objectives by planning, purchasing, and providing health care. As per the New Zealand Public Health and Disability Act 2000, DHBs need to provide appropriate, effective, and timely services with a focus on reducing health disparities, "to the extent that they are *reasonably achievable* within the funding provided" (italics added).

A similar focus on inequalities is observed in England. The National Health Service (NHS) is a tax-funded system that covers all residents, largely free at the point of use, "except in limited circumstances sanctioned by the Parliament." [19] Its scope is not a priori set out in legislation. The promotion of equality and fairness is clearly outlined in its guiding principles, as is the importance of value for money and sustainability. The latter two elements point toward certain limits (see discussion of the cost-effectiveness threshold in Section 3.3).

In Germany, the broad contents of the benefit package are underpinned by law in Book V of the Social Code (SGB V), but specifics are decided by the Federal

---

18. Schreyögg et al., "Defining the Health Benefit Basket in Nine European Countries."

19. Department of Health, *The NHS Constitution: The NHS Belongs to Us All* (London: Department of Health, 2013), 1–15.

Joint Committee (Gemeinsamer Bundesausschuss, G-BA), which is the highest decision-making body in the joint self-governance of physicians, dentists, hospitals, and health insurance funds. Article 3 of the SGB V stipulates that to be covered by statutory health insurance, services must be "*sufficient*, appropriate and efficient; they are not allowed to surpass the measure of necessity" (italics added). In terms of wording, this approach perhaps resembles the concept of sufficiency most closely.

The Dutch system was designed to minimize direct government involvement in the provision of acute care, as stipulated in the 2006 Health Insurance Act. The government only lays down broad legal requirements for what entitlements cover and when entitlements exist (so-called "functional entitlements"). This should entail "*essential care*," as tested against its demonstrable effect, cost-effectiveness, and need for collective financing.[20] This also means that the insurers receive great latitude in contracting care and thus interpreting the functional entitlements. The legal framework could be viewed as reflecting a sufficientarian approach, with defined essential benefits where there is a need for collective financing (because risk cannot be borne individually), on the one hand, and the option to purchase complementary and voluntary insurance packages, on the other hand.

Thus, although sufficiency is rarely invoked explicitly in the examples described previously, some concepts and ideas resembling a sufficiency notion can be traced.

3.2. Breadth of Coverage

In the WHO definition, universal health coverage implicitly encompasses all three dimensions of coverage, namely breadth, depth, and height ("all people receiving quality health services that meet their needs without exposing them to financial hardship in paying for them").[21] However, in everyday discourse, it is usually the breadth of coverage (i.e., the percentage of the population covered by the statutory scheme) that is first considered when the question arises, "Is coverage in system X universal?" There are, perhaps, two main questions in regard to breadth of coverage when one considers the sufficientarian notion "as long as everyone has enough": Who is "everyone"? and Should "enough" be understood differently for different population groups according to entitlement? In fact, in most countries

---

20. Ministry of Health Welfare and Sports, "Health Insurance in The Netherlands," accessed April 4, 2015, http://www.government.nl/documents-and-publications/leaflets/2012/09/26/health-insurance-in-the-netherlands.html.

21. World Health Organization, *The World Health Report: Research for Universal Health Coverage*.

listed in Table 13.1, entitlement is connected to either citizenship or residence, thus covering the vast majority of the population. Temporary residents or short-term visitors (e.g., tourists) are covered to a variable degree, usually for emergency services.

The most notable exception in terms of breadth of coverage among high-income countries can be seen in the United States. The US health care system developed largely through the private sector and combines high levels of funding with limited government involvement. Most Americans are covered by private health insurance, usually through plans negotiated by their employer. Public coverage programs are in place for people older than age 65 years, with certain disabilities or end-stage renal disease (Medicare), or low-income populations (Medicaid and the Children's Health Insurance Program). In 2012, before important new provisions of the Affordable Care Act (ACA) took effect, more than one-fifth of the population did not have any form of health insurance. The main systemic change brought about by ACA is the expansion of private and public insurance coverage. For private insurance, a requirement to take out policies was introduced for individuals not covered by their employers and for employers with more than 50 employees. ACA further makes provisions to increase the breadth of Medicaid coverage.[22] Hospitals, however, are obligated under federal law to provide emergency services to anyone needing such care, including uninsured and many undocumented migrants. In addition, several community health centers provide emergency care.[23] Latest coverage numbers in the United States show a notable decrease to an uninsurance rate of 13.2%.[24]

Even in systems in which breadth of coverage is near universal, vulnerable groups usually have limited or no access to services provided by the statutory system.[25] Notable examples are the Roma (as is the case in several eastern European countries) and undocumented migrants. For example, in Norway, undocumented migrants only have access to emergency acute care but are obliged to pay the full costs if possible, whereas some preventive care is free of charge. In Germany,

22. Thomas Rice et al., "United States of America: Health System Review," *Health Systems in Transition* 15, no. 3 (2013).

23. Ewout van Ginneken and Bradford Gray, "Coverage for Undocumented Migrants Becomes More Urgent," *Annals of Internal Medicine* 158, no. 5 (2013): 347–348.

24. Office of the Assistant Secretary for Planning and Evaluation, "Health Insurance Coverage and the Affordable Care Act," accessed March 17, 2015, https://aspe.hhs.gov/health/reports/2015/uninsured_change/ib_uninsured_change.cfm.

25. Ewout van Ginneken and Bradford Gray, "European Policies on Healthcare for Undocumented Migrants," in *The Palgrave International Handbook of Healthcare Policy and Governance*, ed. Ellen Kuhlmann et al. (Basingstoke, UK: Palgrave Macmillan, 2015), 631–648.

undocumented migrants have a right to health services beyond emergency care, but the procedure to reimburse the cost of nonemergency care involves public officials with a duty to report to immigration authorities, which prevents access in practice because it will lead to deportation. England provides access to primary health care free of charge (including general practitioners or local health centers). In The Netherlands, undocumented migrants have to pay the full cost of treatment unless they are unable to do so, in which case there is compensation available. This, however, may create an administrative burden and in practice a great deal of legal ambiguity, both for undocumented migrants and for providers.[26]

It is clear that even when coverage can in theory be considered universal, as is the case in the majority of high-income countries, vulnerable groups often face substantial barriers to accessing care. Therefore, one cannot unequivocally conclude that "everyone" is covered, and the application of a sufficiency principle thus seems to be compromised.

3.3. Depth of Coverage

As previously mentioned, depth of coverage is usually decided at two levels. The areas of care to be covered are decided at a higher (legislative) level and may show similarities between countries. For example, some areas of care are almost always included, such as primary care and acute inpatient care. Others, such as dental care and cosmetic surgery, are among the most likely to be excluded. However, the exact range of services contained in the benefit package is variable and subject to decision-making at the regulatory level. Benefit packages can be more or less explicitly defined.[27]

Decision-making processes leading to more explicitly defined packages and the criteria that underpin them are system-specific, but a commonality is that they are increasingly adopting evidence-based approaches. To name a few examples, the Medicare Benefit Schedule (MBS) in Australia is a concrete listing of services subsidized by the government under the Medicare Benefit Scheme. The Health Insurance Act 1973 stipulates that to be covered, services need to be clinically relevant ("generally accepted in the medical profession as necessary for the appropriate treatment of the patient") and listed on the MBS. The government is advised about which services to cover by the Medical Services Advisory Committee, which provides independent expert advice on all new and amended MBS services regarding

26. Ewout Van Ginneken, "Health Care Access for Undocumented Migrants in Europe Leaves Much to Be Desired," *Eurohealth* 20, no. 4 (2014): 11–14.

27. Schreyögg et al., "Defining the Health Benefit Basket in Nine European Countries."

their comparative safety, effectiveness, cost-effectiveness, and total cost.[28] In New Zealand, the Pharmaceutical Management Agency (PHARMAC) is responsible for the assessment and prioritization of pharmaceuticals to be included in the national formulary, medical devices, and vaccines under the New Zealand Medicines System, which is a subset of the health system. PHARMAC uses nine criteria to assess technologies, which include the health needs of all New Zealanders with particular attention to the Maori and Pacific people, availability, clinical benefit and risk, cost-effectiveness, budgetary impact and direct costs, as well as their position within government health priorities.[29]

In The Netherlands, the government defines a list of "essential" benefits, which health insurers are legally required to provide, based on recommendations from the National Health Care Institute (Zorginstituut Nederland). As a general rule, services that have been found to be effective after evidence-based evaluations are recommended for inclusion. Whereas all pharmaceuticals and medical aids are evaluated, evaluation of other categories (e.g., health services, technologies, and products) must be requested by a letter from a stakeholder. The Zorginstituut considers the following four criteria when evaluating a given intervention: necessity (severity of condition and ability of patients to pay for treatment themselves), efficacy, cost-effectiveness, and feasibility (including sustainability considerations).[30] As previously mentioned, insurers have important leeway in contracting care; as a result, differences occur between insurers in the content of contracted care benefits.

In Germany, the Federal Joint Committee (Gemeinsamer Bundesausschuss, G-BA) issues directives determining or modifying the explicit benefit catalog of the statutory health insurance funds, thus specifying which services are to be reimbursed. The general approach toward coverage is different based on the level of care: In inpatient care, services can be offered (and reimbursed) unless explicitly excluded by the G-BA (*Verbotsvorbehalt*); in ambulatory care, they need to be explicitly included in the benefit package to be reimbursed (*Erlaubnisvorbehalt*). Decisions in both cases are based on the principles of diagnostic or therapeutic benefit, medical necessity, and cost-effectiveness.[31] The G-BA is supported in

28. Medical Services Advisory Committee, "Medical Services Advisory Committee," accessed March 15, 2015, http://www.msac.gov.au.

29. Pharmaceutical Management Agency, "Decision Criteria," accessed March 15, 2015, https://www.pharmac.health.nz/medicines/how-medicines-are-funded/decision-criteria.

30. National Health Care Institute, "Health Care Coverage: A Well-Balanced Basic Health Care Package," accessed March 15, 2015, http://www.zorginstituutnederland.nl/binaries/content/documents/zinl-www/documenten/rubrieken/english/1404-health-care-coverage-a-well-balanced-basic-health-care-package/Health+Care+Coverage+%28A+well-balanced+basic+health+care+package%29.pdf.

31. Reinhard Busse, Miriam Blümel, and Diana Ognyanova, *Das Deutsche Gesundheitssystem: Akteure, Daten, Analysen* (Berlin: Medizinisch Wissenschaftliche Verlagsgesellschaft, 2013).

the scientific assessment of the evidence on medical benefit by the Institute for Quality and Efficiency in Health Care, an independent institute founded in 2004. Although all three criteria are considered in each case, it is mainly (added) benefit that determines inclusion or exclusion from the lists.[32]

In systems with less explicit benefit packages, different approaches to priority-setting for health care are in place. With the goal of promoting "appropriate, necessary and efficient" care, the National Institute for Health and Care Excellence (NICE) in England issues guidance on clinically effective treatments to be provided by the NHS and appraises health technologies with regard to their efficacy and cost-effectiveness. Technologies that are positively evaluated are made available by the NHS. Explicit rationing and prioritization have been largely rejected in the NHS context; however, NICE does employ a concrete threshold when deciding on a technology's cost-effectiveness, ranging between £20,000 and £30,000 per quality-adjusted life-year (QALY) gained.[33] Nevertheless, final NICE decisions are based not just on comparative cost-effectiveness but, rather, include other considerations, such as fair distribution of resources.[34] Finally, when issuing a recommendation, NICE can recommend that use of an intervention be restricted to a particular group of people within the population only if there is clear evidence about increased effectiveness in this subgroup or there are other reasons relating to fairness in society or relevant legal requirements.[35]

Norway does not have an explicit list of approved benefits for statutory coverage. Parliament decides about the areas of care to be covered under the publicly funded system along with criteria for cost-sharing and its caps. The necessity of certain treatments, such as elective surgery, is to be determined by the treating physician before they qualify for public reimbursement. Although the range (and budget) of services is set at the municipal level, some prioritized services, such as pediatric care, are mandatory for all municipalities. Priority-setting criteria (severity of condition, effectiveness, and cost-effectiveness) are used differently for different types of service categories. There is neither an official QALY valuation nor a

32. Federal Joint Committee, "Aufgabe des G-BA" [Task of the Federal Joint Committee], accessed June 12, 2014, https://www.g-ba.de/institution/themenschwerpunkte/methoden-bewertung/aufgabe.

33. Karl Claxton et al., "Methods for the Estimation of the National Institute for Health and Care Excellence Cost-Effectiveness Threshold," *Health Technology Assessment* 19, no. 14 (2015): 1–542.

34. National Institute for Health and Clinical Excellence, "Social Value Judgements: Principles for the Development of NICE Guidance, Second Edition," accessed April 5, 2015, https://www.nice.org.uk/proxy/?sourceurl=http://www.nice.org.uk/aboutnice/howwework/social-valuejudgements/socialvaluejudgements.jsp.

35. National Institute for Health and Clinical Excellence, "Social Value Judgements."

set threshold value for cost-effectiveness decisions; however, certain set amounts are sometimes used for comparisons or estimations (e.g., NOK 500,000—or $60,355—per QALY gained). [36] The Norwegian Knowledge Centre for the Health Services carries out economic evaluations of interventions on behalf of the Ministry of Health and Care Services, the health trusts, the Norwegian Directorate of Health, the Norwegian Medicines Agency, and the National Council for Priority Setting in Health Care.

Similarly, covered services in the Swedish system vary throughout the country due to the decentralized nature of financing and provision. Decisions on what care to prioritize given a finite health care budget rest on guidelines adopted by the Swedish Parliament (Riksdag) in 1997 in the bill "Priority Setting in Healthcare" 1996/97:60. The bill introduced the so-called "ethics platform" upon recommendation of the Parliamentary Priorities Commission. The platform is based on the principles of human dignity, need and solidarity, and cost-effectiveness in descending order of significance. The National Model for Transparent Prioritisation in Swedish Health Care (last revised in 2011) is based on those principles and is meant for prioritization decisions by all types of publicly funded health care providers, within county councils, municipalities, and privately managed health care. [37]

As perhaps expected, the definition of depth of coverage is complex and variable across countries. Interestingly, a group of core criteria seems to be similar across countries—namely that services need to be necessary and effective with a certain consideration of costs. This reflects the recognition that when the full range cannot be covered, there is merit to first eliminating those services that do not bring (added) value. However, certain criteria used in some countries bear more resemblance to specific interpretations of sufficiency. For example, the Dutch approach toward services that are easily payable by patients (not covered) is reminiscent of Crisp's position that a low (or no) priority applies to "cases concerning trivial benefits below the threshold" just as to those above the threshold. [38] The prioritization of need (Sweden) or severity of condition (Norway), on the other hand, are closer to the position that the situation is worse (and therefore to be prioritized) "the further from a sufficient level a person is." [39]

36. Norwegian Ministry of Finance, "Valuation of Life: Official Norwegian Report Nr. 10," accessed March 12, 2015, http://omega.regjeringen.no/nb/dep/fin/dok/nouer/2012/nou-2012-16-2/11/6/1.html?id=713616.

37. Mari Broqvist et al., *National Model for Transparent Prioritisation in Swedish Health Care* (Linköping: National Center for Priority Setting in Healthcare, 2011).

38. Crisp, "Equality, Priority, and Compassion."

39. Robert Huseby, "Sufficiency: Restated and Defended," *Journal of Political Philosophy* 18, no. 2 (2010): 178–197.

3.4. Height of Coverage

User charges (cost-sharing) are often used to (1) control expenditure by means of limiting (ideally unnecessary) utilization of care and (2) generate additional revenue from private sources. Although cost-sharing can introduce barriers to care for patients with lower ability to pay or make patients forgo necessary care, it may also be used to promote the efficient use of health services. The range of services for which cost-sharing requirements apply, their manner of calculation (e.g., as copayment (fixed), co-insurance (percentage), or deductible (amount to be borne before insurer will reimburse)), as well as amounts due vary considerably across systems (Table 13.1).

Height of coverage seems to be easier to modify in times of systemic changes compared to the other two dimensions. A comprehensive study by the European Observatory on Health Systems and Policies on system responses to the 2007–2008 financial crisis found that 14 countries reduced user charges or improved protection, whereas 13 increased charges to generate revenue.[40] Changes to the basis for entitlement and range of services covered in the statutory package were comparatively less common.

User charges may pose a conceptual problem from a sufficientarian viewpoint: If the goal is to provide sufficient health care (in order to ensure a sufficiently good life) for everyone irrespective of an individual's ability to pay, do OOP payments become unjustifiable? On the reverse side of the argument, if user charges promote efficiency, strengthen the financial sustainability of the system, and take vulnerable groups into consideration by means of expenditure caps and exemptions, they may contribute to the provision of a sufficient level of care for all. It is interesting to note that lower overall OOP spending in a given country does not necessarily predicate a lower likelihood that the population foregoes care due to financial reasons, at least prima facie (Table 13.1). However, it is intuitive that cost-sharing will have a more severe impact on vulnerable populations, unless these are explicitly protected in the system, thus likely detracting from a sufficiency approach.[41]

3.5. Notable Priority-Setting Initiatives

Some of the country approaches illustrated in previous sections are the result of long deliberation and experimentation with the concept of priority-setting. For

---

40. Sarah Thomson et al., *Economic Crisis, Health Systems and Health in Europe: Impact and Implications for Policy* (Maidenhead, UK: Open University Press, 2014).

41. See Govind Persad and Harald Schmidt's chapter in this volume for further discussion of the height of coverage and sufficiency (Chapter 14).

example, Norway is a pioneer with regard to priority-setting for resource allocation at different levels. The first public committee on prioritization issues, most widely known after its Chair as the Lønning I Committee, was established in 1985 and proposed an approach to priority-setting for different sectors based almost exclusively on severity of condition. A decade later, a second committee (the Lønning II Committee) was appointed and revised these criteria, adding effectiveness and cost-effectiveness of the intervention as guiding principles and stressing that the strength of underlying evidence also should be taken into account. The criteria outlined by the Lønning committees were codified in health legislation (Patients' Rights Act 1999) and several regulations. The Lønning II criteria are still observed today. A new public commission on priority-setting was formally established in June 2013, with the purpose of revising existing criteria in the contemporary context and considering if and how they should be amended and/or extended. It presented its first report to the Minister of Health in November 2014, proposing that future priority-setting be based on four principles: achieving the most and most fairly distributed healthy life-years for all; clarity of criteria; focus on a systematic, transparent, and participatory manner of application; and using a complete set of effective tools.[42]

Another renowned example of priority-setting based on the formulation of general criteria is that of the Dunning Committee in The Netherlands. The committee was assembled in 1990 and tasked with discussing principles and methods of priority-setting for the Dutch health care system. The underlying logic was that in order to be able to ensure that necessary services are readily provided, nonessential and/or ineffective services should be removed from public coverage (an approach that has since been adopted in several systems, as demonstrated previously). The idea, therefore, was for the four principles of necessity, effectiveness, efficiency, and individual responsibility to be applied successively, thus narrowing the pool of eligible services step by step (funnel approach). The committee's system was only partially implemented, largely due to the unclear definition of the four substantive criteria, which were found difficult to apply in practice.[43] The committee's first three criteria were used to guide the development of a new decision framework for priority-setting in coverage decision-making in the Dutch system, called "proportional shortfall." The proportional shortfall model assumes that priority should be given to those patients who are likely to lose the highest

---

42. Ånen Ringard and Ingrid Sperre Saunes, January 29, 2015. "Update on New Official Norwegian Report on Priority Setting in Health Care Presented," *Online HiT for Norway— HSPM*, http://www.hspm.org/countries/norway08012014/livinghit.aspx?Section=2.7%20 Health%20information%20management&Type=Section.

43. Sabik and Lie, "Priority Setting in Health Care."

proportion of health expectancy if their condition remains untreated. As with the application of the Dunning principles in the 1990s, the implementation of the model is not straightforward and remains largely theoretical despite broad acceptance.[44]

One of the most explicit and most controversial efforts to prioritize services for coverage took place in the United States. Among the goals of the 1989 health reform in Oregon was to expand the Medicaid coverage of the Oregon Health Plan (OHP) to include all Oregonians who fell below 100% of the federal poverty line. To be able to afford this expansion, the reform foresaw limiting Medicaid coverage to a package of "basic" services, which were to be prioritized by a body consisting of providers and consumers on the basis of existing evidence on effectiveness and costs, under the coordination of the newly instituted Health Services Commission.[45] The idea was that based on the budget assigned to Medicaid every 2 years, the state legislature would draw a concrete line in a prioritized list of services and Oregon Medicaid would pay for all services above it and only those. To create this ranked list of services, the Oregon Health Services Commission initially used the Quality of Well-Being Scale, a quantified tool that ranked condition–treatment pairs according to their comparative cost-effectiveness. The resulting rankings elicited substantial public backlash, and the scale was subsequently abandoned in favor of more flexible criteria, which allowed for intuitive decisions by the commissioners and the incorporation of consumer values.[46] Oregon's current approach rank orders general categories of health services based on relative importance. For example, as of 2008, a more explicit focus has been placed on preventive services and chronic conditions. Within these general categories, individual condition–treatment pairs are prioritized according to impact on health and effectiveness. Cost is used as an additional criterion when two pairs score identical on the previous two. In 2012, the Health Evidence Review Commission replaced the Health Services Commission, but the mandate and approach with regard to priority-setting have been maintained. Despite the fact that the OHP has faced both fiscal instability and enrolment issues,[47] it estimates that approximately

---

44. Liesbet van de Wetering et al., "Balancing Equity and Efficiency in the Dutch Basic Benefits Package Using the Principle of Proportional Shortfall," *European Journal of Health Economics* 14 (2013): 107–115.

45. Rice et al., "United States of America: Health System Review."

46. Sabik and Lie, "Priority Setting in Health Care."

47. Jonathan Oberlander, "Health Reform Interrupted: The Unraveling of the Oregon Health Plan," *Health Affairs* 26, no. 1 (2007): 96–105.

1.5 million people have gained health coverage due to the expanded access made possible by explicitly prioritizing health services.[48]

In combination, the previously discussed examples may point to an important issue regarding the implementation of an explicitly sufficientarian approach in health care: When it is attempted to guide policymaking using normative criteria that correspond to the principles ideally underpinning "sufficient" care, operationalization is difficult because other elements will (additionally) influence practice, such as political priorities or stakeholder pressure. On the other hand, strictly pragmatic and quantified approaches attempting to achieve "adequate" coverage for a given budget are bound to be heavily opposed because the health care needs of specific groups will be left unaddressed. As a result, the approach itself runs the risk of becoming less sufficientarian and more utilitarian in nature.

4. Conclusion

Although each country has a unique combination of principles that guide coverage decisions, processes to operationalize these principles for practice, and degree of definition of the final benefit package, it seems clear that a certain interpretation of sufficiency is reflected in all applications of two-tiered approaches aiming at universal coverage. In this respect, one could, for the purpose of describing coverage, interpret the sufficiency threshold in a given country as the volume of the shaded box in Figure 13.1. Thus, each country's approach and the trade-offs made would be reflected in the volume (e.g., how much in terms of revenue is allocated) and shape (e.g., assuming universal coverage is already achieved, how far is the range of services (i.e., depth) prioritized over cost-sharing (i.e., height)). It is evident that these trade-offs greatly depend on the country's economic, political, and cultural context. Such an interpretation also suggests that making changes in any of the three dimensions could impact the level of sufficiency of coverage and that the comprehensiveness of the benefit package alone is not an adequate indicator. For example, even with a very comprehensive benefit package, some groups may have limited coverage (e.g., Roma and undocumented migrants), or certain services may still be inaccessible due to high cost-sharing requirements, especially for vulnerable groups.

The WHO Consultative Group on Equity and Universal Health Coverage issued strategic recommendations for achieving universal coverage goals in May

---

48. Bob DiPrete and Darren Coffman, *A Brief History of Health Services Prioritization in Oregon* (March 2007), available from http://www.oregon.gov/oha/OHPR/HSC/docs/prioritizationhistory.pdf.

2014, suggesting a stepwise approach.[49] The proposed strategy entails explicit prioritization of services as a first step; the idea is to ensure that high-priority services (controlling depth) are covered for everyone (increasing breadth) with minimal cost-sharing (increasing height). This is to a certain degree reminiscent of the primary goal of the Oregon Health Plan initiative, which preferred guaranteeing "fewer services to more people rather than more services to fewer people."[50]

The need to prioritize is clearly endorsed in some of the countries with universal coverage described previously, reflecting a clear concession that not all services can be covered for everyone under a publicly funded system. This practice seems to correspond to what is likely to be required by a sufficiency principle, albeit not necessarily an explicit one. For example, in its document on social value judgments, NICE remarks that "deciding which treatments to recommend involves balancing the needs and wishes of individuals and the groups representing them against those of the wider population."[51] On the other hand, in Germany, there was both a political reluctance to openly admit to resource constraints and a corresponding mentality among the population that "everything for everybody will be made available."[52] Finally, the new guiding principles suggested by the Norwegian commission on priority-setting take the necessity for priority-setting as a given but reinforce the notion that it is to be carried out with the aim of maximizing health gains for all. In any case, explicit prioritization initiatives are not necessarily straightforward (e.g., Oregon) or uniformly translated in final coverage decisions.[53]

Experience with past and current approaches further demonstrates that the notion of sufficiency would be particularly difficult to conceptualize and implement in practice. Substantive criteria underlying statutory coverage decisions are not identical between or uncontested within countries. Necessity and effectiveness are almost always among the first considerations, even if the decision on what constitutes a "necessary" service is taken at different levels (e.g., in the form of an explicit service list or left to individual providers). The decisiveness of and approach

---

49. World Health Organization, *Making Fair Choices on the Path to Universal Health Coverage: Final Report of the WHO Consultative Group on Equity and Universal Health Coverage* (Geneva: World Health Organization, 2014).

50. Somnath Saha, Darren D. Coffman, and Ariel K. Smits, "Giving Teeth to Comparative Effectiveness Research: The Oregon Experience," *New England Journal of Medicine* 362 (2010): e18.

51. National Institute for Health and Clinical Excellence, "Social Value Judgements."

52. Corina Klingler et al., "Regulatory Space and the Contextual Mediation of Common Functional Pressures: Analyzing the Factors That Led to the German Efficiency Frontier Approach," *Health Policy* 109, no. 3 (2013): 270–280.

53. Sabik and Lie, "Priority Setting in Health Care."

toward cost-related elements, on the other hand, vary considerably. Even in countries in which fixed cost-effectiveness thresholds are not adopted, quantifying approaches have been developed to operationalize abstract criteria in a concrete way (e.g., proportional shortfall in The Netherlands and indicative benchmark amounts in Norway). Conversely, the fact that cost-effectiveness cannot be the only consideration in certain cases is understood even where fixed thresholds are in place.[54] Thus, it seems that frameworks aiming to provide a general guideline for prioritization are more likely to stipulate (un)acceptable principles or trade-offs to be made than prescribe normative approaches in a one-size-fits-all manner.[55] Taking all these aspects into account, the potential contribution of HTA for countries that are in the process of setting up mechanisms to achieve universal coverage is substantial,[56] as is the consideration of approaches (or elements thereof) that have already been attempted or instituted in more established systems.

In the absence of a consensus on substantive principles, due process becomes indispensable for fair decision-making. In their framework of "accountability for reasonableness," Norman Daniels and James Sabin set out the key elements for fair process (publicity, relevance, appeals, and enforcement).[57] Perhaps unsurprisingly, all structured approaches toward prioritizing health services attempted so far entail an element of public input and participation, be it in the form of preference elicitation or fair representation of stakeholders in decision-making processes.[58] However, this does not mean that all coverage-related processes are transparent or subject to open deliberation. In fact, formal decision-making processes for pharmaceutical coverage were found to be largely intransparent in many European countries.[59] The aforementioned strategy for achieving universal

---

54. National Institute for Health and Clinical Excellence, "Social Value Judgements"; cf. Michael Rawlins, David Barnett, and Andrew Stevens, "Pharmacoeconomics: NICE's Approach to Decision-Making," *British Journal of Clinical Pharmacology* 70, no. 3 (2010): 346–349.

55. World Health Organization, *Making Fair Choices*; see also Alex Voorhoeve, Trygve Ottersen, and Ole F. Norheim, "Making Fair Choices on the Path to Universal Health Coverage: A Précis," *Health Economics, Policy and Law* 11 (2016): 1–7.

56. Kalipso Chalkidou et al., "Health Technology Assessment in Universal Health Coverage," *Lancet* 382 (2013): e48–e49.

57. Norman Daniels and James Sabin, "The Ethics of Accountability in Managed Care Reform," *Health Affairs* 17, no. 5 (1998): 50–64; Norman Daniels, "Accountability for Reasonableness: Establishing a Fair Process for Priority Setting Is Easier Than Agreeing on Principles," *British Medical Journal* 321 (2000): 1300–1301.

58. Sabik and Lie, "Priority Setting in Health Care."

59. Dimitra Panteli, Helene Eckhardt, Alexandra Nolting, Reinhard Busse, Michael Kulig, "From market access to patient access: overview of evidence-based approaches for the

coverage proposed by WHO endorses the accountability for reasonableness frame-work and underlines the importance of public participation.[60]

Finally, it is even more challenging to determine when, after all, the coverage provided is actually sufficient, leading to a population with sufficient *health*. Not until valid and reliable information on the three dimensions of coverage is col-lected according to internationally agreed standards and an internationally agreed taxonomy of benefits can anything meaningful be said on the differences in access to health care between countries.[61] Furthermore, in order to be able to determine whether these benefits actually provide value-added and sufficient health, an overarching, common understanding of both normative sufficiency criteria and the flexibility of their implementation in real-world scenarios would have to be reached.

Acknowledgments

We thank Carina Fourie, Annette Rid, and Reinhard Busse for their support.

---

reimbursement and pricing of pharmaceuticals in 36 European countries," *Health Res Policy Syst* 13(2015):39; doi: 10.1186/s12961-015-0028-5.

60. World Health Organization, *Making Fair Choices*.

61. Even then, international comparisons can be particularly challenging and controversial, as demonstrated by the backlash to the health system ranking in World Health Organization, *The World Health Report: Health Systems: Improving Performance* (Geneva: World Health Organization, 2000).

14

Sufficiency, Comprehensiveness
of Health Care Coverage, and
Cost-Sharing Arrangements
in the Realpolitik of Health Policy

Govind Persad and Harald Schmidt

1. Introduction

Sufficientarian approaches to distributive justice aim to ensure that everyone has "enough" of morally relevant goods or services.[1] One aspect of determining what constitutes "enough" in the health care arena involves deciding which interventions comprise a decent minimum basket of preventative, curative, or rehabilitative health care benefits—that is, a basket that enables the realization of normative conceptions of sufficiency that may be based on notions of a minimally decent life, a life of dignity, or a life of genuine political equality in a democracy.[2] In practice, some countries have more comprehensive benefit packages than others.[3] Theoretical accounts can provide an independent "moral yardstick" that helps determine the extent to which international variation, rather than convergence, is acceptable.

In this chapter, we focus on a different aspect of sufficiency—namely what price individuals can be asked to pay for an otherwise sufficient basket of benefits.

1. Harry Frankfurt, "Equality as a Moral Ideal," *Ethics* 98, no. 1 (1987): 21–43.

2. Dean T. Jamison et al., "Global Health 2035: A World Converging Within a Generation," *Lancet* 382, no. 9908 (2013): 1898–1955; Carina Fourie, Chapter 1 in this volume.

3. Dimitra Panteli and Ewout van Ginneken, Chapter 13 in this volume.

A well-designed minimum package is useless if accessing it entails exorbitant costs to potential beneficiaries.[4] Out-of-pocket costs (OOPCs), such as user fees, point-of-service charges, copayments, or co-insurance, represent one category of such costs and are part of many health care systems. Policymakers are increasingly interested in directing users to effective services, which can involve raising OOPCs for less effective interventions. Insurance premiums represent another type of cost to beneficiaries. To ensure affordability, the use of an income-related cost ceiling—or sometimes several thresholds—that demarcates acceptable from unacceptable cost-sharing typically represents a cornerstone of any sufficientarian approach, regardless of how that approach is anchored in normative terms and even though approaches differ regarding where exactly the threshold should be set. As such, health care costs pose two questions: What should be the threshold for the costs individuals are asked to bear? and What should be the relationship between costs and benefits (because benefits might be designed more generously if costs are higher, and, conversely, costs might be reduced if benefits are less comprehensive)?[5]

Broader movement toward universal health coverage (UHC) has recently brought the cost of health care into sharper focus.[6] The World Health Organization (WHO) first formally endorsed UHC in 2005, calling on states to provide "access to [necessary] promotive, preventive, curative and rehabilitative health interventions for all at an affordable cost."[7] In 2015, the United Nations' General Assembly adopted the Sustainable Development Goals (SDGs) successors to the Millennium Development Goals SDG Goal 3 is concerned with health, and it includes as a target "universal health coverage ... including financial risk protection, access to quality essential health care services, and access to safe, effective, quality, and affordable essential medicines and vaccines for all."[8]

---

4. Institute of Medicine, *Essential Health Benefits: Balancing Coverage and Cost* (Washington, DC: National Academies Press, 2012), 12.

5. A third question is, of course, Who is to be covered? In principle, reducing (or not increasing) the number of people eligible for health care can allow for more generous benefit packages and/or lower OOPCs. Although the eligibility of noncitizens and others for health care is the topic of substantial debate, we bypass this issue in the following and make the simplifying assumption that policymakers seek to enable access to the widest group of people.

6. Thomas O'Connell, Kumanan Rasanathan, and Mickey Chopra, "What Does Universal Health Coverage Mean?" *Lancet* 383, no. 9913 (2014): 277–279.

7. World Health Organization, *World Health Assembly 58, Resolution 33, Sustainable Health Financing, Universal Coverage and Social Health Insurance*, http://apps.who.int/iris/bitstream/10665/20383/1/WHA58_33-en.pdf

8. Jamison et al., "Global Health 2035," 1898–1955.

Both the 2005 and the characterizations of UHC refer explicitly to cost. However, the relationship between "financial risk protection," which has become the primary yardstick for assessing the financial aspects of UHC, and thresholds for costs to individuals is complex. Levels of financial risk protection are typically measured using two indicators: the incidence of so-called "catastrophic" health expenditures (where OOPCs exceed some percentage of household resources) and the incidence of impoverishment due to out-of-pocket health payments (where OOPCs push households below the poverty line).[9] The health economists Adam Wagstaff and Eddy van Doorslaer define catastrophic expenditures as those exceeding 40% of income after accounting for expenditures on food.[10]

Should efforts to ensure that individual health care costs fall below a manageable threshold focus on protecting individuals against the costs of expensive, one-time interventions? A report by the Lancet Commission on investing in health succinctly set out some of the principal problems with such an approach:

> The most obvious administrative difficulty with the use of public funds for catastrophic coverage is that the definition of catastrophic for individual patients depends on their income. Therefore, means testing at all income levels must be enforced or, more typically, catastrophic coverage is defined at such a high level that many expenses that are catastrophic for poor people remain uncovered. As the health economist Austin Frakt has argued, "almost any cost is catastrophic if you are poor." A second difficulty is that the natural response of providers and patients will be to avoid less costly interventions in favour of more costly ones in order to receive coverage. Third, and most important, ... evidence suggests that coverage of only high-cost procedures might be an inefficient way to buy financial protection.[11]

Instead, the commission advocated an alternative approach termed "progressive universalism," which can be realized in two subforms: by subsidizing interventions frequently used by poor people, or by exempting poor people from insurance premiums and copayments.[12]

---

9. Jennifer Prah Ruger, "An Alternative Framework for Analyzing Financial Protection in Health," *PLoS Medicine* 9, no. 8 (2012), accessed June 4, 2015, doi:10.1371/journal. pmed.1001294.

10. Adam Wagstaff and Eddy van Doorslaer, "Catastrophe and Impoverishment in Paying for Health Care: With Applications to Vietnam 1993–1998," *Health Economics* 12, no. 11 (2003): 921–934.

11. Jamison et al., "Global Health 2035," 1936.

12. Jamison et al., "Global Health 2035," 1898–1955.

In this chapter, we illustrate how individual health care costs pose the issue of a fair threshold for medical costs by reviewing the introduction of essential health benefits (EHBs) as part of the Affordable Care Act (ACA),[13] the major health reform measure recently adopted in the United States. Among the questions debated as part of this reform were which services should be covered and what cost-sharing arrangements are appropriate. We argue that many health insurance plans, particularly those with significant copayments, may not protect individuals from health care costs that threaten their access to a decent minimum of care, and that individuals may be encouraged to purchase insurance at levels that are inadequate if they become ill, leading to insufficient access to otherwise sufficient care. In particular, because financial burdens that impoverish people are incompatible with a minimally decent life, ensuring that people remain above a decent minimum, however defined, after paying for health care is a desideratum for health system design, including cost-sharing.

2. Essential Health Benefits in the Affordable Care Act

Currently, as has been the case historically, the United States lacks uniform national standards for EHBs. In part, the absence of national standards reflects the complex mix of private and public providers through which health care is organized:

1. Private, employer-sponsored health insurance covers 48% of the population, with larger employers offering their own programs and smaller ones purchasing in groups from insurers.
2. Medicare (covering 16%) and Medicaid and the Children's Health Insurance program (covering 14%) are financed by federal and state governments. These organizations provide services for people older than age 65 years, the least well-off, and individuals who meet special criteria, such as patients with end-stage renal disease.
3. Tricare provides services for active military personnel, and the Veterans Health Administration provides services for former servicemen and -women (3% are covered in this way).
4. Four percent of the population purchases insurance privately on the market.[14]

---

13. Patient Protection and Affordable Care Act, 42 U.S.C. §18001 et seq.

14. Kenneth Finegold, *New Census Estimates Show 3 Million More Americans Had Health Insurance Coverage in 2012 (ASPE Issue Brief)* (Washington, DC: US Department of Health

Until recently, the United States had no universal medical coverage, and in 2010, when the Patient Protection and Affordable Care Act (ACA) was passed, approximately 60 million people completely lacked health insurance.[15] ACA implemented an individual mandate that required people to either purchase insurance or incur a tax penalty.[16] ACA also introduced insurance exchanges to enable purchasers to select policies from providers that have undergone quality screening and offer a set of EHBs, which all providers participating in the exchanges (as well as outside of them) were required to cover from 2014 onward.

3. The Affordable Care Act's Benefit Package

US legislators first addressed the question of what levels of benefits should be covered when Congress established Medicaid in 1965. Congress required that Medicaid participants have access to "medically necessary care," but did not define what this meant.[17] Although some private plans developed working definitions and the subject became the matter of lawsuits, it was not until the 2010 health reform that it was revisited on a broader scale.

ACA's provisions regarding EHBs are relatively brief and apply to health plans sold in the individual and small-group markets, as well as to Medicaid coverage. They do not apply to self-insured health plans, those in the large-group market (typically companies with more than 100 employees), or grandfathered health plans (those in existence when ACA was passed). Section 1302 of ACA requires that plans provide services in at least 10 categories: (1) ambulatory patient services; (2) emergency services; (3) hospitalization; (4) maternity and newborn care; (5) mental health and substance use disorder services, including behavioral health treatment; (6) prescription drugs; (7) rehabilitative and habilitative services and devices; (8) laboratory services; (9) preventive and wellness services and chronic disease management; and (10) pediatric services, including oral and vision care. Within these categories, benefits must be equal to the scope of benefits covered in "a typical employer plan."[18] The content of EHBs became the subject of intense

and Human Services, 2013); See also Thomas Rice et al., "United States of America: Health System Review," *Health Systems in Transition* 15, no. 3 (2013): 1–431.

15. Jacob Molyneux, "The Top Health Care News Story of 2010: Health Insurance Dominated the Year," *American Journal of Nursing* 111, no. 1 (2011): 14–15.

16. Elenora E. Connors and Lawrence O. Gostin, "Health Care Reform—A Historic Moment in US Social Policy," *JAMA* 303, no. 24 (2010): 2521–2522.

17. Daniel Callahan, "Medical Futility, Medical Necessity. The-Problem-Without-a-Name," *Hastings Center Report* 21, no. 4 (1991): 30–35.

18. Patient Protection and Affordable Care Act, 42 U.S.C. §18002(b)(2)(A).

lobbying from numerous interest groups, including patient groups, large employers, and health plans, during ACA's passage through Congress and in subsequent stages.[19]

ACA required the US Department of Health and Human Services (DHHS) to commission a report from the Institute of Medicine (IOM) that would recommend a process for defining and updating EHBs. Addressing the definition of "typical employer," the report noted difficulties in narrowing down the concept: If a "typical employer" should be representative of most employers, then the term refers to a small employer because 98% of all employer firms are classified as small. By contrast, if the term refers, then the "typical employer" is large, since large employers cover 65% of all employees.[20] Reviewing the scope of benefits and premiums offered by small and large employers, the report found them to be broadly similar. However, benefit design differed frequently, with smaller employers more frequently having higher deductibles. Ultimately, the report suggested a focus on the health plans of small employers because most growth was expected in this sector.

The report considered two approaches to formulating a list of benefits. One strategy would specify a set of benefits first and consider cost later; another would establish a cost threshold first and then decide which benefits to include. IOM was unequivocal that the latter approach was superior. It proposed to take as a point of departure the national average premium (approximately $6,000) that small employers would have paid in 2014 for a mid-level single-person plan, had ACA not been enacted.

IOM's recommended method for defining EHBs was pragmatic and process driven, and the institute did not set out a "shopping list" of "best buy" items. Its report focused on specifying criteria for determining the content of the aggregate EHB package and criteria for specific components (Table 14.1). It recommended starting with a typical small employer plan, developing a preliminary service list, and then applying the criteria to adjust the list as appropriate. Overall cost would be incorporated from the outset. It then proposed using public deliberation processes and other public participatory processes to provide further guidance, before issuing final guidance on inclusions and permissible exclusions of services.

IOM's proposal received a cold response. Its bold attempt to tackle rising health care costs by starting with a cost target smacked too much of unacceptable

---

19. Ezekiel J. Emanuel, *Reinventing American Health Care: How the Affordable Care Act Will Improve Our Terribly Complex, Blatantly Unjust, Outrageously Expensive, Grossly Inefficient, Error Prone System* (New York: PublicAffairs, 2014).

20. Institute of Medicine, *Essential Health Benefits*.

Table 14.1 Criteria for Determining EHBs

In the aggregate, the EHB package must
- Be affordable for consumers, employers, and taxpayers.
- Maximize the number of people with insurance coverage.
- Protect the most vulnerable by addressing their needs.
- Encourage better care practices by promoting the right care to the right patient in the right setting at the right time.
- Advance stewardship of resources: maximize high-value services, minimize low-value services. Value is defined as outcomes relative to cost.
- Address the medical concerns of greatest importance to enrollees in EHB-related plans, as identified through a public deliberative process.
- Protect against the greatest financial risks due to catastrophic events or illnesses.

Specific components (individual services, devices, or drugs) must
- Be safe—expected benefits should be greater than expected harms.
- Be medically effective, supported by a sufficient evidence base, or in the absence of evidence on effectiveness, a credible standard of care is used.
- Demonstrate meaningful improvement over current services/treatments.
- Be a medical service, not serving primarily a social or educational function.
- Be cost-effective so that the health gain for individuals and the population is sufficient to justify the additional cost to taxpayers and consumers.

Caveats
- Failure to meet any of the criteria should result in exclusion/significant limits on coverage.
- Each component is still subject to the aggregate EHB package criteria.

EHBs, essential health benefits.
Source: Adapted from IOM (2010); Institute of Medicine, *Essential Health Benefits: Balancing Coverage and Cost* (Washington, DC: National Academies Press, 2012), 55.

rationing for both consumer and provider groups.[21] Due to concerns about political pressure, DHHS also did not go along with the key elements. Instead, in what has been described as "passing the buck,"[22] DHHS announced that there would be no national set of benefits but that states individually would need to identify

---

21. David Himmelstein, "Response to the Institute of Medicine's Recommendation That Cost Determine Insurance Policies' 'Essential Benefits'," *International Journal of Health Services* 42, no. 3 (2012): 571–573.

22. Noam N. Levey, "Passing the Buck—Or Empowering States? Who Will Define Essential Health Benefits?" *Health Affairs (Millwood)* 31, no. 4 (2012): 663–666.

EHBs, working from a benchmark plan. The benchmark could be (1) one of the three largest small-group plans in the state by enrollment, (2) one of the three largest state employee health plans by enrollment, (3) one of the three largest federal employee health plans by enrollment, or (4) the largest health maintenance organization plan offered in the state's commercial market by enrollment.[23]

ACA gave IOM no space to propose a way forward regarding the financial impact on users, which was set out clearly in Section 1302 of ACA. Coverage was to be provided under four "metal" tiers. Plans in different tiers do not differ in content—all cover the same interventions—but they differ in cost-sharing. ACA stipulates that a bronze-level health plan will cover 60% of health care costs, with 40% to be met by the user. Plans cover 70% of health care costs in the silver level, 80% in gold, and 90% in platinum, with users responsible for the respective remainder. In addition, insurers may offer a plan with lower actuarial value than that of the bronze plan to individuals under 30 years of age and to those who are otherwise exempt from the insurance mandate because available coverage is unaffordable or enrolment would constitute a hardship. Insurers selling plans on the exchanges are not obliged to cover all four levels, but they must offer one silver and one gold plan.

ACA also adopted several measures to reduce the financial impact on insured individuals. For all tiers, ACA caps the extent of cost-sharing achieved through OOPCs, requiring health plans to cover OOPCs that exceed the cap amount. In 2014, the OOPC cap was approximately $6,000 for an individual and $12,000 for a family. Where insurance is purchased through an exchange, people with incomes below 400% of the federal poverty level (FPL)—defined as $11,490 for a single-person household and $23,550 for a four-person household in 2014—can further reduce the OOPC cap to as low as approximately $2,000 (Table 14.2). All preventive care is exempt from OOPCs. In addition, ACA provided refundable tax credits to individuals below 400% of the FPL, which aimed to offset the financial burdens of premiums on lower-income households by reducing their tax burden or even making their tax burden negative.[24]

For example, an individual with an income of $17,235 (150% of FPL in 2014) would be expected to pay no more than 6.3% ($1,086) of her income per year for the second-lowest-cost silver plan. The remainder of the plan's cost would be covered by tax credits. In addition, her OOPCs could not exceed $2,167 (the OOPC cap of $6,350 minus her two-thirds subsidy of $4,233). In the period of October 1, 2013—March 1, 2014, 18% of those who selected a marketplace plan opted for

---

23. Levy, "Passing the Buck—Or Empowering States?" 665.

24. For a useful overview of these credits, see Center for Budget and Policy Priorities, "Premium Tax Credits: Answers to Frequently Asked Questions," accessed January 24, 2015, http://www.cbpp.org/sites/default/files/atoms/files/QA-on-Premium-Credits.pdf.

Table 14.2 Premium Tax Credits and OOPC Subsidies for EHBs

Household Income (% FPL)[a]	Expected Contribution (% of Household Income)	OOPC Subsidies (Reduction of Maximum OOPC)
Up to 133	2	Two-thirds
133–150	3–4	
150–200	4–6.3	
200–250	6.3–8.05	One-half
250–300	8.05–9.5	
300–400	9.5	One-third

[a]FPL in 2014 was $11,490 for a single-person household and $23,550 for a four-person household.
EHBs, essential health benefits; FPL, federal poverty level; OOPC, out-of-pocket costs.
Source: US Department of Health and Human Services, Office of the Assistant Secretary for Planning and Evaluation, "2014 Poverty Guidelines," accessed January 24, 2015. https://aspe.hhs.gov/poverty/14poverty.cfm.

the bronze level, with 63% opting for silver, 11% for gold, and 6% for platinum. [25] Eighty-three percent of those selecting a plan on an exchange chose one for which they received financial assistance; 93% of those selecting a silver plan are eligible for federal premium assistance.

ACA's subsidy provisions function, although never explicitly, as protection against costs that exceed a threshold. The OOPC limits and premium subsidies serve to protect households against excessive medical costs incurred after they have purchased a plan that, at least in principle, secures access to sufficient medical care. In so doing, they reduce the number of households that fall below the poverty line as a result of seeking care.

4. Financial Thresholds and Health Care Costs

Health care costs—including insurance premiums and OOPCs—can worsen households' financial positions. Ill health can have similar effects, whereas good health can improve financial position. Although policymakers frequently set thresholds at levels different from the theoretical literature, both policymakers and sufficientarian philosophers share a commitment to thresholds. Some policy

---

25. US Department of Health and Human Services, "Health Insurance Marketplace: March Enrollment Report; For the Period: October 1, 2013–March 1, 2014," accessed January 24, 2015, https://aspe.hhs.gov/health/reports/2014/marketplaceenrollment/mar2014/ib_2014mar_enrollment.pdf.

proposals employ an *absolute* threshold of resources below which no individual should fall—for instance, the $1.25/day global poverty line adopted by the World Bank. Others employ a *societally relative* threshold, such as the European Union's definition of poor households as those falling below 60% of the median income in their society. Adopting a societally relative threshold means that a household whose income is above the threshold in a less-developed country might fall below the threshold if it emigrates to a wealthier nation. It also entails that any society with substantial inequality, no matter how high the median income, is likely to have members who fall below the threshold. Still others use a *individually relative* threshold: As economists Olivia Mitchell and Gary Fields state, "A standard of relative adequacy might be adopted where adequacy could be judged relative to one's level of consumption prior to the event precipitating economic insecurity."[26] Adopting this approach entails that two households in the same society could have the same income or same net worth but fall on different sides of the threshold depending on their prior income.

We suggest that the individually relative threshold is least defensible. Although wealthier households may privately prefer to insure their current level of consumption, insuring such consumption is not a high-priority use of public funds. Nor is it morally appealing to ignore the plight of households experiencing chronic medical costs that are small in individually relative terms but, over time, lead to growing disadvantage and social exclusion. In contrast, protecting households against the detrimental effects of expenses that threaten to exclude them from participation in society is widely agreed, not only by sufficientarians but also by theorists ranging from egalitarians to classical liberals, to be a public priority.[27] This provides support both for the societally relative threshold and for the absolute threshold.

Different approaches to health care financing can affect not only households' physical health but also their financial health. An entirely publicly funded health care system that does not require individuals to devote income toward premiums or significant OOPCs, such as the UK's National Health Service, will not drop households below a threshold because of excessive health care costs. However, if a publicly funded system can offer only a limited package of benefits, households may fall below a threshold because of ill health that prevents work.

---

26. Gary S. Fields and Olivia S. Mitchell, "Reforming Social Security and Social Safety Net Programs in Developing Countries," in *Development Issues: Presentations to the 47th Meeting of the Development Committee*, ed. P. Mountfield (Washington, DC: The World Bank, 1993), 116.

27. See Rawls, *Justice as Fairness* (Cambridge: Belknap Press, 2001), 132; Matt Zwolinski, "Libertarianism and the Welfare State," forthcoming in *The Routledge Handbook of Libertarianism*, eds. Jason Brennan, Bas van der Vossen, and David Schmidtz (forthcoming 2016).

ACA's approach to health care provision, particularly the cap on OOPCs and the subsidy for premiums, helps to limit health care costs. However, ACA's caps and subsidies still allow some individuals to fall below a poverty threshold due to health care costs. Even reaching the cap of approximately $2,000 in OOPCs to which a family near the poverty line is exposed under ACA would almost certainly drop a household near the poverty line into poverty. The same is true, although to a lesser extent, for premium costs. Although households can be exempted from ACA's requirement to purchase insurance and pay premiums if the payments would cause hardship or exceed 8% of income,[28] exemption simply leaves a household uninsured, exposing it to potentially unlimited OOPCs. The same is true for the choice to make the fee payment for failing to purchase insurance.

By providing health care coverage without premiums and with limited OOPCs to households below 138% of the poverty line, ACA's initially intended expansion of Medicaid would have substantially reduced the danger of households near the poverty line becoming impoverished by OOPCs and premiums. However, the Supreme Court made the Medicaid expansion voluntary, and nearly half of US states have refused to expand Medicaid for adults without dependent children, with many of these states providing Medicaid only to adults with dependents who fall substantially below the poverty line.[29] Furthermore, even in those states that expanded Medicaid, households above the poverty line can be subjected to cost-sharing requirements up to 5% of yearly income, which means that households within Medicaid could still be impoverished by OOPCs.[30]

In addition, the design of the metal tiers, with the same coverage but different levels of cost-sharing, when combined with the choice to design the subsidies to cover a silver plan, raises the risk that poorer households will be exposed to high OOPCs. Households can receive the OOPC subsidies only if they choose silver plans,[31] and they receive tax credits toward premiums that are based on purchasing a silver plan. A silver plan provides the exact same benefits as a platinum plan, but it has lower premiums and is actuarially predicted to involve higher OOPCs.

28. US Department of Health and Human Services, "Exemptions from the Fee for Not Having Health Coverage," accessed January 24, 2015, https://www.healthcare.gov/fees-exemptions/exemptions-from-the-fee.

29. Kaiser Family Foundation, "Medicaid Income Eligibility Limits for Adults at Application, as of August 28, 2014 (Table)," accessed January 24, 2015, http://kff.org/state-category/medicaid-chip/medicaidchip-eligibility-limits.

30. Kaiser Commission on Medicaid and the Uninsured, *Premiums and Cost-Sharing in Medicaid (Policy Brief)* (Menlo Park, CA: Kaiser Family Foundation, 2013), 2.

31. Kaiser Family Foundation, *Focus Health Reform: Patient Cost-Sharing Under the Affordable Care Act* (Menlo Park, CA: Kaiser Family Foundation, 2012).

For many other goods, such as food, clothing, transportation, and housing, poorer households ensure that they preserve financial sufficiency by making functional but less luxurious purchases. The uniformity of the metal tiers excludes the possibility of purchasing insurance that covers fewer interventions. Although there may be good arguments for not differentiating coverage by tier, related to concerns about adverse selection and about underinsured households imposing costs on hospitals and physicians, the choice not to subsidize cost-sharing for plans at the gold or platinum level seems to assume that poorer households should accept the silver plan's comparatively higher level of cost-sharing. This is so even though poorer households are frequently less able to self-insure, making the purchase of gold or platinum insurance—which is actuarially predicted to cover a larger share of health care expenses—more rational for them.

Meanwhile, ACA provides subsidies even to households in little danger of falling below any morally significant threshold. OOPCs totaling $9,000 for a four-person household at 400% of poverty—one making more than $90,000 per year—would not drop that household below an absolute or a societally relative threshold. Indeed, even individually relative thresholds do not regard a household that incurs OOPCs amounting to 10% of income as in danger of financial insufficiency. Furthermore, preventing people from falling below a decent social minimum is a morally more urgent priority than providing subsidies that protect better-off households against income fluctuations. The US tax code does not permit taxpayers younger than age 65 to deduct OOPCs from their taxable income until the OOPCs exceed 10% of income.[32] Although middle-class and wealthy households may well wish to insure themselves against such OOPCs, such insurance is not a priority for public spending. Indeed, allowing households who can afford higher OOPCs without risk of poverty to choose higher OOPCs might help to encourage greater cost awareness in the market for medical services.

5. Limiting Costs Within the Affordable Care Act's Framework

How might ACA evolve to better promote the goal of keeping citizens above a threshold? Perhaps the most important evolution would be the broadening of access to Medicaid. The judicially imposed decision to give states discretion whether to expand Medicaid exposed many lower-income households to burdensome OOPCs and premiums. If more states expand Medicaid access, households near the poverty line will be insured while being protected against potentially

---

32. 26 U.S.C. § 213(a), (f).

impoverishing OOPCs and insurance premiums. States can and should also choose to further reduce the OOPCs within the Medicaid program. Although nominal OOPCs may serve an important gatekeeping function, they should not expose households to poverty. To the extent that financial incentives to choose cost-effective interventions are desirable, paying patients to choose those interventions, rather than imposing OOPCs, would prevent the risk of imposing excessive costs.[33]

Another evolution would be a shift in the OOPC subsidies. The current structure of the OOPC subsidies lacks a defensible foundation: They leave poorer households exposed to impoverishment despite being insured while arguably being too generous to better-off households. They also contain sharp "cliffs"—the transitions between different subsidies and out of the subsidy program—that are difficult to justify. A better design for the OOPC subsidies would cover all but nominal OOPCs for individuals up to 138% of the poverty line—the Medicaid access cutoff—and would phase OOPC subsidies out in a continuous, rather than stepwise, manner after that. Ending the subsidy before 400% of FPL could allow the increased coverage at lower incomes to be revenue-neutral. Another alternative to OOPC subsidies for wealthier households would be access to loans that enable them to spread the costs of one-time medical expenses over several years.

Extending OOPC subsidies to lower-income households receiving premium tax credits who choose to purchase gold or platinum plans instead of silver plans would also help to ensure financial sufficiency. Purchasing a gold or platinum plan—despite these metals' evocations of luxury—simply involves making larger prepayments for the exact same package of interventions in exchange for a reduced actuarial probability of high OOPCs. It does not make sense to deny households who choose to minimize their downside risk an OOPC subsidy, particularly because such a subsidy will likely be less costly given the reduced OOPCs in gold and platinum plans.

Moving from OOPCs to premiums, the increased premiums permitted under ACA for subgroups of the population (tobacco users, overweight individuals, and older people) should be designed so that they do not threaten financial sufficiency.[34] Premiums should be such that no household, regardless of medical risk factors, risks being impoverished by purchasing insurance. The exemption that permits individuals whose insurance would exceed 8% of income to go uninsured

33. Harald Schmidt and Ezekiel J. Emanuel, "Lowering Medical Costs Through the Sharing of Savings by Physicians and Patients: Inclusive Shared Savings," *JAMA Internal Medicine* 174, no. 12 (2014): 2009–2013.

34. Kristin Madison, Harald Schmidt, and Kevin G. Volpp, "Smoking, Obesity, Health Insurance, and Health Incentives in the Affordable Care Act," *JAMA* 310, no. 2 (2013): 143–144.

without paying a penalty represents another major gap that allows health care costs to threaten financial sufficiency. It would be preferable to mandate that these individuals purchase a plan that protects them against health care costs that would leave them below a threshold while ensuring that they can access such a plan without impoverishment.

Finally, IOM's suggestion that EHBs protect against financial risks should be reconceived. Rather than subsidizing access to one-time, high-cost interventions such as high-cost chemotherapy that would be prohibitively expensive without insurance, EHB design should put the highest priority on ensuring access to interventions that help to sustain and improve households' ability to maintain financial sufficiency in the long term, particularly among lower-income households. ACA's subsidies for preventive care are congruent with this goal, but curative interventions can also help in achieving financial sufficiency. For example, interventions to help individuals quit smoking, overcome substance abuse, and deal with mental illnesses can ensure that earners stay in the workforce and continue earning income for their households. The same is true for interventions that address chronic childhood conditions such as learning disabilities and autism.

ACA represents an important step toward a health care system that ensures that every US citizen has access to a decent quantum of health care. However, whether it can do so while also ensuring that citizens receiving such care do not fall below a decent financial standard depends on how its financing structure evolves. A design that places greater emphasis on preventing impoverishment due to OOPCs and premiums, and that finances the achievement of that goal by reducing unnecessary subsidies to better-off households, would better accord with a sufficientarian approach to health care. Reducing impoverishment caused by ill health or lack of funds for health care helps to ensure that citizens can secure minimally decent lives.

Acknowledgments

We are grateful for feedback on previous versions of the chapter by Anne Barnhill, Ezekiel Emanuel, and Jen Ruger and to Francis Terpening for editorial assistance. The usual caveats apply, and all errors are the authors' alone.

15

Applying the Capability Approach in Health Economic Evaluations

A SUFFICIENT SOLUTION

Paul Mark Mitchell, Tracy E. Roberts, Pelham M. Barton, and Joanna Coast

1. Introduction

Economic evaluation is an analytic approach used to weigh the costs and consequences of interventions competing for the same resources. It provides a systematic way of dealing with scarcity, a core economic concept meaning that there are an unlimited number of wants to provide within a finite amount of resources. In health care, scarcity plays an important role, with limits on how many doctors, nurses, hospitals, and interventions can be provided within available resources. Economic evaluations in health have evolved in the past half century to help achieve the aims of a health care system in an efficient manner. Specifying the aims of a health care system and determining the meaning of efficiency for each health care system, however, involve normative judgments that are likely to vary across jurisdictions and societies. Although the standard health economic evaluation approach focuses on an objective that aims to maximize population health, there is enduring debate as to the appropriateness of this objective. A new approach emerging as an alternative is the use of the capability approach, developed by Amartya Sen. In this chapter, we aim to show how economic evaluation in health has developed over time, and we discuss its core tenets and underlying assumptions. We then present a new way of conducting economic evaluation based on people's capabilities. We call this alternative the sufficient capability approach and present an illustrative example of the approach. Although the work presented in this chapter has been primarily developed in the UK context, the potential application of the sufficient capability approach is not restricted to any jurisdiction.

2. Health Economics and Health Economic Evaluation: Overview

The study of the economics of health and health care has grown significantly in approximately the past 50 years, ever since Kenneth Arrow wrote his seminal paper on the welfare economics of medical care in 1963, setting out the need for a different approach in economic analysis when assessing the provision of health care.[1] Health economics has developed a number of unique methods for measuring the benefits of health interventions, which are, for the most part, focused on the quantification of health benefits from interventions.

The role of health economic evaluations in aiding decision-making has grown significantly in approximately the past 15 years, with increasing application of economic evaluations in developing countries as well.[2] This can be partly attributed to the foundation of the English advisory body for health guidance, the National Institute for Health and Care Excellence (NICE), in 1999. Since then, NICE has stipulated the requirement for economic evaluations for selected new interventions to be conducted before they can be recommended for use within the National Health Service.[3] This requirement has led to a significant increase in the use of economic evaluations within the United Kingdom, and the use of health economic evaluations is increasing globally also.[4]

2.1. Theories Underpinning Health Economic Evaluation

2.1.1. Welfarism

Alongside the numerous definitions used to define economics, welfarism is a term that has many interpretations, and it has hence been applied in a variety of

---

1. Kenneth J. Arrow, "Uncertainty and the Welfare Economics of Medical Care," *American Economic Review* 53, no. 5 (1963): 941–973.

2. Peter J. Neumann et al., "The Changing Face of the Cost-Utility Literature, 1990–2012," *Value in Health* 18, no. 2 (2015): 271–277.

3. NICE, *Developing NICE Guidelines: The Manual* (London: National Institute for Health and Care Excellence, 2014).

4. Neumann et al. "The Changing Face."

ways. When referring to welfarism, welfarist, or welfare economics, we mean the interpretation as noted by Sen as a focus on individual utilities only, in terms of desire and satisfaction based on people's preferences.[5] Welfare economics is the standard theoretical framework in areas such as environmental economics and transport economics,[6] and it is the theoretical basis for the majority of economic evaluations applied in public policy by the UK government.[7]

There are four key principles on which welfarism attempts to achieve economic efficiency.[8] The first principle is known as *utilitarianism*. Utilitarianism assumes that each individual in society is a rational agent. Under utilitarianism, individuals order their options so that they achieve their optimum or highest possible level of utility or preferences.

The second principle of welfarism is *individualism*. Under individualism, individuals themselves are thought to be the best judges of how to maximize their utility, with a laissez-faire approach from the state that permits utility maximization by individuals.

Consequentialism is the third principle. Under consequentialism, the outcome of choices made by individuals is the only consideration for assessing their goodness. The means by which the ends or outcomes are reached are deemed irrelevant.

The final principle is *welfarism*. Welfarism can be defined in many different ways, but the principal tenet of welfarism is concerned with the judgment that the goodness of states be based only on the aggregation of individual utility.

The main type of economic evaluation arising from the theoretical basis of welfare economics is cost–benefit analysis (CBA). The main aim of CBA is to compare interventions by valuing the costs and benefits of different interventions or treatments, usually in monetary terms.[9] CBA plays a major role in

---

5. Amartya Sen, *Inequality Reexamined* (Oxford: Oxford University Press, 1992), 12–30.

6. See, for example, Nick Hanley and Edward B. Barbier, *Pricing Nature: Cost–Benefit Analysis and Environmental Policy* (Cheltenham, UK: Elgar 2009); Kenneth Button, *Recent Development in Transport Economics* (Cheltenham, UK: Elgar, 2003).

7. HM Treasury, *"The Green Book: Appraisal and Evaluation in Central Government"* (London: The Stationary Office, 2003).

8. Four principles of welfarism are drawn from Jeremiah Hurley, "Welfarism, Extra-welfarism and Evaluative Economic Analysis," in *Health, Healthcare and Health Economics: Perspectives on Distribution*, ed. Morris L. Barer, Thomas E. Getzen, and Greg L. Stoddart (Chichester, UK: Wiley, 1998), 373–395; Jeremiah Hurley, "An Overview of the Normative Economics of the Health Sector," in *Handbook of Health Economics Vol. 1, Part A*, ed. Anthony J. Culyer and Joseph P. Newhouse (Oxford: North-Holland, 2000), 55–118.

9. Michael F. Drummond et al., *Methods for the Economic Evaluation of Health Care Programmes* (Oxford: Oxford University Press, 2005), 211–214.

aiding decision-making in areas concerning transport and other areas across the public sector, such as environment and education projects.[10] The use of CBA in health care, however, remains somewhat on the periphery of decision-making, due at least in part to the difficulty attached to the direct monetary valuation of a life.[11,12]

CBA focuses on allocative efficiency—that is, the overall impact of a project across the society in which resources are being allocated. This means that when CBA is applied within the health service, all health and non-health-related costs and benefits are, in welfarist theory, accounted for within monetary outcomes known as willingness to pay (WTP). Assuming costs are the same for providing different interventions, the option that produces the highest net benefit, judged by how much people are willing to pay for different interventions, is the option that produces the optimal allocation. Allocative efficiency allows for comparison of welfare across multiple interventions for different population groups.[13] Practical examples of allocative efficiency studies linked with the CBA framework within health care include comparing helicopter ambulance services, heart operations and hip replacements,[14] and mental health care compared to cancer and elderly care.[15]

A major issue with the application of CBA within a health care setting is the monetary valuation of the benefits of health improvements to human life, thereby directly or indirectly leading to a monetary value on a human life.[16] However, many economists believe it is the best way of evaluating outcomes because it is grounded within welfare economic theory, the predominant theory of economic

10. Amiram Gafni, "Economic Evaluation of Health-Care Programmes: Is CEA Better Than CBA?" *Environmental & Resource Economics* 34, no. 3. (2006): 407–418.

11. Joanna Coast, "Is Economic Evaluation in Touch with Society's Health Values," *British Medical Journal* 329, no. 7476 (2004): 1234.

12. For recent developments in CBA for health, see Emma McIntosh et al., *Applied Methods of Cost–Benefit Analysis in Health Care* (Oxford: Oxford University Press, 2010).

13. Stephen Palmer and David J. Torgerson, "Definitions of Efficiency," *British Medical Journal* 318, no. 7191 (1999): 1136.

14. Jan A. Olsen and Cam Donaldson, "Helicopters, Hearts and Hips: Using Willingness to Pay to Set Priorities for Public Sector Health Care Programmes," *Social Science & Medicine* 46, no. 1 (1998): 1–12.

15. Eamon O'Shea, Brenda Gannon, and Brendan Kennelly, "Eliciting Preferences for Resource Allocation in Mental Health Care in Ireland," *Health Policy* 88, no. 2–3 (2008): 359–370.

16. James C. Robinson, "Philosophical Origins of the Economic Valuation of Life," *Milbank Quarterly* 64, no. 1 (1986): 133–155.

practice. New methods of valuing improvements in health in monetary terms continue to be made to further develop this type of evaluation for health care.[17]

2.1.2. Extra-welfarism

The application of the normative theoretical framework of welfarism to a health care setting is controversial because there are a number of principles in welfarism that arguably conflict with the nature of health care. The principle underlying welfarism that has been most strongly challenged within health economics is that of utilitarianism—that is, relying solely on utility information to judge individual well-being. The theoretical critique of welfarism for use in health care has been drawn primarily from the critique of utility as a basis for assessing societal welfare by Amartya Sen.[18] In his critique of welfare economics, Sen referred to capturing additional information beyond individual utility as extra-welfarist. From this critique, and from Culyer's subsequent developments in the health context,[19] the term extra-welfarist has become associated with the health economics alternative to welfarism.

Brouwer and colleagues identified four ways in which extra-welfarism can be distinguished from welfare economic theory.[20] First, extra-welfarism permits the use of non-utility outcomes. Given that the focus in the health care sector is on improving health, Brouwer and colleagues argue that a sole focus on utility is too narrow for health analysis and in theory attempts to complement utility with non-utility information. The primary normative framework for extra-welfarism in health economics is mainly based on incorporating information beyond utility into outcome measurement for health care provision, although in practice the focus is on health status,[21] such as the quality-adjusted life-year (QALY), a composite measure of health and duration (see Section 3).

Second, extra-welfarism allows for the valuation of outcomes from those not directly affected by the outcome of interest. Within extra-welfarism, a number of different population groups could be considered relevant for valuing outcomes and not, as within the welfarist tradition, just the individuals directly affected. Such alternative values can be appropriate within state provision of health care.

---

17. McIntosh et al., *Applied Methods.*

18. Amartya Sen, "Social Choice Theory: A Re-examination," *Econometrica* 45, no. 1 (1977): 53–89.

19. Anthony J. Culyer, "The Normative Economics of Health Care Finance and Provision," *Oxford Review of Economic Policy* 5, no. 1 (1989): 34–58.

20. Werner B. F. Brouwer et al., "Welfarism vs. Extra-welfarism," *Journal of Health Economics* 27, no. 2 (2008): 325–338.

21. Culyer, "The Normative Economics," 34–58.

For example, where the general population is funding the treatment of those who receive treatment, it could be argued that they are stakeholders in the benefit obtained from such interventions and should be involved in the valuation of outcomes.[22]

Third, Brouwer and colleagues consider extra-welfarism to be different from welfarism because it allows the weighting of outcomes to be based on factors other than individual preferences. For example, different weights could be applied based on sociodemographic characteristics of the individuals receiving the intervention, or additional weight could be added if priority was advocated for a particular patient group (e.g., children).

Finally, extra-welfarism is different from welfarism because it permits interpersonal comparison in a number of dimensions of well-being. This means that, for example, this framework allows comparisons between the health (or well-being) of different people.

Although it has been argued that there are a number of differences between the extra-welfarist and welfarist frameworks, a number of similarities in the applications of the two theories remain. The objective within the extra-welfarist framework remains consequential in evaluation, in terms of maximization, mirroring the same form of consequentialism as applied in welfarism. The only difference is what is maximized, with the maximization of utility in welfarism replaced with the maximization of health in extra-welfarism.[23] Whereas the extra-welfarist framework argues for the multidimensionality of outcomes to be accounted for within evaluation, the practical application of extra-welfarism focuses on a single dimension—that is, health status.[24] This is particularly true within the extra-welfarist theoretical framework currently applied within health economics, in which the objective of the maximization of health using health-related outcomes is the primary objective of interest.[25]

Cost–utility analysis (CUA) is a type of economic evaluation that focuses attention particularly on health-related outcomes for health care treatments (note that the terminology here is at odds with the nature of the analysis).[26] CUA is the main evaluation framework of the extra-welfarist theory for health care as developed by

---

22. Marthe R. Gold et al., *Cost-Effectiveness in Health and Medicine* (Oxford: Oxford University Press, 1996), 1–303.

23. Jeremiah Hurley, "Welfarism, Extra-welfarism," 373–395.

24. Jeremiah Hurley, "Welfarism, Extra-welfarism," 373–395; Joanna Coast, Richard D. Smith, and Paula Lorgelly, "Welfarism, Extra-welfarism and Capability: The Spread of Ideas in Health Economics," *Social Science & Medicine* 67, no. 7 (2008): 1190–1198.

25. Anthony J. Culyer, "The Normative Economics," 34–58.

26. Drummond et al., *Economic Evaluation*, 137–139.

Culyer. Culyer believed that the maximand (what is to be maximized) for evaluation conducted under extra-welfarism should be health.[27] Although utility is referred to within the title of CUA, it is not utility as is commonly interpreted within welfare economics. Measures of generic health-related quality of life (HRQoL) rely on preferences of individuals to value a generic health state in comparison to the anchors of full health and a state equivalent to being dead.[28] The index scores generated from HRQoL questionnaires are then combined with length of time to form a QALY, which is used as the outcome of benefit from economic evaluation and provides the reference case outcome measure for NICE evaluations.[29]

The CUA evaluation framework requires a consistent HRQoL outcome measure to be applied across all interventions evaluated so that decisions can be made that address not only technical efficiency between treatment options for the same health condition but also allocative efficiency across interventions so that funding can be justified in comparison with any other treatment across the health service.[30] This is of particular importance in a publicly funded health care system in which decisions should ensure that resources are appropriately allocated to different areas of the health service so that taxpayers are getting value for money.[31]

3. Extra-welfarism in Practice

The extra-welfarist framework has become synonymous with one health outcome measure in particular: the quality-adjusted life-year. The QALY as it was defined first in 1977[32] has changed relatively little over time.[33] The QALY takes account of quality of life in terms of both health (quality or Q) and length of life (i.e., life-years or LY). The quality part of the QALY is measured on a scale with the common anchoring of full health anchored to 1 and health states equivalent to being dead anchored to 0.[34] The quality part of the QALY is collected over time and combined

---

27. Anthony J. Culyer, "The Normative Economics," 54–55.

28. Paul Dolan et al., *A Social Tariff for EuroQol: Results from a UK General Population Survey* (York, UK: Centre for Health Economics, 1995).

29. NICE, *Developing NICE Guidelines*, 123.

30. Palmer and Torgerson, "Definitions of Efficiency," 1136.

31. Karen Gerard, "Setting Priorities in the New NHS: Can Purchasers Use Cost–Utility Information," *Health Policy* 25, no. 1–2 (1993): 109–125.

32. Milton C. Weinstein and William B. Stason, "Foundations of Cost-Effectiveness Analysis for Health and Medical Practices," *New England Journal of Medicine* 296, no. 3 (1977): 716–721.

33. F. Reed Johnson, "Moving the QALY Forward or Just Stuck in Traffic?" *Value in Health* 12, no. s1 (2009): 38–39.

34. Drummond et al., *Economic Evaluation*, 14.

with time spent in each health state to measure QALYs, where 1 QALY is equivalent to 1 year in full health. When applied to patient populations, the QALY seeks to find the additional health benefit of receiving a new treatment in comparison to an alternative by measuring the change in quality and quantity of life if a new treatment were introduced.[35]

To determine the quality part of the QALY, two questions need to be answered: What attributes of quality need to be valued? and How are these attributes to be valued?[36] Both of these are addressed next.

3.1. What Attributes to Value?

To calculate what is to be valued in the QALY, a generic measure of health status is usually collected from patients. The main method recommended by NICE for measuring quality for QALYs is the EuroQol (EQ-5D).[37] The EQ-5D is a five-item questionnaire of health status that assesses mobility, self-care, usual activities, pain/discomfort, and anxiety/depression.[38] The dimensions on the EQ-5D were originally developed on three levels (no problems, some problems, and a lot of problems on a given dimension). The EQ-5D has been expanded to a five-level version, the EQ-5D-5L.[39]

3.2. How Are the Attributes Valued?

Generic health status instruments need to be valued. NICE stipulates that the method for valuing between different health states must be choice based.[40] Thus, rating scales of health such as the EuroQol Visual Analogue Scale (EQ-VAS), a scale of 0 (worst health state imaginable) to 100 (best health state imaginable), cannot be used to value health states because respondents are not presented with a choice (i.e., preference of one health state over another) in the task. Preferences

---

35. Milton C. Weinstein, George Torrance, and Alistair McGuire, "QALYs: The Basics," *Value in Health* 12, no. s1 (2009): 5–9.

36. Paul Dolan et al., "Valuing Health Directly," *British Medical Journal* 339 (2009): b2577.

37. NICE, *Developing NICE Guidelines*, 123.

38. Richard Brooks, "EuroQol: The Current State of Play," *Health Policy* 37, no. 1 (1996): 53–72.

39. Michael Herdman et al., "Development and Preliminary Testing of the New Five-Level Version of EQ-5D (EQ-5D-5L)," *Quality of Life Research* 20, no. 10 (2011): 1727–1736.

40. NICE, *Guide to the Methods of Technology Appraisal* (London: National Institute for Health and Care Excellence, 2013), 43.

for health states are used to compare different interventions to represent a societal value of changes in health status.[41]

For the EQ-5D-3L, the values associated with each of the 245 possible health states (3^5 or 243 health states and 2 additional health states for "unconscious" and "dead") were generated in the United Kingdom by Dolan from a representative sample of the general UK adult population.[42] These preferences were elicited using the time trade-off (TTO) technique developed by Torrance and colleagues to generate health preferences between quality and quantity of life. The TTO method asks participants how much quantity of life they are willing to trade off in a worse state of full health (i.e., <1) to improve their quality of life to its optimum level of full health.[43]

Once a health status questionnaire has been completed to give a profile of an individual for a given condition, values are then assigned to the patient profile to generate an index score for that state of being.[44] Index scores for individual health states can then be combined with the length of period a given individual spends within this health state to calculate the QALY. For example, an individual who scores an EQ-5D score of 0.5 and is in this health state for 1 year generates 0.5 QALY.

A number of alternatives to the QALY have been suggested within the health economics literature. The most well-known of these is the disability-adjusted life-year (DALY), which has been the measure of choice for assessing the global burden of disease by the World Health Organization (WHO) since the early 1990s.[45] The calculation of QALYs and that of DALYs are somewhat similar. However, the objective of maximizing health within the QALY approach is substituted in the DALY approach by minimizing disease burden through reducing DALYs lost. The DALY has been developed to assess population health primarily within developing countries, which is easier to measure where information on HRQoL may not be easily accessible. The DALY provides more information than mortality data alone. Relatively

41. Drummond et al., *Economic Evaluation*, 143–147.

42. Paul Dolan, "Modeling Valuations for EuroQol Health States," *Medical Care* 35, no. 11 (1997): 1095–1108.

43. George W. Torrance, Warren H. Thomas, and David L. Sackett, "A Utility Maximisation Model for Evaluation of Health Care Programs," *Health Services Research* 7, no. 2 (1972): 118–133.

44. Drummond et al., *Economic Evaluation*, 155–156.

45. Christopher Murray and Alan Lopez, *The Global Burden of Disease: A Comprehensive Assessment of Mortality and Disability from Diseases, Injuries and Risk Factors in 1990 and Projected to 2020* (Cambridge, MA: Harvard University Press, 1996).

recently, new economic evaluation guidelines have been developed to improve the reporting of economic evaluations in developing countries.[46]

3.3. Decision Rules

A number of decision rules can, in theory, be used to aid health care decision-making. Decision rules are generally based on aiding decision-making as to whether new interventions are worth the additional cost burden to the funding or implementing body in question (e.g., hospital and regional or national provision). For NICE, QALY scores are aggregated for the population under consideration, with the costs and benefits combined by calculating a cost-effectiveness ratio or cost per QALY gained. To compare differences between costs and effects for competing interventions, the incremental cost-effectiveness ratio (ICER) is applied to measure the cost per additional QALY gained for the more expensive and/or effective treatments.[47] The ICER for a given treatment is then compared with a shadow price for the budget of interest. This is known as the threshold ICER rule. For new interventions to be recommended by NICE, the willingness to pay for an additional QALY must fall within or below the threshold range of £20,000–£30,000. However, in exceptional circumstances, the willingness to pay for QALY gains is sometimes raised above the £30,000 threshold.[48] A recent study suggested that 82% of NICE decisions can be predicted by the prevailing threshold ICER rule of less than £30,000 per QALY gain.[49] However, a number of health economists have argued that the NICE threshold is too high and should instead be set at £13,000 per QALY gain.[50]

Another alternative for decision-making using these ICERs is the "QALY league table," in which interventions with the lowest ICERs are recommended until no more resources are available.[51] This approach has been previously applied within the United States.[52] However, the league table approach came under heavy

---

46. Karl Claxton et al., *The Gates Reference Case for Economic Evaluation* (Seattle, WA: The Bill and Melinda Gates Foundation, 2014).

47. Michael F. Drummond et al., *Economic Evaluation*, 40.

48. NICE, *Developing NICE Guidelines*, 146.

49. Helen Dakin et al., "The Influence of Cost-Effectiveness and Other Factors on NICE Decisions," *Health Economics* 24, no.10 (2015), 1256-1271.

50. Karl Claxton et al., "Methods for the Estimation of the National Institute for Health and Care Excellence Cost-Effectiveness Threshold," *Health Technology Assessment* 19, no. 14 (2015): 73–78.

51. Stephen Birch and Ariman Gafni, "Decision Rules in Economic Evaluation," in *The Elgar Companion to Health Economics*, ed. Andrew Jones (Cheltenham, UK: Elgar, 2006), 492–502.

52. David C. Hadorn, "Setting Health Care Priorities in Oregon: Cost-Effectiveness Meets the Rule of Rescue," *JAMA* 216, no. 17 (1991): 2218–2225.

scrutiny,[53] which led to the ICER threshold rule as the current dominant method for comparing interventions in health economics. The aim of both approaches, however, is to maximize QALY gains for the scarce resources available, irrespective of distributional concerns.

4. Critiquing the QALY

The QALY has faced a number of criticisms since it was developed concerning both the theoretical assumptions underpinning the outcome measure[54] and the considerations that are overlooked within the measure.[55]

There are a number of theoretical arguments against the use of the QALY outcome for measuring the benefits from health interventions. One such argument is the focus on changes in individual health status only, rather than a more holistic measure of individual welfare that would capture the broader benefits to individual well-being from health care. The health QALY also limits the generalizability to compare the benefits to society with other public interventions, such as education, justice, and transport. Even if it accepted that health maximization is an intuitive objective for health services, there are many practical examples concerning social care,[56] end-of-life care,[57] process of care,[58] and complex interventions[59] in which QALY maximization proves problematic. Indeed, there is doubt as to how much the objective of QALY maximization is reflective of societal values.[60]

---

53. For example, see Michael Drummond, George Torrance, and James Mason, "Cost-Effectiveness League Tables: More Harm Than Good?" *Social Science & Medicine* 37, no. 1 (1993): 33–40; Karen Gerard and Gavin Mooney, "QALY League Tables: Handle with Care," *Health Economics* 2, no. 1 (1993): 59–64.

54. For example, see Roy A. Carr-Hill, "Assumptions of the QALY Procedure," *Social Science & Medicine* 29, no. 3 (1989): 469–477; Graham Loomes and Lynda McKenzie, "The Use of QALYs in Health Care Decision Making," *Social Science & Medicine* 29, no. 3 (1989): 299–308.

55. Erik Nord, *Cost–Value Analysis in Health Care: Making Sense Out of QALYs* (Cambridge, UK: Cambridge University Press, 1999).

56. Hareth Al-Janabi, Terry N. Flynn, and Joanna Coast, "QALYs and Carers," *Pharmacoeconomics* 29, no. 12 (2011): 1015–1023.

57. Charles Normand, "Measuring Outcomes in Palliative Care: Limitations of QALYs and the Road to PaLYs," *Journal of Pain and Symptom Management* 38, no. 1 (2009): 27–31.

58. Victoria K. Brennan and Simon Dixon, "Incorporating Process Utility into Quality Adjusted Life Years: A Systematic Review of Empirical Studies," *Pharmacoeconomics* 31, no. 8 (2013): 677–691.

59. Katherine Payne, Marion McAllister, and Linda M. Davies, "Valuing the Economic Benefits of Complex Interventions: When Maximising Health Is Not Sufficient," *Health Economics* 22, no. 3 (2013): 258–271.

60. Paul Dolan et al., "QALY Maximisation and People's Preferences: A Methodological Review of the Literature," *Health Economics* 14, no. 2 (2005): 197–208.

An alternative proposal to the welfarist (through WTP) and extra-welfarist (through HRQoL and QALYs) approaches to measuring benefits is the capability approach. The capability approach, developed originally by Amartya Sen,[61] is a prominent critique of standard welfare economic theory. Sen argues that standard welfare economic theory is used to evaluate societal well-being through a narrow focus on a person's utility levels.

The first attempt following Culyer to incorporate the capability approach within a health economic evaluation format was by Cookson, although it has been previously suggested as an alternative to HRQoL measures. Cookson and, recently, Bleichrodt and Quiggin have argued for a formulation of QALYs as a measure that reflects the capability approach.[62] However, others have argued that the objectives of maximizing health and measuring "more than health" are key rationales for moving away from the current QALY approach in health economics.[63] Specific areas in which health care resources are allocated that have argued for a broader assessment than health include social care,[64] public health,[65] mental health,[66] palliative care,[67] and chronic pain.[68]

---

61. Although there are numerous writings by Sen on the capability approach, see Amartya Sen, *The Idea of Justice* (London: Lane, 2009); see also chapters in this volume by Fourie (Chapter 10) and Ram-Tiktin (Chapter 8) for more detailed discussion on the theory underpinning the capability approach.

62. Richard Cookson, "QALYs and the Capability Approach," *Health Economics* 14, no. 8 (2005): 817–829; Han Bleichrodt and John Quiggin, "Capabilities as Menus: A Non-welfarist Basis for QALY Evaluation," *Journal of Health Economics* 32, no. 1 (2013): 128–137.

63. Paul Anand, "Capabilities and Health," *Journal of Medical Ethics* 31 (2005): 299–303; Joanna Coast, Richard Smith, and Paula Lorgelly, "Should the Capability Approach Be Applied in Health Economics?" *Health Economics* 17, no. 6 (2008): 667–670.

64. Ini Grewal et al., "Developing Attributes for a Generic Quality of Life Instrument for Older People: Preferences or Capabilities? *Social Science and Medicine* 62, no. 8 (2006): 1891–1901; Ann Netten et al., "Outcome of Social Care for Adults: Developing a Preference Weighted Measure," *Health Technology Assessment* 16, no. 16 (2012): 1–166.

65. Paula Lorgelly et al., "Outcome Measurement in Economic Evaluation of Public Health Interventions: A Role for the Capability Approach?" *International Journal of Environmental Research and Public Health* 7, no. 5 (2010): 2274–2289.

66. Judit Simon et al., "Operationalising the Capability Approach for Outcome Measurement in Mental Health Research," *Social Science & Medicine* 98 (2013): 187–196.

67. Joanna Coast, "Strategies for the Economic Evaluation of End-of-Life Care: Making a Case for the Capability Approach," *Expert Review of Pharmacoeconomics & Outcomes Research* 14, no. 4 (2014): 473–482.

68. Philip Kinghorn, Angela Robinson, and Richard D. Smith, "Developing a Capability-Based Questionnaire for Assessing Well-Being in Patients with Chronic Pain," *Social Indicators Research* 120, no. 3 (2015): 897–916.

Table 15.1 Capability Measures Developed to Aid Health Decision-Making

First Author	Publication Year	Population	Targeted Interventions
Coast	2008	Older people	Health and social care
Anand	2009	General adult	Generic
Al-Janabi	2012	General adult	Generic
Netten	2012	Older people	Social care
Simon	2013	Mental health	Mental health
Ferrer	2014	Obese/diabetic	Physical activity and diet
Sutton	2014	End of life	Palliative care
Kinghorn	2015	Chronic pain	Chronic pain
Lorgelly	2015	General adult	Public health

The use of the capability approach directly in the health economics field has so far largely focused on the development of capability questionnaires (Table 15.1).[69] Indeed, capability measures have been recommended for use in social care interventions in the most recent NICE economic evaluation reference case.[70] Less progress has been made with regard to how such questionnaires, once fully developed and validated, can or should be used within an economic evaluation framework to aid priority-setting in health care for advisory bodies such as NICE.

5. The Capability Approach as an Alternative Theoretical Basis for Economic Evaluation

The capability approach, most prominently developed by Amartya Sen and philosopher Martha Nussbaum, is an alternative theory of assessing individual's advantage compared to the utilitarian tradition in welfare economics.[71] The capability perspective has been identified by a number of researchers in the health field as a promising alternative,[72] with some researchers conceptualizing the approach to

69. For more details on these capability measures, see Joanna Coast, Philip Kinghorn, and Paul Mitchell, "The Development of Capability Measures in Health Economics: Opportunities, Challenges and Progress," *The Patient* 8, no. 2 (2015): 119–126.

70. NICE, *Developing NICE Guidelines*, 123.

71. For the most current accounts of the capability approach, see Sen, *The Idea*; and Martha C. Nussbaum, *Creating Capabilities: The Human Development Approach* (London: Belknap, 2011).

72. M. A. Verkerk, J. J. V. Busschbach, and E. D. Karssing, "Health-Related Quality of Life Research and the Capability Approach of Amartya Sen," *Quality of Life Research* 10, no. 1 (2001): 49–55; Anand, "Capabilities and Health," 299–303; Coast et al., "Should the

health in particular.[73] However, one of the difficulties with the capability approach is its underspecified nature (e.g., there is no explicit capability list appropriate for all policy decisions or common objective in capability evaluations).[74] Although also viewed as an advantage in that the approach can be adapted to address particular policy concerns, this poses a challenge in offering a coherent practical application of the capability approach as an alternative, for example, to the current methods of economic evaluation in health care. Indeed, the capability approach has been used to justify a move away from traditional welfare economic practice toward extra-welfarist QALYs and DALYs. However, both QALYs and DALYs are primarily concerned with health as opposed to capability more generally.[75]

A literature review of health studies attempting to measure capability found that none of the studies focused on health status alone to capture capability.[76] The review of capability applications also found that although there is no consensus in the objective of capability-based evaluations, a large proportion of studies were concerned with an objective related to sufficiency of capabilities. Predominantly, this is due to the application of the capability approach in developing countries and the need to alleviate the insufficiency of basic capabilities in these impoverished scenarios. Following from this, research has led to the development of methods for generating capability outcomes reflective of the findings from the literature review of the objective of sufficiency of capabilities.

5.1. Sufficient Capability Outcomes

Drawing on methodology from the multidimensional poverty literature, which also draws its theoretical basis from the capability perspective,[77] and health economic

Capability," 667–670; Iain Law and Heather Widdows, "Conceptualising Health: Insights from the Capability Approach," *Health Care Analysis* 16, no. 4 (2008): 303–314; Vikki A. Entwistle and Ian S. Watt, "Treating Patients as Persons: A Capabilities Approach to Support Delivery of Person-Centred Care," *American Journal of Bioethics* 13, no. 8 (2013): 29–39.

73. Jennifer Prah Ruger, *Health and Social Justice* (Oxford: Oxford University Press, 2010); Sridhar Venkatapuram, *Health Justice: An Argument from the Capabilities Approach* (Cambridge, UK: Polity, 2011).

74. Robert Sugden, "Welfare, Resources and Capabilities: A Review of *Inequality Reexamined* by Amartya Sen," *Journal of Economic Literature* 31, no. 4 (1993): 1947–1962.

75. Michael Drummond et al., "Towards a Consensus on the QALY," *Value in Health* 12, no. s1 (2009): 31–35; Erik Nord, "Disability Weights in the Global Burden of Disease 2010: Unclear Meaning and Overstatement of International Agreement," *Health Policy* 111, no. 1 (2013): 99–104.

76. Paul M. Mitchell et al., "Applications of the capability approach in the health field: a literature review," *Social Indicators Research*, (2016): doi:10.1007/s11205-016-1356-8.

77. Sabina Alkire and James Foster, "Counting and Multidimensional Poverty Measurement," *Journal of Public Economics* 95, no. 7–8 (2011): 476–487.

outcomes, we developed a methodology for calculating a composite measure of sufficient capability and time.[78] Multidimensional poverty measurement is based on capturing multiple deprivations beyond income, and the approach uses a capability perspective to allow for a richer evaluative space on deprivation through a multidimensional lens. Using an example from the United States, Alkire and Foster demonstrate how focusing on income can give a distorted view of how poverty is portrayed within a community and who should be targeted by policy decisions.[79]

The approach developed by us is based on an outcome called years of sufficient capability (YSC). Instead of focusing on the absolute gains of capability across a population (i.e., capability maximization), the YSC targets those who fall below a threshold level of sufficient capability, with the aim being to improve capability to sufficient levels for those who are "capability poor."[80]

To demonstrate the use of YSC, we use a newly developed capability index for the general adult UK population, the ICEpop (Investigating Choice Experiments for the Preferences of Older People) CAPability measure for Adults (ICECAP-A).[81] The ICECAP-A research team conducted qualitative research with members of the UK population to identify the most important capabilities for adults aged 18 years or older. Through thematic analysis of semistructured interviews with the UK general population, Al-Janabi and colleagues found five capabilities of most importance:

Stability—"ability to feel settled and secure"
Attachment—"an ability to have love, friendship, and support"
Autonomy—"an ability to be independent"
Achievement—"an ability to achieve and progress in life"
Enjoyment—"an ability to experience enjoyment and pleasure"

The ICECAP-A instrument was developed using these five attributes after an iterative process was used to test the understanding of questions, making sure that questions were interpreted in the same way as the original conceptual attributes

78. Paul M. Mitchell et al., "Assessing Sufficient Capability: A New Approach to Economic Evaluation," *Social Science & Medicine* 139 (2015): 71-79.

79. Alkire and Foster, "Counting and Multidimensional," 483–484.

80. Mitchell et al., "Assessing Sufficient Capability."

81. Hareth Al-Janabi, Terry N. Flynn, and Joanna Coast, "Development of a Self-Report Measure of Capability Wellbeing for Adults: The ICECAP-A," *Quality of Life Research* 21, no. 1 (2012): 167–176; Terry N. Flynn et al., "Scoring the ICECAP-A Capability Instrument: Estimation of a UK Population Tariff," *Health Economics* 24, no. 3 (2015): 258–269.

developed. This resulted in five attributes of capability across four levels, ranging from no capability to full capability for each attribute (Table 15.2).[82] The focus on capability in the ICECAP-A offers an alternative method for measuring the impact of health interventions to measures focused on health status.

Values for the ICECAP-A capability index were generated for a representative sample of the UK adult population through a method called best–worst scaling. Best–worst scaling presents scenarios to participants whereby, for the ICECAP-A, they are asked to state their most and least favored attribute from the five options presented to them (i.e., one from each attribute). For example, a person could be asked to choose the best and worst capability states when the ICECAP-A stability and attachment attributes are at their highest levels, autonomy is at the second highest level, and both achievement and enjoyment attributes are at their lowest levels. The best–worst scaling approach is favored by the ICECAP team due to the fact that this method of valuation does not necessarily rely on individual preferences because individuals are not directly asked to choose between two different scenarios.[83] Values are anchored on a no capability–full capability (0–1) scale.[84] To score 1, a person must have the highest levels of all ICECAP-A attributes. To score 0, a person would need to have the lowest levels on each of the ICECAP-A attributes.

Because the ICECAP-A is a relatively new measure, limited studies have assessed its validity in patient groups. However, in a general adult UK population sample, capability differences were found between health and socioeconomic groups, showing that it can distinguish between groups that can be considered disadvantaged.[85] The ICECAP-A has also been tested and has demonstrated reliability and face validity in the UK population.[86]

In Table 15.2, we present the ICECAP-A questionnaire format and sufficient capability values, with sufficient capability thresholds set at "33333" and "22222" for illustration.[87] What this means in practice is that for someone to be classed as

---

82. Al-Janabi et al., "The ICECAP-A," 167–176.

83. Joanna Coast et al., "Valuing the ICECAP Capability Index for Older People," *Social Science & Medicine* 67, no. 5 (2008): 874–882.

84. Flynn et al., "Scoring the ICECAP-A," 258–269.

85. Hareth Al-Janabi et al., "An Investigation of the Construct Validity of the ICECAP-A Capability Measure," *Quality of Life Research* 22, no. 7 (2013): 1831–1840.

86. Hareth Al-Janabi et al., "Test–Retest Reliability of Capability Measurement in the UK General Population," *Health Economics* 24, no. 5 (2014): 625–630; Hareth Al-Janabi et al., "Can Capabilities Be Self-Reported? A Think Aloud Study," *Social Science & Medicine* 87 (2013): 116–122.

87. The original ICECAP-A valuation can be obtained from Flynn et al., "Scoring the ICECAP-A," 265.

Table 15.2 ICECAP-A Questions and Values: Sufficient Capability Thresholds[a]

	Attribute	"33333"	"22222"
	Stability		
4	I am able to feel settled and secure in *all* areas of my life.	0.2255	0.2294
3	I am able to feel settled and secure in *many* areas of my life.	0.2255	0.2294
2	I am able to feel settled and secure in *a few* areas of my life.	0.1193	0.2294
1	I am *unable* to feel settled and secure in *any* areas of my life.	−0.0009	−0.0018
	Attachment		
4	I can have *a lot* of love, friendship, and support.	0.2225	0.2183
3	I can have *quite a lot* of love, friendship, and support.	0.2225	0.2183
2	I can have *a little* love, friendship, and support.	0.1135	0.2183
1	I *cannot* have *any* love, friendship, and support.	−0.0281	−0.0541
	Autonomy		
4	I am able to be *completely* independent.	0.1837	0.1894
3	I am able to be independent in *many* things.	0.1837	0.1894
2	I am able to be independent in *a few* things.	0.0984	0.1894
1	I am *unable* at all to be independent.	0.0074	0.0143
	Achievement		
4	I can achieve and progress in *all* aspects of my life.	0.1870	0.2059
3	I can achieve and progress in *many* aspects of my life.	0.1870	0.2059
2	I can achieve and progress in *a few* aspects of my life.	0.1070	0.2059
1	I *cannot* achieve and progress in *any* aspects of my life.	0.0247	0.0476
	Enjoyment		
4	I can have *a lot* of enjoyment and pleasure.	0.1813	0.1570
3	I can have *quite a lot* of enjoyment and pleasure.	0.1813	0.1570
2	I can have *a little* enjoyment and pleasure.	0.0816	0.1570
1	I *cannot* have *any* enjoyment and pleasure.	−0.0031	−0.0059

[a]To see the original ICECAP-A questionnaire layout, see Al-Janabi, Hareth, Terry N. Flynn, and Joanna Coast, "Development of a Self-Report Measure of Capability Wellbeing for Adults: The ICECAP-A," *Quality of Life Research* 21, no. 1 (2012): 167–176.

having sufficient capability for threshold "33333," he or she needs to answer the questionnaire level 3 or higher for each attribute to be classed as having sufficient capability (e.g., level 3 for the ICECAP-A stability attribute would read, "I am able to feel settled and secure in many areas of my life").[88]

5.2. Illustrative Example

A decision-maker has to decide which of two mutually exclusive interventions to provide. Both interventions cost $1 million, and both treat 100 patients with similar sociodemographic characteristics. Intervention A is a medicine to improve a mild health problem and is clinically effective. Intervention B is an intervention that requires fewer hospital visits and stays for moderate health problems, although it has less clinical effectiveness than intervention A. The decision-maker is presented with information about health gain (arbitrarily estimated here for illustrative purposes to calculate a likely health state score on a measure such as EQ-5D), full capability gain, and sufficient capability gain. Intervention A improves the autonomy attribute on ICECAP-A by one level for 20 individuals previously at level 1 (i.e., from level 1 to level 2), 40 individuals previously at level 2, and 40 individuals previously at level 3. Intervention B improves the attachment attribute on ICECAP-A for 40 individuals previously at level 1, 40 individuals at level 2, and 20 individuals at level 3. Intervention A improves its population health by twice as much as intervention B. We assume that these gains are kept for 1 year following intervention. The results of this illustrative example are presented in Table 15.3.

The first matter to note is that in this example, we present a situation in which change in full and sufficient capability may differ from change in health status. Although this is unlikely to always be the case, this would be the first reason for considering moving from a focus on health status to capability because it may result in a change in how resources are allocated. The second matter is that in this example, all capability outcomes point to intervention B. However, of most importance is the effect that focusing on sufficient capability could have on deciding what intervention to choose. Compared to considering full capability gain, using a threshold of "22222" means that improvements from level 1 to level 2 are valued much more highly, whereas improvements above level 2 are not valued at all. In the case of intervention B, the higher valuation of the gains from level 1 to level 2 outweighs the fact that the gains by the other 60 individuals are now valued at 0, so the valuation of the overall gain increases from 0.09 to 0.11. This contrasts with intervention A, in which only 20 individuals' gains are valued more highly,

---

88. For further details on the sufficient capability methodology, see Mitchell et al., "Assessing Sufficient Capability."

Table 15.3 Comparing Health Gain, Capability Gain,
and Sufficient Capability Outcomes[a]

Benefit	Treatment A	Treatment B
Health gain	*0.10*	0.05
Capability gain	0.06	*0.09*
Threshold "33333"	0.05	*0.10*
Threshold "22222"	0.04	*0.11*

[a]Numbers in italics represent optimum strategy based on different objectives.

whereas 80 individuals' gains are not weighted at all, with the result that the valuation of the overall gain decreases from 0.06 to 0.04. Therefore, one can imagine a situation in which two interventions focusing on capability may give different results if the focus is on maximum capability gain across a population versus a focus on the improvement of capability below a sufficient threshold. This illustrative example shows the potential for developing an approach for implementing capability measures in a framework to aid decision-making linked to an objective of sufficient capability.

6. Discussion

In this chapter, we highlighted how a sufficient capability approach may lead to different decisions being made with regard to the provision of health care interventions. The development of capability measures and the lack of reliance on health status as a sole indicator of welfare in capability studies indicate a need to move beyond measures focused purely on a person's health state when adopting a capability perspective. Although no clear consensus exists with regard to the objective of a capability-based evaluation, we argue that, based on how most studies are applying the approach[89] and the need to offer a coherent alternative to welfare economic practice, there is appeal in some form of merging of ideas between concepts related to sufficiency and capability. We presented an example of how the use of the YSC outcome could lead to different decisions than those based on the current application of health QALY maximization.

A number of criticisms have been made of the QALY approach. Many of these criticisms concern people who may be considered to be disadvantaged by taking a singular approach to assessing all interventions. Most of these critiques have been

---

89. Mitchell et al., "Applications of the capability approach."

based on claims to different groups, most notably those who are most severely ill[90] but also others.[91] For example, NICE has given additional weight to interventions that meet end-of-life criteria. Most tweaks to the QALY have been based on these claims, although health status has remained central within this calculation. Instead of tweaking the QALY, we argue that it is necessary to redesign the evaluative space to focus on individual capabilities.

There has been one notable attempt in the health economics literature to align economic evaluation with a sufficiency criterion. Alan Williams argued for "fair innings" for everyone so that once one reaches one's "fair innings" of years lived (Williams argued this to be 70 years), priority should be shifted to those who have yet to reach their sufficient number of years alive.[92] Although we also adopt sufficiency principles, our approach is different. We suggest that interventions should be targeted at those who fall below a sufficient level of capability—the level of capability to live a life someone has reason to value—without making any further claims on who should be prioritized.

How to define a sufficient threshold of capability needs to be considered further. One approach would be to conduct qualitative research using participatory methods to assign a sufficient threshold for a given population.[93] Alternatively, quantitative research could be conducted to assign sufficient thresholds, similar to an approach taken in the poverty literature to assign "core poverty" thresholds.[94] Although we have argued for and justified the rationale for adopting a sufficient capability approach, the same methodology could, of course, be used to reach a sufficient level of health. Such an approach would require a similar justification as the one presented for sufficient capability. Here, however, our attention focuses on people's capabilities more broadly and setting an objective that is reflective of practical capability studies.[95]

90. Nord, *Cost–Value Analysis*.

91. Dolan et al., "QALY Maximisation," 197–208.

92. Alan Williams, "Intergenerational Equity: An Exploration of the 'Fair Innings' Argument," *Health Economics* 6, no. 2 (1997): 117–132.

93. Joanna Coast, "The Appropriate Uses of Qualitative Methods in Health Economics," *Health Economics* 8, no. 4 (1999): 345–353.

94. David A. Clark and Mozaffar Qizilbash, "Core Poverty, Vagueness and Adaptation: A New Methodology and Some Results from South Africa," *Journal of Development Studies* 44, no. 4 (2008): 519–544.

95. Mitchell et al., "Applications of the capability approach."

Acknowledgments

The work presented in this chapter was primarily undertaken during a School of Health and Population Sciences PhD studentship at the Health Economics Unit, University of Birmingham, United Kingdom. Writing of the chapter was supported by a Wellcome Trust fellowship, "Capabilities Theory and Global Population-Level Bioethics," (WT094245) led by Sridhar Venkatapuram at the Department of Social Science, Health & Medicine, King's College London. We are grateful for the helpful comments provided by Annette Rid and Carina Fourie in the compilation of this chapter.

Bibliography

Albertsen, Andreas, and Carl Knight. "A Framework for Luck Egalitarianism in Health and Healthcare." *Journal of Medical Ethics* 41, no. 2 (2015): 165–169.

Al-Janabi, Hareth, Terry N. Flynn, and Joanna Coast. "QALYs and Carers." *Pharmacoeconomics* 29, no. 12 (2011): 1015–1023.

Al-Janabi, Hareth, Terry N. Flynn, and Joanna Coast. "Development of a Self-Report Measure of Capability Wellbeing for Adults: The ICECAP-A." *Quality of Life Research* 21, no. 1 (2012): 167–176.

Al-Janabi, Hareth, Terry N. Flynn, Tim J. Peters, Stirling Bryan, and Joanna Coast. "Test–Retest Reliability of Capability Measurement in the UK General Population." *Health Economics* 24, no. 5 (2014): 625–630.

Al-Janabi, Hareth, Thomas Keeley, Paul Mitchell, and Joanna Coast. "Can Capabilities Be Self-Reported? A Think Aloud Study." *Social Science & Medicine* 87 (2013): 116–122.

Al-Janabi, Hareth, Tim J. Peters, John Brazier, Stirling Bryan, Terry N. Flynn, Sam Clemens, et al. "An Investigation of the Construct Validity of the ICECAP-A Capability Measure." *Quality of Life Research* 22, no. 7 (2013): 1831–1840.

Alkire, Sabina, and James Foster. "Counting and Multidimensional Poverty Measurement." *Journal of Public Economics* 95, no. 7–8 (2011): 476–487.

Altman, Lawrence. "Cost of Treating AIDS Patients is Soaring." *New York Times*, July 23, 1992. Accessed June 11, 2014, http://www.nytimes.com/1992/07/23/us/cost-of-treating-aids-patients-is-soaring.html.

Alvarez, Allen Andrew A. "Threshold Considerations in Fair Allocation of Health Resources: Justice Beyond Scarcity." *Bioethics* 21 (2007): 426–438

Amundson, Ron. "Disability, Handicap, and the Environment." *Journal of Social Philosophy* 23, no. 1 (1992): 105–119.

Anand, Paul. "Capabilities and Health." *Journal of Medical Ethics* 31, no. 5 (2005): 299–303.

Anand, Paul, Graham Hunter, Ian Carter, Keith Dowding, Francesco Guala, and Martin Van Hees. "The Development of Capability Indicators." *Journal of Human Development and Capabilities* 10, no. 1 (2009): 125–152.

Anderson, Elizabeth. "What Is the Point of Equality?" *Ethics* 109, no. 2 (1999): 287–337.

Anderson, Elizabeth. "Justifying the Capabilities Approach to Justice." In *Measuring Justice Primary Goods and Capabilities*, edited by Harry Brighouse and Ingrid Robeyns. New York: Cambridge University Press, 2010.

Anell, Anders, Anna H. Glenngård, and Sherry Merkur. *Sweden: Health System Review 2012*, Health Systems in Transition, vol. 14, no. 5. Brussels, Belgium: European Observatory on Health Systems and Policies, 2012. http://www.euro.who.int/en/about-us/partners/observatory/publications/health-system-reviews-hits/countries-and-subregions/sweden-hit-2012.

Arneson, Richard. "Equality and Equal Opportunity for Welfare." *Philosophical Studies* 56 (1989): 77–93.

Arneson, Richard. "Liberalism, Distributive Subjectivism, and Equal Opportunity for Welfare." *Philosophy and Public Affairs* 19 (1990): 158–193.

Arneson, Richard J. "Egalitarianism and Responsibility." *Journal of Ethics* 3, no. 3 (1999): 225–247.

Arneson, Richard J. "Equality of Opportunity for Welfare Defended and Recanted." *Journal of Political Philosophy* 7 (1999): 488–497.

Arneson, Richard J. "Why Justice Requires Transfers to Offset Income and Wealth Inequalities." *Social Philosophy and Policy* 19, no. 1 (2002): 172–200.

Arneson, Richard J. "Distributive Justice and Basic Capability Equality." In *Capabilities Equality: Basic Issues and Problems*, edited by Alexander Kaufman. New York: Routledge, 2006.

Arrhenius, Gustaf. "An Impossibility Theorem for Welfarist Axiologies." *Economics and Philosophy* 16, no. 2 (2000): 247–266.

Arrhenius, Gustaf. *Population Ethics*. Oxford: Oxford University Press, Forthcoming.

Arrow, Kenneth J. "Uncertainty and the Welfare Economics of Medical Care." *American Economic Review* 53, no. 5 (1963): 941–973.

Arrow, Kenneth J. "Some Ordinalist–Utilitarian Notes on Rawls's Theory of Justice." *Journal of Philosophy* 70, no. 9 (1973): 245–263.

Asada, Yukiko. *Health Inequality: Morality and Measurement*. Toronto: University of Toronto Press, 2007.

Axelsen, David V. *Global Redistributive Obligations in the Face of Severe Poverty*. Aarhus, Denmark: Politica, 2014.

Axelsen, David. V., and Lasse Nielsen. "Sufficiency as Freedom from Duress." *Journal of Political Philosophy* 23, no. 4 (2015): 406–426.

Barrett, Scott. "Eradication Versus Control: The Economics of Global Infectious Disease Policies." *Bulletin of the World Health Organization* 82, no. 9 (2004): 683–687.

Beauchamp, Tom L., and James F. Childress. *Principles of Biomedical Ethics*, 7th ed. New York: Oxford University Press, 2013.

Benbaji, Yitzhak. "The Doctrine of Sufficiency: A Defence." *Utilitas* 17, no. 3 (2005): 310–332.

Benbaji, Yitzhak. "Sufficiency or Priority?" *European Journal of Philosophy* 14, no. 3 (2006): 327–348.

Berkman, Lisa F., Ichiro Kawachi, and M. Maria Glymour, eds. *Social Epidemiology*, 2nd ed. Oxford: Oxford University Press, 2014.

Bielinski, S., J. Olson, J. Pathak, et al. "Preemptive Genotyping for Personalized Medicine: Design of the Right Drug, Right Dose, Right Time—Using Genomic Data to Individualize Treatment Protocol." *Mayo Clinic Proceedings* 89 (2014): 25–33.

Birch, Stephen, and Ariman Gafni. "Decision Rules in Economic Evaluation." In *The Elgar Companion to Health Economics*, edited by Andrew Jones, 492–502. Cheltenham, UK: Elgar, 2006.

Blake, Michael. "Distributive Justice, State Coercion, and Autonomy." *Philosophy & Public Affairs* 30, no. 3 (2001): 257–296.

Bleichrodt, Han, and John Quiggin. "Capabilities as Menus: A Non-welfarist Basis for Economic Evaluation." *Journal of Health Economics* 32, no. 1 (2013): 128–137.

Boorse, Christopher. "On the Distinction Between Disease and Illness." *Philosophy and Public Affairs* 5, no. 1 (1975): 49–68.

Boorse, Christopher. "Health as a Theoretical Concept." *Philosophy of Science* 44, no. 4 (1977): 542–573.

Boorse, Christopher. "A Rebuttal on Health." In *What Is Disease? Biomedical Ethics Reviews*, edited by James M. Humber and Robert F. Almeder, 3–134. Totowa, NJ: Humana Press, 1997.

Brennan, Victoria K., and Simon Dixon. "Incorporating Process Utility into Quality Adjusted Life Years: A Systematic Review of Empirical Studies." *Pharmacoeconomics* 31, no. 8 (2013): 677–691.

Brett, Allen S. "Two-Tiered Health Care: A Problematic Double Standard." *Archives of Internal Medicine* 167 (2007): 430–432.

Brighouse, Harry, and Adam Swift. "Equality, Priority, and Positional Goods." *Ethics* 116, no. 3 (2006): 471–497.

Brock, Dan. "Ethical Issues in the Use of Cost-Effectiveness Analysis for the Prioritization of Health Care Resources." In *Public Health, Ethics, and Equity*, edited by Sudhir Anand, Fabienne Peter, and Amartya Sen, 201–224. New York: Oxford University Press, 2006.

Brock, Gillian. "Sufficiency and Needs-Based Approaches to Distributive Justice." In *Oxford Handbook of Distributive Justice*, edited by Serena Olsaretti. New York: Oxford University Press, Forthcoming.

Brooks, Richard. "EuroQol: The Current State of Play." *Health Policy* 37, no. 1 (1996): 53–72.

Broome, John. "Measuring the Burden of Disease by Aggregating Well-Being." In *Summary Measures of Population Health: Concepts, Ethics, Measurement and Applications*, edited by Christopher J. L. Murray, Joshua A. Salomon, Colin D. Mathers, and Alan D. Lopez, 91–113. Geneva: World Health Organization, 2002.

Broqvist, Maria, Maria Branting Elgstrand, Per Carlsson, Kristina Eklund, and Anders Jakobsson *National Model for Transparent Prioritisation in Swedish Health Care*. Linköping, Sweden: National Center for Priority Setting in Healthcare, 2011.

Brouwer, Werner B. F., Anthony J. Culyer, N. Job A. van Exel, and Frans Rutter. "Welfarism vs. Extra-welfarism." *Journal of Health Economics* 27, no. 2 (2008): 325–338.

Brown, Campbell. "Priority or Sufficiency . . . or Both?" *Economics and Philosophy* 21, no. 2 (2005): 199–220.

Buchanan, Allen. "The Right to a Decent Minimum of Health Care." *Philosophy and Public Affairs* 13 (1984): 55–78.

Buchanan, Allen. "Public and Private Responsibilities in the U.S. Health Care System." In *Justice and Health Care: Selected Essays*, edited by Allen Buchanan, 77–88. New York: Oxford University Press, 2009. [Origin work published 1992]

Buchanan, Allen. "The Right to a Decent Minimum in Health Care." In *Justice and Health Care: Selected Essay*, edited by Allen Buchanan, 17–36. New York: Oxford University Press, 2009.

Buchanan, Allen, ed. *Justice and Health Care: Selected Essays*. New York: Oxford University Press, 2009.

Busse, Reinhard, Miriam Blümel, and Diana Ognyanova. *Das Deutsche Gesundheitssystem: Akteure, Daten, Analysen*. Berlin: Medizinisch Wissenschaftliche Verlagsgesellschaft, 2013.

Busse, Reinhard, and Sophia Schlette. *Health Policy Developments 7/8: Focus on Prevention, Health and Ageing and Human Resources*. Gütersloh, Germany: Verlag Bertelsmann Stiftung, 2007.

Button, Kenneth. *Recent Development in Transport Economics*. Cheltenham, UK: Elgar, 2003.

Callahan, Daniel. *What Kind of Life: The Limits of Medical Progress*. New York: Simon & Schuster, 1990.

Callahan, Daniel. "Medical Futility, Medical Necessity. The-Problem-Without-a-Name." *Hastings Center Report* 21, no. 4 (1991): 30–35.

Caney, Simon. "Just Emissions." *Philosophy & Public Affairs* 40 (2012): 255–300.

Carr-Hill, Roy A. "Assumptions of the QALY Procedure." *Social Science & Medicine* 29, no. 3 (1989): 469–477.

Casal, Paula. "Why Sufficiency Is Not Enough." *Ethics* 117, no. 2 (2007): 296–326.

Center for Budget and Policy Priorities. "Premium Tax Credits: Answers to Frequently Asked Questions." Accessed January 24, 2015. http://www.cbpp.org/sites/default/files/atoms/files/QA-on-Premium-Credits.pdf.

Centers for Medicare and Medicaid Services. "National Health Expenditures 2012–22." Accessed June 11, 2014. http://www.cms.gov/Research-Statistics-Data-and-Systems/Statistics-Trends-and-Reports/NationalHealthExpendData/downloads/proj2012.pdf.

Chalkidou, Kalipso, Robert Marten, Derek Cutler, Tony Culyer, Richard Smith, Yot Teerawattananon, et al. "Health Technology Assessment in Universal Health Coverage." *Lancet* 382 (2013): E48–E49.

Claassen, Rutger, and Marcus Düwell. "The Foundations of Capability Theory: Comparing Nussbaum and Gewirth." *Ethical Theory and Moral Practice* 16, no. 3 (2013): 493–510.

Clark, David A., and Mozaffer Qizilbash. "Core Poverty, Vagueness and Adaptation: A New Methodology and Some Results from South Africa." *Journal of Development Studies* 44, no. 4 (2008): 519–544.

Claxton, Karl, Steve Martin, Marta Soares, Nigel Rice, Eldon Spackman, Sebastian Hinde, et al. "Methods for the Estimation of the National Institute for Health and Care Excellence Cost-Effectiveness Threshold." *Health Technology Assessment* 19, no. 14 (2015): 1–542.

Claxton, Karl, P. Revill, M. Sculpher, T. Wilkinson, J. Cairns, and A Briggs. *The Gates Reference Case for Economic Evaluation.* Seattle, WA: The Bill & Melinda Gates Foundation, 2014.

Clouser, Danner K., Charles M. Culver, and Bernard Gert. "Malady." In *What Is Disease? Biomedical Ethics Reviews*, edited by James M. Humber and Robert F. Almeder, 175–217. Totowa, NJ: Humana Press, 1997.

Coast, Joanna. "The Appropriate Uses of Qualitative Methods in Health Economics." *Health Economics* 8, no. 4 (1999): 345–353.

Coast, Joanna. "Is Economic Evaluation in Touch with Society's Health Values?" *British Medical Journal* 329, no. 7476 (2004): 1233–1236.

Coast, Joanna. "Strategies for the Economic Evaluation of End-of-Life Care: Making a Case for the Capability Approach." *Expert Review of Pharmacoeconomics & Outcomes Research* 14, no. 4 (2014): 473–482.

Coast, Joanna, Terry N. Flynn, Lucy Natarjan, Kerry Sproston, Jane Lewis, Jordan J. Louviere, et al. "Valuing the ICECAP Capability Index for Older People." *Social Science & Medicine* 67, no. 5 (2008): 874–882.

Coast, Joanna, Philip Kinghorn, and Paul Mitchell, "The Development of Capability Measures in Health Economics: Opportunities, Challenges and Progress." *The Patient* 8, no. 2 (2015): 119–126.

Coast, Joanna, Richard D. Smith, and Paula Lorgelly. "Should the Capability Approach Be Applied in Health Economics?" *Health Economics* 17, no. 6 (2008): 667–670.

Coast, Joanna, Richard D. Smith, and Paula Lorgelly. "Welfarism, Extra-welfarism and Capability: The Spread of Ideas in Health Economics." *Social Science & Medicine* 67, no. 7 (2008): 1190–1198.

Cohen, G. A. "On the Currency of Egalitarian Justice." *Ethics* 99 (1989): 906–944.

Connors, Elanora E., and Lawrence O. Gostin. "Health Care Reform—A Historic Moment in US Social Policy." *Journal of the American Medical Association* 303, no. 24 (2010): 2521–2522.

Cookson, Richard. "QALYs and the Capability Approach." *Health Economics* 14, no. 8 (2005): 817–829.

Crisp, Roger. "Egalitarianism and Compassion." *Ethics* 114, no. 1 (2003): 119–126.

Crisp, Roger. "Equality, Priority, and Compassion." *Ethics* 113, no. 4 (2003): 745–763.

Culyer, Anthony J. "The Normative Economics of Health Care Finance and Provision." *Oxford Review of Economic Policy* 5, no. 1 (1989): 34–58.

Dakin, Helen, Nancy Devlin, Yan Feng, Nigel Rice, Phill O'Neill, and David Parkin. "The Influence of Cost-Effectiveness and Other Factors on NICE Decisions." *Health Economics*, Early View (2014): doi: 10.1002/hec.3086.

Daly, Herman. *Beyond Growth: The Economics of Sustainable Development*. Boston: Beacon Press, 1996.

Daniels, Norman. *Just Health Care*. Cambridge, UK: Cambridge University Press, 1985.

Daniels, Norman. *Am I My Parents' Keeper? An Essay on Justice Between the Young and the Old*. New York: Oxford University Press, 1988.

Daniels, Norman. "Rationing Fairly: Programmatic Considerations." *Bioethics* 7 (1993): 224–233.

Daniels, Norman. "Accountability for Reasonableness: Establishing a Fair Process for Priority Setting is Easier Than Agreeing on Principles." *British Medical Journal* 321 (2000): 1300–1301.

Daniels, Norman. *Just Health: Meeting Health Needs Fairly*. Cambridge, UK: Cambridge University Press, 2008.

Daniels, Norman. "Justice, Health, and Health Care." In *Medicine and Social Justice: Essays on the Distribution of Health Care*, edited by Rosamond Rhodes, Margaret Battin, and Anita Silvers, 2nd ed., 17–33. New York: Oxford University Press, 2012.

Daniels, Norman. "Justice and Access to Health Care." In *The Stanford Encyclopedia of Philosophy*, edited by Edward N. Zalta, Spring 2013 edition. Accessed May 25, 2015. http://plato.stanford.edu/archives/spr2013/entries/justice-healthcareaccess.

Daniels, Norman, and James Sabin. "The Ethics of Accountability in Managed Care Reform." *Health Affairs* 17, no. 5 (1998): 50–64.

De la Croix, David, and Vincent Vandenberghe. "Human Capital as a Factor of Growth and Employment at the Regional Level: The Case of Belgium," Report to the European Commission, Employment and Social Affairs, 2004.

Department of Health. *The NHS Constitution: The NHS Belongs to Us All*. London: Department of Health, 2013.

DiPrete, Bob, and Darren Coffman. "A Brief History of Health Services Prioritization in Oregon," March 2007. Accessed March 25, 2015. http://www.oregon.gov/oha/OHPR/HSC/docs/prioritizationhistory.pdf.

Dolan, Paul. "Modeling Valuations for EuroQol Health States." *Medical Care* 35, no. 11 (1997): 1095–1108.

Dolan, Paul, Claire Gudex, Paul Kind, and Alan Williams. *A Social Tariff for EuroQol: Results from a UK General Population Survey.* York, UK: Centre for Health Economics, 1995.

Dolan, Paul, Henry Lee, Dominic King, and Robert Metcalfe. "Valuing Health Directly." *British Medical Journal* 339 (2009): b2577.

Dolan, Paul, Rebecca Shaw, Aki Tsuchiya, and Alan Williams. "QALY Maximisation and People's Preferences: A Methodological Review of the Literature." *Health Economics* 14, no. 2 (2005): 197–208.

Dorsey, Dale. "Toward a Theory of the Basic Minimum," *Politics, Philosophy and Economics* 7, no. 4 (2008): 432–445.

Dorsey, Dale. "Equality-Tempered Prioritarianism." *Politics, Philosophy & Economics* 13, no. 1 (2014): 45–61.

Drummond, Michael, Diana Brixner, Marthe Gold, Paul Kind, Alistair McGuire, Erik Nord, et al. "Towards a Consensus on the QALY." *Value in Health* 12, no. s1 (2009): 31–35.

Drummond, Michael F., Mark J. Sculpher, George W. Torrance, Bernie O'Brien, and Greg L. Stoddart. *Methods for the Economic Evaluation of Health Care Programmes.* Oxford: Oxford University Press, 2005.

Drummond, Michael, George Torrance, and James Mason. "Cost-Effectiveness League Tables: More Harm Than Good?" *Social Science & Medicine* 37, no. 1 (1993): 33–40.

Dworkin, Ronald. *Taking Rights Seriously.* London: Bloomsbury, 1977.

Dworkin, Ronald. "The Original Position." In *Reading Rawls: Critical Studies on Rawls' A Theory of Justice*, edited by Norman Daniels, 16–53. Stanford, CA: Stanford University Press, 1989.

Dworkin, Ronald. "Justice and the High Cost of Health." In *Sovereign Virtue: The Theory and Practice of Equality*, 307–319. Cambridge, MA: Harvard University Press, 2000.

Dworkin, Ronald. *Sovereign Virtue: The Theory and Practice of Equality.* Cambridge, MA: Harvard University Press, 2000.

Dworkin, Ronald. *Justice for Hedgehogs.* Cambridge, MA: Belknap, 2013.

Economist Intelligence Unit. *The Future of Health Care in Europe (2011–2030).* Accessed November 1, 2014. http://www.janssen-emea.com/sites/default/files/The-Future-Of-Healthcare-In-Europe.pdf.

Eddy, David M. "What Care Is 'Essential'? What Services Are 'Basic'?" *Journal of the American Medical Association* 265 (1991): 786–788.

Emanuel, Ezekiel. *Reinventing American Health Care: How the Affordable Care Act Will Improve Our Terribly Complex, Blatantly Unjust, Outrageously Expensive, Grossly Inefficient, Error Prone System.* New York: Public Affairs, 2014.

Engelhardt, H. Tristram, Jr. *Foundations of Bioethics*, 2nd ed., 398–402. New York: Oxford University Press, 1996.

Entwistle, Vikki A., and Ian S. Watt. "Treating Patients as Persons: A Capabilities Approach to Support Delivery of Person-Centered Care." *American Journal of Bioethics* 13, no. 8 (2013): 29–39.

Eyal, Nir, Samia A. Hurst, Ole F. Norheim, and Dan Wikler, eds. *Inequalities in Health: Concepts, Measures, and Ethics.* New York: Oxford University Press, 2013.

Fabre, Cécile. *Justice in a Changing World.* Cambridge, UK: Polity Press, 2007.

Faden, Ruth, and Madison Powers. "Sufficiency, Relational Egalitarianism, and Health." Unpublished manuscript, May 8, 2012.

Federal Joint Committee. "Aufgabe des G-BA" [Task of the Federal Joint Committee]. Accessed June 12, 2014. https://www.g-ba.de/institution/themenschwerpunkte/methodenbewertung/aufgabe.

Fenton, Elizabeth. "Mind the Gap: Ethical Issues of Private Treatment in the Public Health System." *New Zealand Medical Journal* 124 (2011): 89–96.

Ferrer, Robert L., Inez Cruz, Sandra Burge, Bryan Bayles, and Martha I. Castilla. "Measuring Capability for Healthy Diet and Physical Activity." *Annals of Family Medicine* 12, no. 1 (2014): 46–56.

Fields, Gary S., and Olivia S. Mitchell. "Reforming Social Security and Social Safety Net Programs in Developing Countries." In *Development Issues. Presentations to the 47th Meeting of the Development Committee,* edited by P. Mountfield, 113–119. Washington, DC: The World Bank, 1993.

Finegold, Kenneth. *New Census Estimates Show 3 Million More Americans Had Health Insurance Coverage in 2012 (Aspe Issue Brief).* Washington, DC: US Department of Health and Human Services, 2013.

Fleck, Leonard. *Just Caring: Health Care Rationing and Democratic Deliberation.* New York: Oxford University Press, 2009.

Fleck, Leonard. "Just Caring: Defining a Basic Benefit Package." *Journal of Medicine and Philosophy* 36 (2011): 589–611.

Fleck, Leonard. "Just Caring: Health Care Rationing, Terminal Illness, and the Medically Least Well Off." *Journal of Law, Medicine, and Ethics* 39 (2011, Summer): 156–171.

Fleck, Leonard. "Just Caring: Can We Afford the Ethical and Economic Costs of Circumventing Cancer Drug Resistance?" *Journal of Personalized Medicine* 3, no. 3 (2013): 124–143.

Fleck, Leonard. "The Ethical Challenges Raised by Hepatitis C Drugs." http://msubio-ethics.com/2014/10/23/hepatitis-c/?utm_source=Center+Newsletters&utm_campaign=6db5c63009-Bioethics_in_the_News10_2014&utm_medium=email&utm_term=0_ebda7a82a0-6db5c63009-158359345.

Fleurbaey, Marc, Marie-Louise Leroux, and Grégory Ponthière. "Compensating the Dead." *Journal of Mathematical Economics* 51 (C) (2014): 28–41.

Flynn, Terry N., Elisabeth Huynh, Tim J. Peters, Hareth Al-Janabi, Sam Clemens, Alison Moody, et al. "Scoring the ICECAP-A Capability Instrument: Estimation of a UK Population Tariff." *Health Economics* 24, no. 3 (2015): 258–269.

Foster, James E. "On Economic Poverty: A Survey of Aggregate Measures." *Advances in Economietrics* 3 (1984): 215–251.

Foster, James E., Joel Greer, and Erik Thorbecke. "A Class of Decomposable Poverty Measures." *Econometrica* 52, no. 3 (1984): 761–766.

Foster, James E., and Anthony F. Shorrocks. "Subgroup Consistent Poverty Indices." *Econometrica* 59, no. 3 (1991): 687–709.

Foubister, Thomas, Sarah Thomson, Elias Mossialos, and Alistair L. McGuire. *Private Medical Insurance in the United Kingdom.* Geneva: World Health Organization Regional Office for Europe, and European Observatory on Health Systems and Policies, 2006. http://apps.who.int//iris/handle/10665/107741.

Fourie, Carina. "What Do Theories of Social Justice Have to Say About Health Care Rationing? Well-Being, Sufficiency, and Explicit Age-Rationing." In *Rationing Health Care: Hard Choices and Unavoidable Trade-Offs,* edited by Andre den Exter and Martin Buijsen, 65–86. Antwerp: Maklu, 2012.

Fourie, Carina. "What Is Social Equality? An Analysis of Status Equality as a Strongly Egalitarian Ideal." *Res Publica* 18, no. 2 (2012): 107–126.

Fourie, Carina. "To Praise and to Scorn: The Problem of Inequalities of Esteem for Social Egalitarians." In *Social Equality: On What It Means to Be Equals,* edited by Carina Fourie, Fabian Schuppert, and Ivo Wallimann-Helmer, 87–106. New York: Oxford University Press, 2015.

Frankfurt, Harry. "Necessity and Desire." *Philosophy and Phenomenological Research* 45, no. 1 (1984): 1–13.

Frankfurt, Harry. "Equality as a Moral Ideal." *Ethics* 98, no. 1 (1987): 21–43.

Frankfurt, Harry. "Equality and Respect." *Social Research* 64, no. 1 (1997): 3–15.

Frankfurt, Harry. "The Moral Irrelevance of Equality." *Public Affairs Quarterly* 14, no. 2 (2000): 87–103.

Freimann, Christopher. "Why Poverty Matters Most: Towards a Humanitarian Theory of Social Justice." *Utilitas* 24, no. 1 (2012): 26–40.

Gafni, Amiram. "Economic Evaluation of Health-Care Programmes: Is CEA Better Than CBA?" *Environmental & Resource Economics* 34, no. 3. (2006): 407–418.

Gaspart, Frédéric, and Axel Gosseries. "Are Generational Savings Unjust?" *Politics, Philosophy & Economics* 6, no. 2 (2007): 193–217.

Gerard, Karen. "Setting Priorities in the New NHS: Can Purchasers Use Cost-Utility Information." *Health Policy* 25, no. 1–2 (1993): 109–125.

Gerard, Karen, and Gavin Mooney. "QALY League Tables: Handle with Care." *Health Economics* 2, no. 1 (1993): 59–64.

Gheaus, Anca. "Could There Ever Be a Duty to Have Children?" In *Permissible Progeny?* edited by Samantha Brennan, Sarah Hannan & Richard Vernon. New York: Oxford University Press, 2015.

Gold, Marthe R., Joanna E. Siegel, Louise B. Russell, and Milton C. Weinstein. *Cost-Effectiveness in Health and Medicine.* Oxford: Oxford University Press, 1996.

Goldberger, J., B. Anirban, and R. Boineau. "Risk Stratification for Sudden Cardiac Death: A Plan for the Future." *Circulation* 129 (2014): 516–526.

Goodin, Robert. "Egalitarianism, Fetishistic and Otherwise." *Ethics* 98, no. 1 (1987): 44–49.

Gosseries, Axel. "Are Seniority Privileges Unfair?" *Economics & Philosophy* 20, no. 2 (2004): 279–305.

Gosseries, Axel. "On Future Generations' Future Rights." *Journal of Political Philosophy* 16, no. 4 (2008): 446–474.

Gosseries, Axel. "Theories of Intergenerational Justice: A Synopsis." *Surveys and Perspectives Integrating Environment and Society* 1, no. 1 (2008): 61–71.

Gosseries, Axel. "Three Models of Intergenerational Reciprocity." In *Intergenerational Justice,* edited by A. Gosseries and L. Meyer, 119–146. Oxford: Oxford University Press, 2009.

Gosseries, Axel. "A Justiça Intergeracional e a Metáfora do Refúgio de Montanha." *Philosophica (Lisbon)* 38 (2011): 121–141.

Gosseries, Axel. "Qu'est-ce que le suffisantisme?" *Philosophiques* 38, no. 2 (2011): 465–492.

Gosseries, Axel. "Nations, Generations and Climate Justice." *Global Policy* 5, no. 1 (2014): 96–102.

Gosseries, Axel. "Reply to My Critics." *Diacritica* 28, no. 2 (2014): 343–348.

Gosseries, Axel. "What Makes Age Discrimination Special? A Philosophical Look at the ECJ Case Law. *Netherlands Journal of Legal Philosophy* 43, no. 1 (2014): 59–80.

Gosseries, Axel. "Les Générations, le Fleuve et l'océan." *Philosophiques* 42, no. 1 (2015).

Grewal, Ini, Jane Lewis, Terry Flynn, Jackie Brown, John Bond, and Joanna Coast. "Developing Attributes for a Generic Quality of Life Measure for Older People: Preferences or Capabilities?" *Social Science & Medicine* 62, no. 8 (2006): 1891–1901.

Gusmano, Michael K. "Is It Reasonable to Deny Older Patients Treatment for Glioblastoma?" *Journal of Law, Medicine, and Ethics* 42, no. 2 (2014): 183–189.

Hadorn, David C. "Setting Health Care Priorities in Oregon: Cost-Effectiveness Meets the Rule of Rescue." *Journal of the American Medical Association* 216, no. 17 (1991): 2218–2225.

Hall, Mark A. *Making Medical Spending Decisions: The Law, Ethics, and Economics of Rationing Mechanisms.* New York: Oxford University Press, 1997.

Hanley, Nick, and Edward B. Barbier. *Pricing Nature: Cost–Benefit Analysis and Environmental Policy.* Cheltenham, UK: Elgar, 2009.

Harman, Elizabeth. "Can We Harm and Benefit in Creating?" *Philosophical Perspectives* 18, no. 1 (2004): 89–113.

Harris, John. *The Value of Life.* Oxford: Routledge & Kegan Paul, 1985.

Harris, John. "QALYfying the Value of Life." *Journal of Medical Ethics* 13, no. 3 (1987): 117–123.

Herdman, Michael, C. Gudex, A. Lloyd, M. F. Jansses, P. Kind, D. Parkin, et al. "Development and Preliminary Testing of the New Five-Level Version of EQ-5D (EQ-5D-5L)." *Quality of Life Research* 20, no. 10 (2011): 1727–1736.

Himmelstein, David. "Response to the Institute of Medicine's Recommendation That Cost Determine Insurance Policies' 'Essential Benefits'." *International Journal of Health Services* 42, no. 3 (2012): 571–573.

Hirose, Iwao. *Equality, Priority, and Aggregation*. St. Andrews, UK: University of St. Andrews, 2004.

Hirose, Iwao. *Egalitarianism*. London: Routledge, 2015.

HM Treasury. *The Green Book: Appraisal and Evaluation in Central Government*. London: The Stationary Office, 2003.

Hoffmann, Christine, and Reinhard Busse. "Priorisierung in Anderen Gesundheitssystemen; Was Kann Deutschland lernen?" *Bundesgesundheitsblatt*, 53 (2010): 882–889.

Holtug, Nils. *Persons, Interests, and Justice*. Oxford: Oxford University Press, 2010.

Holtug, Nils. "The Cosmopolitan Strikes Back: A Critical Discussion of Miller on Nationality and Global Equality." *Ethics & Global Politics* 4, no. 3 (2011): 147–163.

Howarth, Richard. "Towards an Operational Sustainability Criterion." *Ecological Economics* 63 (2007): 656–663.

Hucklenbroich, Peter. "'Disease Entity' as the Key Theoretical Concept of Medicine." *Journal of Medicine and Philosophy* 39, no. 6 (2014): 609–633.

Huikiri, Heikki. "Prediction of Benefits from Implantable Cardioverter Defibrillators." *Journal of the American College of Cardiology* 63 (2014): 2270–2271.

Hume, David. *A Treatise of Human Nature*, book III, part II, section II.

Hurley, Jeremiah. "Welfarism, Extra-Welfarism and Evaluative Economic Analysis." In *Health, Healthcare and Health Economics: Perspectives on Distribution*, edited by Morris L. Barer, Thomas E. Getzen, and Greg L. Stoddart, 373–395. Chichester, UK: Wiley, 1998.

Hurley, Jeremiah. "An Overview of the Normative Economics of the Health Sector." In *Handbook of Health Economics Vol. 1, Part A*, edited by Anthony J. Culyer and Joseph P. Newhouse, 55–118. Oxford: North-Holland, 2000.

Huseby, Robert. "Sufficiency: Restated and Defended." *Journal of Political Philosophy* 18, no. 2 (2010): 178–197.

Huseby, Robert. "Sufficiency and Population Ethics." *Ethical Perspectives* 19 (2012): 187–206.

Institute of Medicine. *Essential Health Benefits: Balancing Coverage and Cost*. Washington, DC: National Academies Press, 2012.

Jamison, Dean T., Lawrence H. Summers, George Alleyne, Kenneth J. Arrow, Seth Berkley, Agnes Binagwaho, et al. "Global Health 2035: A World Converging within a Generation." *Lancet* 382, no. 9908 (2013, December 7): 1898–1955.

Johnson, F. Reed. "Moving the QALY Forward or Just Stuck in Traffic?" *Value in Health* 12, no. s1 (2009): 38–39.

Johnson, Matthew. "Towards a Theory of Cultural Evaluation." *Critical Review of Social and Political Philosophy* 17, no. 2 (2014): 145–167.

Kaiser Commission on Medicaid and the Uninsured. *Premiums and Cost-Sharing in Medicaid (Policy Brief)*. Menlo Park, CA: Kaiser Family Foundation, 2013.

Kaiser Family Foundation. *Focus Health Reform: Patient Cost-Sharing under the Affordable Care Act*. Menlo Park, CA: Kaiser Family Foundation, 2012.

Kaiser Family Foundation. "Medicaid Income Eligibility Limits for Adults at Application, as of August 28, 2014 (Table)." Accessed January 24, 2015. http://kff.org/state-category/medicaid-chip/medicaidchip-eligibility-limits.

Kaiser, Jocelyn. "New Cystic Fibrosis Drug Offers Hope." *Science* 335 (2012, February 10): 645.

Keehan, S., G. Cuckler, A. Sisko, A. Madison, S. Smith, D. Stone, et al. "National Health Expenditure Projections, 2014–2024: Spending Growth Faster Than Recent Trends." *Health Affairs* 34, no. 8 (2015): 1407–1417.

Kelleher, J. Paul. "Health Inequalities and Relational Egalitarianism" (n.d.).

Kinghorn, Philip, Angela Robinson, and Richard D. Smith. "Developing a Capability-Based Questionnaire for Assessing Well-Being in Patients with Chronic Pain." *Social Indicators Research* 120, no. 3 (2015): 897–916.

Kingma, Elselijn. "What Is It to Be Healthy?" *Analysis* 67, no. 294 (2007): 128–133.

Klingler, Corina, Sarah Shah, Anthony Barron, and John Wright. "Regulatory Space and the Contextual Mediation of Common Functional Pressures: Analyzing the Factors That Led to the German Efficiency Frontier Approach." *Health Policy* 109, no. 3 (2013): 270–280.

Knight, Carl. "Enough Is Too Much." Unpublished manuscript (n.d.).

Knight, Carl. *Luck Egalitarianism: Equality, Responsibility, and Justice*. Edinburgh, UK: Edinburgh University Press, 2009.

Korsgaard, Christine M. "Two Distinctions in Goodness." *Philosophical Review* 92, no. 2 (1983): 169–195.

Krohmal, Benjamin J., and Ezekiel J. Emanuel. "Access and Ability to Pay: The Ethics of a Tiered Health Care System." *Archives of Internal Medicine* 167 (2007): 433–437.

Krohmal, Benjamin J., and Ezekiel J. Emanuel. "Tiers Without Tears: The Ethics of a Two-Tier Health Care System." In *The Oxford Handbook of Bioethics*, edited by Bonnie Steinbock, 175–189. New York: Oxford University Press, 2007.

Law, Iain, and Heather Widdows. "Conceptualising Health: Insights from the Capability Approach." *Health Care Analysis* 16, no. 4 (2008): 303–314.

Lazenby, Hugh. "Mistakes and the Continuity Test." *Politics, Philosophy, and Economics* 15, no. 2 (2016):190-205.

Levey, Noam N. "Passing the Buck—or Empowering States? Who Will Define Essential Health Benefits." *Health Affairs (Millwood)* 31, no. 4 (2012): 663–666.

Lewis, David. "Finkish Dispositions." *Philosophical Quarterly* 47, no. 187 (1997): 143–158.

Lippert-Rasmussen, Kasper. "The Insignificance of the Distinction Between Telic and Deontic Egalitarianism." In *Egalitarianism: New Essays on the Meaning and Value of Equality*, edited by Nils Holtug and Kasper Lippert-Rasmussen, 101–124. Oxford: Oxford University Press, 2007.

Lippert-Rasmussen, Kasper. "Justice and Bad Luck." *The Stanford Encyclopedia of Philosophy*, edited by Edward N. Zalta (Summer 2014 edition). http://plato.stanford.edu/archives/sum2014/entries/justice-bad-luck.

Littmann, Jasper. *Antibiotic Resistance and Distributive Justice*, PhD thesis. London: University College London.

Loomes, Graham, and Lynda McKenzie. "The Use of QALYs in Health Care Decision Making." *Social Science & Medicine* 29, no. 3 (1989): 299–308.

Lorgelly, Paula K., Kenny D. Lawson, Elisabeth A. L. Fenwick, and Andrew H. Briggs. "Outcome Measurement in Economic Evaluations of Public Health Interventions: A Role for the Capability Approach?" *International Journal of Environmental Research and Public Health* 7, no. 5 (2010): 2274–2289.

Lorgelly, P. et al. "Operationalising the capability approach as an outcome measure in public health: the development of the OCAP-18." *Social Science & Medicine* 142 (2015), 68–81.

Lucas, J. R. "Against Equality." *Philosophy* 40, no. 154 (1965): 296–307.

Lucas, J. R. "Against Equality Again." *Philosophy* 52, no. 201 (1977): 255–280.

Madison, Kristin, Harald Schmidt, and Kevin G. Volpp. "Smoking, Obesity, Health Insurance, and Health Incentives in the Affordable Care Act." *Journal of the American Medical Association* 310, no. 2 (2013, July 10): 143–144.

Mantone, Joe. "Even with Insurance, Hospital Stay Can Cost a Million." *The Wall Street Journal*, November 29, 2007. Accessed June 11, 2014. http://blogs.wsj.com/health/2007/11/29/even-with-insurance-hospital-stay-can-cost-a-million.

Marmot, M., R. Fuhrer, S. L. Ettner, N. F. Marks, L. L. Bumpass, and C. D. Ryff. "Contribution of Psychosocial Factors to Socioeconomic Differences in Health." *Milbank Quarterly* 76, no. 3 (1998): 403–448.

Marmot, Michael. "Social Determinants of Health Inequalities." *Lancet* 365, no. 9464 (2005, March 19): 1099–1104.

Marmot, Michael. *The Status Syndrome: How Social Standing Affects Our Health and Longevity*. New York: Holt, 2005.

Marmot, Michael, and Richard Wilkinson, eds. *Social Determinants of Health*, 2nd ed. New York: Oxford University Press, 2005.

Martin, A., M. Hartmann, L. Whittle, A. Caitlin, and the National Health Accounts Expenditure Team. "National Health Spending in 2012: Rate of Health Spending Growth Remained Low for the Fourth Consecutive Year." *Health Affairs* 33, no. 1 (2014): 67–77.

Mason, Andrew. *Living Together as Equals: The Demands of Citizenship*. Oxford: Oxford University Press, 2012.

Mason, Andrew. "Justice, Respect, and Treating People as Equals." In *Social Equality: On What It Means to Be Equals*, edited by Carina Fourie, Fabian Schuppert, and Ivo Wallimann-Helmer. New York: Oxford University Press, 2015.

McIntosh, Emma, Philip Clarke, Emma J. Frew, and Jordan J. Louviere. *Applied Methods of Cost–Benefit in Health Care*. Oxford: Oxford University Press, 2010.

McKerlie, Dennis. "Equality and Time." *Ethics* 99, no. 3 (1989): 475–491.

McKerlie, Dennis. *Justice Between the Young and the Old*. Oxford: Oxford University Press, 2013.

Medical Services Advisory Committee. "Medical Services Advisory Committee." Accessed March 15, 2015. http://www.msac.gov.au.

Menzel, Paul T. "Determining the Value of Life: Discrimination, Advance Directives, and the Right to Die with Dignity." *Free Inquiry* 25, no. 5 (2005): 39–41.

Menzel, Paul T. "A Cultural Moral Right to a Basic Minimum of Accessible Health Care." *Kennedy Institute of Ethics Journal* 21, no. 1 (2011): 79–120.

Menzel, Paul T. "Justice and Fairness: A Critical Element in U.S. Health System Reform." *Journal of Law, Medicine, and Ethics* 40, no. 3 (2012): 582–597.

Menzel, Paul T. "Justice, Liberty, and the Choice of Health System Structure." In *Medicine and Social Justice*, edited by Rosamond Rhodes, Margaret Battin, and Anita Silvers, 2nd ed., 35–46. New York: Oxford University Press, 2012.

Menzel, Paul T. "Setting Priorities for a Basic Minimum of Accessible Health Care." In *Medicine and Social Justice*, edited by Rosamond Rhodes, Margaret Battin, and Anita Silvers, 2nd ed., 131–141. New York: Oxford University Press, 2012.

Menzel, Paul T. "Statistical and Identified Lives: Why Not to Use the 'R' Word." In *Fair Resource Allocation and Rationing at the Bedside*, edited by Marion Danis, Samia Hurst, Leonard Fleck, Reidun Forde, and Anne Slowther, 238–252. New York: Oxford University Press, 2015.

Menzel, Paul T., Marthe R. Gold, Erik Nord, Jose-Louis Pinto-Prades, Jeff Richardson, and Peter Ubel. "Toward a Broader View of Values in Cost-Effectiveness Analysis of Health." *Hastings Center Report* 29, no. 3 (1999): 7.

Menzel, Paul T., and Bonnie Steinbock. "Advance Directives, Dementia, and Physician-Assisted Death." *Journal of Law, Medicine, and Ethics* 41 (2013): 484–500.

Meulen, Ruud ter. "How 'Decent' Is a Decent Minimum of Health Care?" *Journal of Medicine and Philosophy* 36 (2011): 612–623.

Meyer, Lukas H., and Dominic Roser. "Enough for the Future." In *Intergenerational Justice*, edited by Axel Gosseries and Lukas H. Meyer. Oxford: Oxford University Press, 2009.

Miller, David. *National Responsibility and Global Justice*. Oxford: Oxford University Press, 2007.

Ministry of Health Welfare and Sports. "Health Insurance in The Netherlands." Accessed March 17, 2015. https://www.government.nl/documents-and-publications/leaflets/2012/09/26/health-insurance-in-the-netherlands.html.

Mitchell, Paul M., Tracy E. Roberts, Pelham M. Barton, and Joanna Coast. "Assessing Sufficient Capability: A New Approach to Economic Evaluation." *Social Science & Medicine* 139 (2015): 71–79.

Mitchell, Paul M., Tracy E. Roberts, Pelham M. Barton, and Joanna Coast. "Applications of the Capability Approach in the Health Field: a Literature Review." *Social Indicators Research* (2016): doi: 10.1007/s11205-016-1356-8.

Molyneux, Jacob. "The Top Health Care News Story of 2010: Health Insurance Dominated the Year." *American Journal of Nursing* 111, no. 1 (2011): 14–15.

Mossialos, Elias, Martin Wenzl, Robin Osborn, and Chloe Anderson, eds. *International Profiles of Health Care Systems 2014*. New York: The Commonwealth Fund, 2015.

Murray, Christopher, and Alan Lopez. *The Global Burden of Disease: A Comprehensive Assessment of Mortality and Disability from Diseases, Injuries and Risk Factors in 1990 and Projected to 2020*. Cambridge, MA: Harvard University Press, 1996.

National Conference on Medical Nomenclature, Adaline C. Hayden, Edward T. Thompson, and American Medical Association, eds. *Standard Nomenclature of Diseases and Operations*. New York: McGraw-Hill, 1961.

National Health Care Institute. "Health Care Coverage: A Well-Balanced Basic Health Care Package." Accessed March 15, 2015. http://www.zorginstituutnederland.nl/binaries/content/documents/zinl-www/documenten/rubrieken/english/1506-health-care-coverage-a-well-balanced-basic-health-care-package/Health+Care+Coverage+%28A+well-balanced+basic+health+care+package%29.pdf.

National Institute for Health and Care Excellence (NICE). *Guide to the Methods of Technology Appraisal*. London: NICE, 2013.

National Institute for Health and Care Excellence (NICE). *Developing NICE Guidelines: The Manual*. London: NICE, 2014.

National Institute for Health and Care Excellence. "Social Value Judgements: Principles for the Development of NICE Guidance." Accessed March 17, 2015. https://www.nice.org.uk/media/default/about/what-we-do/research-and-development/social-value-judgements-principles-for-the-development-of-nice-guidance.pdf.

National Institute for Health and Care Excellence. "Social Value Judgements: Principles for the Development of NICE Guidance, Second Edition." Accessed April 5, 2015. https://www.nice.org.uk/media/default/about/what-we-do/research-and-development/social-value-judgements-principles-for-the-development-of-nice-guidance.pdf.

Netten, Ann, Peter Burge, Juliette Malley, Dimitris Potoglou, Ann-Marie Towers, John Brazier, et al. "Outcomes of Social Care for Adults: Developing a Preference-Weighted Measure." *Health Technology Assessment* 16, no. 16 (2012): 1–166.

Neumann, Peter J., Teja Thorat, Jennifer Shi, Cayla J. Saret, and Joshua T. Cohen. "The Changing Face of the Cost–Utility Literature, 1990–2012." *Value in Health* 18, no. 2 (2015): 271–277.

Nielsen, Lasse. "Why Health Matters to Justice: A Capability Theory Perspective." *Ethical Theory and Moral Practice* 18, no. 2 (2014): 403–415.

Nielsen, Lasse. "Sufficiency Grounded as Sufficiently Free: A Reply to Shlomi Segall." *Journal of Applied Philosophy*. doi: 10.1111/japp.12159.

Nielsen, Lasse and David V. Axelsen. "Capabilitarian Sufficiency: Capabilities and Social Justice." *Journal of Human Development and Capabilities*. doi: 10.1080/19452829.2016.1145632.

Nielsen, Lasse, and David V. Axelsen. "Three Strikes Out: Objections to Shlomi Segall's Luck Egalitarian Justice in Health." *Ethical Perspectives* 19, no. 2 (2012): 307–316.

Nord, Erik. *Cost–Value Analysis in Health Care: Making Sense out of QALYs.* Cambridge, UK: Cambridge University Press, 1999.

Nord, Erik. "Disability Weights in the Global Burden of Disease 2010: Unclear Meaning and Overstatement of International Agreement." *Health Policy* 111, no. 1 (2013): 99–104.

Nordenfelt, Lennart. "Concepts of Health and Their Consequences for Health Care." *Theoretical Medicine,* 14 (1993): 277–285.

Nordenfelt, Lennart. "On the Relevance and Importance of the Notion of Disease." *Theoretical Medicine* 14 (1993): 15–26.

Nordenfelt, Lennart. *Quality of Life, Health and Happiness.* Aldershot, UK: Avebury, 1993.

Nordenfeldt, Lennart. *On the Nature of Health.* New York: Springer, 1995.

Nordenfelt, Lennart. *On the Nature of Health—An Action-Theoretical Approach,* 2nd revised and enlarged edition. Dordrecht, The Netherlands: Springer, 1995.

Nordenfelt, Lennart. *Health, Science, and Ordinary Language.* Amsterdam: Rodopi, 2001.

Normand, Charles. "Measuring Outcomes in Palliative Care: Limitations of QALYs and the Road to PALYs." *Journal of Pain and Symptom Management* 38, no. 1 (2009): 27–31.

Norwegian Ministry of Finance. "Cost–Benefit Analysis: Official Norwegian Reports NOU 2012: 16." Accessed March 15, 2015. http://omega.regjeringen.no/nb/dep/fin/dok/nouer/2012/nou-2012-16-2/11/6/1.html?id=713616.

Nussbaum, Martha C. "Nature, Function, and Capability: Aristotle on Political Distribution." *Oxford Studies in Ancient Philosophy* Suppl. Vol. (1988), 145–184.

Nussbaum, Martha C. "Human Functioning and Social Justice." *Political Theory* 20, no. 2 (1992): 202–246.

Nussbaum, Martha C. *Women and Human Development.* New York: Cambridge University Press, 2000.

Nussbaum, Martha C. "Constitutions and Capabilities: 'Perception' Against Lofty Formalism." *Harvard Law Review* 121 (2007): 4–97.

Nussbaum, Martha C. *Frontiers of Justice: Disability, Nationality, Species Membership.* Cambridge, MA: Harvard University Press, 2007.

Nussbaum, Martha C. *Creating Capabilities: The Human Development Approach.* London: Belknap, 2011.

Oberlander, Jonathan. "Health Reform Interrupted: The Unraveling of the Oregon Health Plan." *Health Affairs* 26, no. 1 (2007): 96–105.

O'Connell, Thomas, Kumanan Rasanathan, and Mickey Chopra. "What Does Universal Health Coverage Mean?" *Lancet* 383, no. 9913 (2014): 277–279.

Office of the Assistant Secretary for Planning and Evaluation. "Health Insurance Coverage and the Affordable Care Act." Accessed March 17, 2015. http://aspe.hhs.gov/health/reports/2015/uninsured_change/ib_uninsured_change.cfm.

Olsen, Jan A., and Cam Donaldson. "Helicopters, Hearts and Hips: Using Willingness to Pay to Set Priorities for Public Sector Health Care Programmes." *Social Science & Medicine* 46, no. 1 (1998): 1–12.

Organization for Economic Co-operation and Development (OECD). *OECD Study on Private Health Insurance.* Paris: OECD, 2004.

Organization for Economic Co-operation and Development (OEDC). *Health at a Glance 2013: OECD Indicators.* Paris: OECD, 2013.

Organization for Economic Co-operatoin and Development (OECD), *OECD Health Statistics.* Online database. Paris, OECD, 2014.

O'Shea, Eamon, Brenda Gannon, and Brendan Kennelly. "Eliciting Preferences for Resource Allocation in Mental Health Care in Ireland." *Health Policy* 88, no. 2–3 (2008): 359–370.

Otsuka, Michael, and Alex Voorhoeve. "Why It Matters That Some Are Worse Off Than Others." *Philosophy and Public Affairs* 37 (2009): 171–199.

Ozar, David, T. "What Should Count as Basic Health Care?" *Theoretical Medicine* 4 (1983): 129–141.

Page, Edward. "Justice Between Generations: Investigating a Sufficientarian Approach." *Journal of Global Ethics* 3, no. 1 (2007): 3–20.

Page, Edward. *Climate Change, Justice and Future Generations.* Cheltenham, UK: Elgar, 2007.

Palmer, Stephen, and David J. Torgerson. "Definitions of Efficiency." *British Medical Journal* 318, no. 7191 (1999): 1136.

Panteli, Dimitra, Helene Eckhardt, Alexandra Nolting, Reinhard Busse, and Michael Kulig. "From Market Access to Patient Access: Overview of Evidence-Based Approaches for the Reimbursement and Pricing of Pharmaceuticals in 36 European Countries." Unpublished data.

Parfit, Derek. *Reasons and Persons.* Oxford: Oxford University Press, 1984.

Parfit, Derek. *Equality or Priority? The Lindley Lecture.* Lawrence, KS: University of Kansas, 1995.

Parfit, Derek. "Equality and Priority." *Ratio* 10, no. 3 (1997): 202–221.

Parfit, Derek. "Equality or Priority?" In *The Ideal of Equality*, edited by Matthew Clayton and Andrew Williams, 81–125. Basingstoke, UK: Palgrave Macmillan, 2000.

Parfit, Derek. "Another Defense of the Priority View." *Utilitas* 24 (2012): 399–440.

Patient Protection and Affordable Care Act, 42 U.S.C. §18001 (2010) Et Seq., Sec 1302.

Payne, Katherine, Marion McAllister, and Linda M. Davies. "Valuing the Economic Benefits of Complex Interventions: When Maximising Health Is Not Sufficient." *Health Economics* 22, no. 3 (2013): 258–271.

Pharmaceutical Management Agency. "Decision Criteria." Accessed March 15, 2015. https://www.pharmac.health.nz/medicines/how-medicines-are-funded/decision-criteria.

Phend, Crystal. "ASCO: Targeted Tx Combo Stalls NSCLC." *MedPage Today* (2014, June 3). Accessed June 11, 2014. http://www.medpagetoday.com/MeetingCoverage/ASCO/46127.

Pierson, Ransdell. "Looking for Lessons in Cancer's 'Miracle' Responders." *Reuters*, September 15, 2013. Accessed June 12, 2014. http://www.reuters.com/article/2013/09/15/us-cancer-superresponders-idUSBRE98E07420130915.

Pinchot, Gifford, *The Fight for Conservation*. New York: Doubleday, Page & Company, 1910.

Pogge, Thomas. "A Critique of the Capability Approach." In *Measuring Justice Primary Goods and Capabilities*, edited by Harry Brighouse and Ingird Robeyns. Cambridge, UK: Cambridge University Press, 2010.

Ponthière, Gregory. "Should We Discount Future Generations' Welfare? A Survey of the 'Pure' Discount Rate Debate." Liège: CREPP Working Paper, 2003.

Porter, Eduardo. "Acceleration Is Forecast for Spending on Health." *New York Times*, April 23, 2014, B1–B2.

Powers, Madison, and Ruth Faden. *Social Justice: The Moral Foundations of Public Health and Health Policy*. New York: Oxford University Press, 2006.

President's Commission for the Study of Ethical Problems in Medicine and Biomedical and Behavioral Research. *Securing Access to Health Care: The Ethical Implications of Differences in the Availability of Health Services, Volume One*, 20. Washington, DC: US Government Printing Office, 1983.

Ram-Tiktin, Efrat. "Distributive Justice in Health Care." PhD Dissertation, Bar-Ilan University, 2009. [in Hebrew]

Ram-Tiktin, Efrat. "A Decent Minimum for Everyone as a Sufficiency of Basic Human Functional Capabilities." *American Journal of Bioethics* 11, no. 7 (2011): 24–25.

Ram-Tiktin, Efrat. "The Right to Health Care as a Right to Basic Human Functional Capabilities." *Ethical Theory and Moral Practice* 15, no. 3 (2012): 337–351.

Ram-Tiktin, Efrat. "Fair Equality of Opportunity Versus Sufficiency of Capabilities in Healthcare." Manuscript available from the author.

Rawlins, Michael, David Barnett, and Andrew Stevens. "Pharmacoeconomics: NICE's Approach to Decision-Making." *British Journal of Clinical Pharmacology* 70, no. 3 (2010): 346–349.

Rawls, John. *A Theory of Justice.* Cambridge, MA: Harvard University Press, 1971.

Rawls, John. *Political Liberalism.* New York: Columbia University Press, 1993.

Rawls, John. *A Theory of Justice,* revised edition. Cambridge, MA: Harvard University Press, 1999.

Raz, Joseph. *The Morality of Freedom.* Oxford: Oxford University Press, 1986.

Rechel, Bernd, Sarah Thomson, and Ewout van Ginneken. *Health Systems in Transition: Template for Authors.* Copenhagen: World Health Organization, 2010.

Rhodes, Rosamund, Margaret P. Battin, and Anita Silvers, eds. *Medicine and Social Justice: Essays on the Distribution of Health Care,* 2nd ed. Oxford: Oxford University Press, 2012.

Rice, Thomas, Pauline Rosenau, Lynn Y. Unruh, Andrew J. Barnes, Richard B. Saltman, and Ewout van Ginneken. "United States of America: Health System Review." *Health Systems in Transition* 15, no. 3 (2013): 1–431.

Richardson, Henry S. "Capabilities and the Definition of Health: Comments on Venkatapuram." Bioethics 30, no. 1 (2016): 1–7.

Ridic, Goran, Suzanne Gleason, and Ognjen Ridic. "Comparisons of Health Care Systems in the United States, Germany and Canada." *Materia Socio-Medica* 24, no. 2 (2012): 112–120.

Ringard, Ånen, and Ingrid Sperre Saunes. "Update on New Official Norwegian Report on Priority Setting in Health Care Presented." Online HiT for Norway—HSPM. Accessed March 15, 2015. http://www.hspm.org/countries/norway08012014/livinghit.aspx?Section=2.7%20Health%20information%20management&Type=Section.

Robinson, James C. "Philosophical Origins of the Economic Valuation of Life." *Milbank Quarterly* 64, no. 1 (1986): 133–155.

Roemer, John. "Eclectic Distributional Ethics." *Politics, Philosophy and Economics* 3, no. 3 (2004): 267–281.

Ruger, Jennifer Prah. *Health and Social Justice.* New York: Oxford University Press, 2010.

Ruger, Jennifer Prah. "An Alternative Framework for Analyzing Financial Protection in Health." *PLoS Medicine* 9, no. 8 (2012): e1001294.

Rumbold, Benedict E. "Review Article: The Moral Right to Health: A Survey of Available Conceptions." *Critical Review of International Social and Political Philosophy* (2015): doi: 10.1080/13698230.2014.995505.

Sabik, Lindsay, and Reidar Lie. "Priority Setting in Health Care: Lessons from the Experiences of Eight Countries." *International Journal for Equity in Health* 7, no. 4 (2008): doi: 10.1186/1475-9276-7-4.

Sachs, Benjamin. "Extortion and the Ethics of 'Topping Up'." *Cambridge Quarterly of Healthcare Ethics* 18 (2009): 443–445.

Saha, Somnath, Darren Coffman, and Ariel Smits. "Giving Teeth to Comparative-Effectiveness Research—The Oregon Experience." *New England Journal of Medicine* 362 (2010): e18.

Satz, Debra. "Equality, Adequacy, and Education for Citizenship." *Ethics* 117, no. 4 (2007): 623–648.

Savulescu, Julian. "Justice and Healthcare: The Right to a Decent Minimum, Not Equality of Opportunity." *American Journal of Bioethics* 1 (2001): 1a–3a.

Scanlon, T. M. *What We Owe to Each Other*. Cambridge, MA: Harvard University Press, 1998.

Scanlon, T. M. "The Diversity of Objections to Inequality." In *The Ideal of Equality*, edited by Matthew Clayton and Andrew Williams, 41–59. Basingstoke, UK: Palgrave Macmillan, 2002.

Schmidt, Harald, and Ezekiel J. Emanuel. "Lowering Medical Costs Through the Sharing of Savings by Physicians and Patients: Inclusive Shared Savings." *Journal of the American Medical Association Internal Medicine* 174, no. 12 (2014): 2009–2013.

Schmidt, Harald, Kristin Voigt, and Ezekiel J. Emanuel. "The Ethics of Not Hiring Smokers." *New England Journal of Medicine* 368, no. 15 (2013): 1369–1371.

Schneider, Bryan, Molin Wang, Milan Radovich, et al. "Association of Vascular Endothelial Growth Factor and Vascular Endothelial Growth Factor Receptor-2 Genetic Polymorphisms with Outcome in a Trial of Paclitaxel Compared with Paclitaxel Plus Bevacizumab in Advanced Breast Cancer ECOG 2100." *Journal of Clinical Oncology* 26 (2008): 4672–4678.

Schreyögg Jonas, Tom Stargardt, Marcial Velasco, and Reinhard Busse. "Defining the Health Benefit Basket in Nine European Countries: Evidence from the European Union Health BASKET Project." *European Journal of Health Economics* 6, Suppl. 1 (2005): 2–10.

Schuppert, Fabian. "Distinguishing Basic Needs and Fundamental Interests." *Critical Review of International Social and Political Philosophy* 16, no. 1 (2013): 24–44.

Segall, Shlomi. *Health, Luck and Justice*. Princeton, NJ: Princeton University Press, 2010.

Segall, Shlomi. "Is Health (Really) Special? Health Policy Between Rawlsian and Luck Egalitarian Justice." *Journal of Applied Philosophy* 27, no. 4 (2010): 344–358.

Segall, Shlomi. "What Is the Point of Sufficiency?" *Journal of Applied Philosophy* 33, no. 1 (2016): 36–52.

Sen, Amartya. "Poverty: An Ordinal Approach to Measurement." *Econometrica* 44, no. 2 (1976): 219–231.

Sen, Amartya. "Social Choice Theory: A Re-examination." *Econometrica* 45, no. 1 (1977): 53–89.

Sen, Amartya. "Equality of What?" In *The Tanner Lectures on Human Values: Vol. 1*, edited by Sterling M. McMurrin, 197–220. Salt Lake City, UT: University of Utah Press, 1980.

Sen, Amartya. *Commodities and Capabilities*. Amsterdam: North Holland, 1985.

Sen, Amartya. "Justice: Means Versus Freedom." *Philosophy and Public Affairs* 19, no. 2 (1990): 111–121.

Sen, Amartya. *Inequality Reexamined*. Oxford: Oxford University Press, 1995.

Sen, Amartya. *Development as Freedom*. Oxford: Oxford University Press, 1999.

Sen, Amartya. *The Idea of Justice*. London: Lane, 2009.

Sen, Amartya, "Global Warming Is Just One of Many Environmental Threats That Demand Our Attention." *The New Republic*, August 22, 2014.

Shields, Liam. "The Prospects for Sufficientarianism." *Utilitas* 24, no. 1 (2012): 101–117.

Shields, Liam. "Egalitarianism and Sufficientarianism: A Difficult Relationship." Unpublished manuscript (n.d.).

Shiffrin, Seana Valentine. "Wrongful Life, Procreative Responsibility, and the Significance of Harm." *Legal Theory* 5, no. 2 (1999): 117–148.

Shue, Henry. *Basic Rights*. Princeton, NJ: Princeton University Press, 1980.

Simon, Judit, Paul Anand, Alastair Gray, Jorun Rugkåsa, Ksenija Yeeles, and Tom Burns. "Operationalising the Capability Approach for Outcome Measurement in Mental Health Research." *Social Science & Medicine* 98 (2013): 187–196.

Skorupski, John. "Threshold Justice." In *Ethical Explorations*, 85–102. Oxford: Oxford University Press, 1999..

Stanton, Mark. "The High Concentration of U.S. Health Expenditures" *Research in Action* 19 (2006). Accessed June 11, 2014. http://www.ahrq.gov/research/findings/factsheets/costs/expriach/index.html#diffi.

Steiner, Hillel. *An Essay on Rights*. Oxford: Blackwell, 1996.

Sugden, Robert. "Welfare, Resources and Capabilities: A Review of Inequality Reexamined by Amartya Sen." *Journal of Economic Literature* 31, no. 4 (1993): 1947–1962.

Sutton, Eileen, and Joanna Coast. "Development of a Supportive Care Measure for Economic Evaluation of End of Life Care Using Qualitative Methods." *Palliative Medicine* 28, no. 2 (2014): 152–157.

Temkin, Larry. "Inequality: A Complex, Individualistic, and Comparative Notion." *Philosophical Issues* 11 (2001): 327–353.

Temkin, Larry. "Egalitarianism Defended." *Ethics* 113 (2003): 764–782.

Temkin, Larry. "Equality, Priority, or What?" *Economics and Philosophy* 19 (2003): 61–87.

The Commonwealth Fund, *Commonwealth Fund International Health Policy Survey 2014* (New York: The Commonwealth Fund, 2014).

The State Comptroller of Israel. *Annual Report* 63$_c$ (May 8, 2013): 935 [in Hebrew]. Accessed May 1, 2014. http://www.mevaker.gov.il/he/Reports/Pages/114.aspx.

Thompson, Kimberly, and Radboud Duintjer Tebbens. "Eradication Versus Control for Poliomyelitis: An Economic Analysis." *Lancet* 369 (2007): 1363–1371.

Thomson, Sarah, Josep Figueras, Tamas Evetovits, Matthew Jowett, Philipa Mladovsky, Anna Maresso, et al. *Economic Crisis, Health Systems and Health in Europe: Impact and Implications for Policy*. Maidenhead, UK: Open University Press, 2014.

Torrance, George W., Warren H. Thomas, and David L. Sackett. "A Utility Maximisation Model for Evaluation of Health Care Programs." *Health Services Research* 7, no. 2 (1972): 118–133.

Tuller, David. "A Resisted Pill to Prevent H.I.V." *New York Times*, December 30, 2013. Accessed June 11, 2014. http://www.nytimes.com/2013/12/31/health/a-resisted-pill-to-prevent-hiv.html?_r=0.

Ubel, Peter. *Pricing Human Life: Why It's Time for Health Care Rationing*. Cambridge, MA: MIT University Press, 2000.

United Nations. *The Universal Declaration of Human Rights*, Article 25 (1948). Accessed May 25, 2015. http://www.un.org/en/documents/udhr.

Urban, Thomas, and David Goldstein. "Pharmacogenetics at 50: Genomic Personalization Comes of Age." *Science and Translational Medicine* 6, Issue 220 (2014, January 22). Accessed June 11, 2014. http://stm.sciencemag.org/content/6/220/220ps1.short?rss=1.

US Department of Health and Human Services. "Health Insurance Marketplace: March Enrollment Report; For the Period: October 1, 2013–March 1, 2014." Accessed January 24, 2015. https://aspe.hhs.gov/health/reports/2014/market-placeenrollment/mar2014/ib_2014mar_enrollment.pdf.

US Department of Health and Human Services. "Exemptions from the Fee for Not Having Health Coverage." Accessed January 24, 2015. http://www.healthcare.gov/fees-exemptions/exemptions-from-the-fee.

US Department of Health and Human Services, Office of the Assistant Secretary for Planning and Evaluation. "2014 Poverty Guidelines." Accessed January 24, 2015. https://aspe.hhs.gov/poverty/14poverty.cfm.

US Internal Revenue Service. "Changes to Itemized Deduction for 2013 Medical Expenses." Accessed January 24, 2015. http://www.irs.gov/Individuals/2013-Changes-to-Itemized-Deduction-for-Medical-Expenses.

US Renal Data System. "2013 Atlas of End-Stage Renal Disease." Accessed June 11, 2014. http://www.usrds.org/2013/pdf/v2_00_intro_13.pdf.

Van de Wetering, Liesbet, Elly Stolk, Job van Exel, and Werner Brouwer. "Balancing Equity and Efficiency in the Dutch Basic Benefits Package Using the Principle of Proportional Shortfall." *European Journal of Health Economics* 14 (2013): 107–115.

Van Ginneken, Ewout. "Health Care Access for Undocumented Migrants in Europe Leaves Much to Be Desired." *Eurohealth* 20, 4 (2014): 11–14.

Van Ginneken, Ewout, and Bradford Gray. "Coverage for Undocumented Migrants Becomes More Urgent." *Annals of Internal Medicine* 5, 158 (2013): 347–348.

Van Ginneken, Ewout, and Bradford Gray. "European Policies on Healthcare for Undocumented Migrants." In *The Palgrave International Handbook of Healthcare Policy and Governance*, edited by Ellen Kuhlmann, Robert Blank, Ivy Lynn Bourgeault, and Claus Wendt, 631–648. Basingstoke, UK: Palgrave Macmillan, 2015.

Van Liedekerke, Luc. "Discounting the Future: John Rawls and Derek Parfit's Critique of the Discount Rate." *Ethical Perspectives* 11, no. 1 (2004): 72–83.

Venkatapuram, Sridhar. *Health Justice: An Argument from the Capabilities Approach.* Cambridge, UK: Polity, 2011.

Venkatapuram, Sridhar. "Health, Vital Goals, and Central Human Capabilities." *Bioethics* 27, no. 5 (2013): 271–279.

Verkerk, M. A., J. J. V. Busschbach, and E. D. Karssing. "Health-Related Quality of Life Research and the Capability Approach of Amartya Sen." *Quality of Life Research* 10, no. 1 (2001): 49–55.

Vogel, Lauren. "Medicare on Trial." *Canadian Medical Association Journal* 186, no. 12 (2014): 901.

Voigt, Kristin, and Gry Wester. "Relational Equality and Health." *Social Philosophy and Policy* 31, no. 2 (2015): 204–229.

Voorhoeve, Alex, Trygye Ottersen, and Ole F. Norheim. "Making Fair Choices on the Path to Universal Health Coverage: A Précis." *Health Economics, Policy and Law* 11 (2016): 1–7.

Wagstaff, Adam, and Eddy van Doorslaer. "Catastrophe and Impoverishment in Paying for Health Care: With Applications to Vietnam 1993–1998." *Health Economics* 12, no. 11 (2003): 921–934.

Wakefield, Jerome. "The Concept of Mental Disorder." *American Psychologist* 47 (1992): 373–388.

Walzer, Michael. *Spheres of Justice.* Oxford: Robertson, 1983.

Wasserman, David, Adrienne Asch, Jeffrey Blustein, and Daniel Putnam. "Disability: Definitions, Models, Experience." In *The Stanford Encyclopedia of Philosophy*, edited by Edward N. Zalta (2013). Accessed March 3, 2015. http://plato.stanford.edu/archives/fall2013/entries/disability.

Weinstein, Milton C., and William B. Stason. "Foundations of Cost-Effectiveness Analysis for Health and Medical Practices." *New England Journal of Medicine* 296, no. 3 (1977): 716–721.

Weinstein, Milton C., George Torrance, and Alistair McGuire. "QALYs: The Basics." *Value in Health* 12, no. s1 (2009): 5–9.

White, Joseph. "Gap and Parallel Insurance in Health Care Systems with Mandatory Contributions to a Single Funding Pool for Core Medical and Hospital Benefits for All Citizens in Any given Geographic Area." *Journal of Health Politics, Policy and Law* 34, no. 4 (2009): 543–583.

Widerquist, Karl. "How the Sufficiency Minimum Becomes a Social Maximum." *Utilitas* 22, no. 4 (2010): 474–480.

Wilkinson, Richard G. *Unhealthy Societies.* London: Routledge, 1996.

Wilkinson, Richard, and Michael Marmot, eds. *Social Determinants of Health. The Solid Facts,* 2nd ed. Copenhagen: WHO Europe, 2003.

Williams, Alan. "Intergenerational Equity: An Explanation of the 'Fair Innings' Argument." *Health Economics* 6 (1997): 117–132.

Williams, Andrew. "Liberty, Equality, and Property." In *The Oxford Handbook of Political Theory,* edited by J. Dryzek, B. Honig, and A. Phillips, 488–506. Oxford: Oxford University Press, 2006.

Williams, Bernard. *Ethics and the Limits of Philosophy.* Cambridge, MA: Harvard University Press, 1985.

Wilson, James. "The Ethics of Disease Eradication." *Vaccine* 52 (2014): 7179–7183.

Wolff, Jonathan. "Fairness, Respect, and the Egalitarian Ethos." *Philosophy & Public Affairs* 27, no. 2 (1998): 97–122.

Wolff, Jonathan. *The Human Right to Health.* New York: Norton, 2012.

Wolff, Jonathan, and Avner de-Shalit. *Disadvantage.* Oxford: Oxford University Press, 2007.

World Commission on the Environment and Development. *Our Common Future.* Oxford: Oxford University Press, 1987.

World Health Organization. "Constitution of the World Health Organization." Geneva: World Health Organization, 1948. http://www.who.int/governance/eb/who_constitution_en.pdf.

World Health Organization. *The World Health Report: Health Systems: Improving Performance.* Geneva: World Health Organization, 2000.

World Health Organization. "World Health Assembly 58, Resolution 33. Sustainable Health Financing, Universal Coverage and Social Health Insurance." Presented at the 58th World Health Assembly, Geneva, May 16–25, 2005.

World Health Organization. *The World Health Report: Primary Health Care Now More Than Ever.* Geneva: World Health Organization, 2008.

World Health Organization. *The World Health Report: Health Systems Financing: The Way to Universal Coverage.* Geneva: World Health Organization, 2010.

World Health Organization. *The World Health Report: Research for Universal Health Coverage.* Geneva: World Health Organization, 2013.

World Health Organization. *Making Fair Choices on the Path to Universal Health Coverage: Final Report of the WHO Consultative Group on Equity and Universal Health Coverage.* Geneva: World Health Organization, 2014.

World Health Organization. "What Is Universal Coverage?" Accessed May 25, 2015. http://who.int/health_financing/universal_coverage_definition/en.

World Health Organization. *Global Health Observatory Data, Life Expectancy.* Accessed May 25, 2015. http://who.int/gho/mortality_burden_disease/life_tables/situation_trends/en.

Zwarthoed, Danielle. "Creating Frugal Citizens: The Liberal Egalitarian Case for Teaching Frugality." *Theory and Research in Education* 13, no. 3 (2015): 286–307.

Index

Note: Page numbers followed by "fn" denote a reference to the footnote(s) on the given page

Aas, Sean 30fn
abortion 193
absolutism 77–78, 225, 226, 227
age-related priority 6, 206, 213–214,
    217–222, 232
AIDS 231, 238–239;
    and protease inhibitors 231, 238, 240, 241
Albertsen, Andreas 134fn
Al-Janabi, Hareth 293, 295, 296fn, 297fn
Altman, Lawrence 231fn
Alvarez, Allen Andrew 32fn, 33, 37, 38fn
American Medical Association 169
Amundson, Ron 165, 170, 175fn, 178
Anand, Paul 292fn, 293
Anderson, Elizabeth 11fn, 12fn, 17fn, 21fn,
    69fn, 112fn, 116, 131, 186fn, 201
Anell, Anders 187fn
antibiotics 137–138
appendicitis 231–232
Aristotelian 215
Aristotle 108, 109
Arneson, Richard 15fn, 26, 27fn, 28fn 70fn,
    75, 78fn, 86fn, 93fn, 105fn, 109fn,
    146fn, 190fn, 209fn
Arrhenius, Gustaf 66, 67fn
Arrow, Kenneth 26fn, 28fn, 282
Asada, Yukiko 31fn
aspect pluralism 112–115, 118
asthma 166

Australia 256
autism 280
autonomy 108, 230, 295, 296, 297, 298
Axelsen, David V. 13fn, 17fn, 19fn, 20fn,
    23fn, 97fn, 101fn, 108fn, 111fn
axiological sufficientarianism 51–68

Barbier, Edward B. 283fn
Barrett, Scott 136, 137
basic human functional capability (BHFC)
    5, 149, 150, 152, 153, 155–162, 166–168,
    236, 239
Battin, Margaret P. 31fn
Beauchamp, Tom 31fn, 45fn, 248, 249
Belgium 122, 159
Benbaji, Yitzhak 13fn, 19fn, 22fn, 23fn,
    26fn, 69fn, 71fn, 101, 111, 153fn,
    157fn, 225fn
Berkman, Lisa 30fn
bevacizumab 231, 233, 234, 243, 18fn
Birch, Stephen 290fn
Blake, Michael 106fn, 108fn
Bleichrodt, Han 292, 292fn
Boorse, Christopher 147fn, 165fn, 170–171, 173,
    175, 176, 178, 181fn, 183
Boorsean 172, 173, 176, 178, 179, 180
breast cancer 233–234, 235, 239, 243
Brennan, Victoria K. 291fn
Brighouse, Harry 117fn

Brock, Dan 232fn
Brock, Gillian 17fn, 20fn
Brooks, Richard 288fn
Broome, John 166, 182–183
Broqvist, Mari 259fn
Brouwer, Werner 285, 286
Brown, Campbell 23fn, 51fn
Brundtland, Gro Harlem 125, 126, 127,
    139, 142
Buchanan, Allen 31fn, 43, 44fn–45fn
Busse, Reinhard 251fn, 252fn,
    265fn, 257fn
Button, Kenneth 283fn

Callahan, Daniel 224, 232, 233fn, 271fn
Canada 187, 188, 206, 253
Canada Health Transfer 253
cancer 170, 230, 231–235, 239, 240;
    breast cancer 233–234, 235, 239, 243;
    lung cancer 235, 237
Caney, Simon 133fn
capability approach 32, 33, 36, 39–40, 41,
    42, 85, 115, 124, 125, 126, 128, 142, 144,
    145–163, 166–167, 174, 183, 190, 193–195,
    215, 225, 228, 236–237, 239, 240, 241,
    248, 292–300;
    sufficiency of capabilities approach
    (SCA/SOC) 33, 36–37, 144, 145–163,
    166–167, 185–186, 188–190, 192,
    193–198, 199–204, 282, 292–300
Carr-Hill, Roy A. 291fn
Casal, Paula 13fn, 18fn, 20fn, 27fn, 63,
    70fn, 76fn, 86fn, 88, 92fn, 93fn,
    97fn, 99fn, 102fn, 103fn, 104, 105,
    107, 109fn, 110fn, 153, 226fn, 249fn
Center for Budget and Policy
    Priorities 274fn
Chalkidou, Kalipso 265fn
Childress, James 31fn, 45fn, 248, 249
Claassen, Rutger 113fn
Clark, David A. 300fn
Claxton, Karl 258fn, 290fn
cleronomic approach 126–127, 130, 142
Clouser, Danner K. 148fn

Coast, Joanna 284fn, 286fn, 293,
    296fn, 300fn
Coffman, Darren 263fn
Cohen, G. A. 85fn, 209fn
Commonwealth Fund 252
Connors, Eleonora E. 271fn
contentment 89, 90
contraception 193
Cookson, Richard 292
Copp, David 132fn
Crisp, Roger 13fn, 17fn, 20fn, 21fn, 24fn,
    51fn, 60, 61fn, 71fn, 76fn, 78fn, 88,
    104–105, 107, 112, 153fn, 225, 226,
    249fn, 259;
    and Beverly Hills Case 60, 88, 107,
    112, 249
Culyer, Anthony 285, 286fn, 287, 292
cystic fibrosis 229–230, 235

Dakin, Helen 290fn
Daly, Herman 125
Daniels, Norman 31, 41, 43, 44fn, 147fn,
    213fn, 220fn, 219, 220fn, 227, 241–242,
    265, 265fn
Daniels, Norman 265fn
De la Croix, David 122fn
dementia 157, 213, 237, 239, 241
democratic deliberation 225, 234,
    242–243
democratic egalitarianism 131, 267
deontology 74–75
depression 157, 179, 288
de-Shalit, Avner 117, 202fn
dialysis 38fn, 224, 233
DiPrete, Bob 263fn
disability 5, 164–183, 216, 217, 253, 255,
    280, 289
disability-adjusted life-year (DALY)
    289, 294
discrimination 4, 112–115, 171, 175, 176, 181,
    219, 239
distributive egalitarianism 2, 12–14, 19, 20,
    22, 25–26, 27, 28, 34–35, 38, 69, 75,
    86, 103, 110–112, 153–155, 186fn, 190–191

Dixon, Simon 291fn
Dolan, Paul 287fn, 288fn, 289 289fn,
    291fn, 300fn
Donaldson, Cam 284fn
Dorsey, Dale 92fn, 99fn
Drummond, Michael F. 283fn, 286fn,
    287fn, 289fn, 290fn, 291fn, 294fn
Dunning Committee (Netherlands)
    261–262
Düwell, Marcus 113fn
Dworkin, Ronald 12fn, 85fn, 104, 105fn,
    155fn, 212fn, 227fn

Ebola 170
economic equality 53
egalitarianism 19–21, 25, 34–35, 41, 57, 69,
    70, 74–75, 103, 107, 109, 110, 125, 127,
    129, 144, 153–155, 165, 189, 191, 192, 198,
    200–204, 209, 224, 225, 232, 234, 241,
    242, 248;
    democratic egalitarianism 131;
    leximin egalitarian 127–128, 129, 131, 135, 136;
    maximin egalitarian 131;
    social egalitarian 6, 12, 14fn, 20fn, 22,
    112fn, 185–186, 187fn, 188, 189–191,
    194, 197–204
Egypt 152
Emanuel, Ezekiel 44fn, 45fn, 185fn, 187fn,
    189fn, 197fn, 272fn, 279fn
Engelhardt, Tristram H. Jr 44fn
England 250, 256, 258, 282
enslavement 179
Entwistle, Vikki 294fn
erlotinib 234
Europe 122, 159, 223, 229, 255, 265
European Observatory on Health Systems
    and Policies 260
European Union 276
European Union's Seven Framework
    Programme 47
external pluralism 19, 22
extra-welfarism 285–286, 292, 294

Fabre, Cécile 129fn, 133fn

Faden, Ruth 6, 19fn, 23, 24fn, 26fn, 28fn,
    31fn, 32fn, 33–35, 36, 188fn, 189fn,
    193, 206, 215–218, 219fn, 220, 221,
    236–241
Federal Joint Committee/Gemeinsamer
    Bundesausschuss (Germany)
    253–254, 258fn
Fenton, Elizabeth 44fn, 45fn
Ferrer, Robert 293
Fields, Gary S. 276
Financial crisis 2007–2008 260
Finegold, Kenneth, 270fn
Fleck, Leonard 31fn, 44, 230fn, 234fn,
    235fn, 242fn
Fleurbaey, Marc 123fn
flourishing 108–109, 112–116, 118;
    and health 115, 116, 161, 167, 172, 179,
    215–216, 236
Flynn, Terry N. 295fn, 296fn
Foster, James E. 55fn, 57fn, 59fn, 295
Foubister, Thomas 194fn
Fourie, Carina 17fn, 20fn, 32fn, 33, 45fn,
    191fn, 198fn, 199fn, 220fn, 240fn
Frakt, Austin 269
Frankfurt, Harry 3, 13, 19, 25fn, 52–54, 61,
    67, 88–89, 102–103, 104, 112, 162, 225,
    236, 105fn
freedom 51, 113, 125, 130, 131, 132, 167

Glucose-6-phosphate dehydrogenase
    deficiency 152
Gafni, Amiram 284fn, 290fn
Gaspart, Frédéric 128fn
gender 123
Gerard, Karen 287fn, 291fn
Germany 206, 253–254, 255–256,
    257–258, 264;
    and Federal Joint Committee/
    Gemeinsamer Bundesausschuss
    253–254, 257–258
Gheus, Anca 126fn
Global Polio Eradication Initiative 136fn
Glymour, Maria 30fn
Gold, Marthe R. 286fn

Goldstein, David 234fn
Goodin, Robert 86fn, 103fn
Gosseries, Axel 25fn, 122fn, 123fn, 126fn,
    127fn, 128fn, 129fn, 131fn, 133fn, 137fn
Gostin, Lawrence O. 271fn
Gray, Bradford 255fn
Grewal, Ini 292fn
Gusmano, Michael K. 213fn

Hadorn, David C. 290fn
Hall, Mark 213fn
Hanley, Nick 283fn
Harris, John 239, 172fn
Hawking, Stephen 152
Health Evidence Review Commission
    (United States, state of Oregon) 262
health insurance 2, 8, 31, 186–188, 194, 195f,
    206–214, 219, 252–257, 264, 268–280
Health Services Commission (United
    States, state of Oregon) 262
heart failure 227–228, 230, 231, 232, 237,
    240, 241
Herdman, Michael 288fn
Himmelstein, David 273fn
Hirose, Iwao 12fn, 19fn, 58fn, 63fn
HIV 231, 235, 238;
    and protease inhibitors 231, 238, 240, 241
HM Treasury (United Kingdom) 283fn
Hoffman, Christine 252fn
Holtug, Nils 70, 75, 78fn, 79fn, 80fn, 107fn
Hucklenbroich, Peter 165, 180fn,
    180–181, 182
Hume, David 91fn
Hurley, Jeremiah 283fn, 286fn
Huseby, Robert 13fn, 17fn, 19fn, 21fn, 22fn,
    51fn, 63fn, 65fn, 70fn, 71fn, 72fn, 73fn,
    74fn, 75fn, 101fn, 111fn, 259fn
hybrid sufficiency 18, 19

incremental cost-effectiveness
    ratio 290–291
infertility 148, 180
infliximab 230
Institute for Quality and Efficiency in
    Health Care (Germany) 258

Institute of Medicine (United States)
    268fn, 272–274
intergenerational justice 25, 25fn, 26fn, 121,
    124–126, 129, 132–133, 136–137, 140, 142
in vitro fertilization (IVF) 159–160
ipilimumab 231
isolationist approach 133–134, 140–141, 142, 143
Israel 159–160
ivacaftor 220–230, 235
IVF 159–160

Jamison, Dean T. 267fn, 268fn, 269fn
Johnson, Matthew 117fn

Kaiser, Jocelyn 230fn
Kaiser Commission on Medicaid and the
    Uninsured 277fn
Kaiser Family Foundation 277fn
Kawachi, Ichiro 30fn
Keehan, S. 223fn
Kelleher, Paul J. 197fn
kidney dialysis 224
Kinghorn, Philip 292fn, 293
Klingler, Corina 264fn
Knight, Carl 70, 76fn, 77, 78, 79fn, 80fn,
    133fn–134fn
Korsgaard, Christine 190fn
Krohmal, Benjamin J. 44fn, 45fn, 185fn,
    189fn, 197fn

labor market 82;
    division of labor 101
Lancet Commission for investment in
    health 269
Law, Iain 294fn
Lazenby, Hugh 108fn
Levey, Noam N. 273fn, 274fn
Lewis, David 181fn
leximin egalitarianism 127–128, 131, 135, 136
libertarian 154, 209, 248
Lie, Reidar 250fn, 252fn, 261fn, 262fn,
    264fn, 265fn
Lippert-Rasmussen, Kasper 69fn, 98fn
Littman, Jasper 137fn, 138fn
Lønning I Committee (Norway) 261

Lønning II Committee (Norway) 261
Loomes, Graham 291fn
Lorgelly, Paula 292fn, 293
Lucas, J. R. 19fn
luck egalitarian 98, 110, 129
lung cancer 235, 237

Madison, Kristin 279fn
malaria 170, 181
Mantone, Joe 229fn
Maori 257
Marmot, Michael 30fn, 134fn, 147fn, 198fn
Mason, Andrew 199fn
maximin egalitarianism 131
McIntosh, Emma 284fn, 285fn
McKenzie, Lynda 291fn
McKerlie, Dennis 17fn, 124fn
Medicaid (United States) 255, 262, 270–271,
    277–280
Medical Services Advisory Committee
    (Australia) 256, 257fn
Medicare (United States) 210, 255, 270
Medicare Benefit Schedule (Australia)
    256–257
Menzel, Paul 43, 44, 172fn, 206fn, 207fn,
    211fn, 213fn
Meyer, Lukas 25fn, 132fn
Miller, David 25fn, 106fn, 107fn
Ministry of Health and Care Services
    (Norway) 259
Mitchell, Olivia 276
Mitchell, Paul 17fn, 30fn–31fn, 294fn,
    295fn, 298fn, 299fn, 300fn
Molyneaux, Jacob 271fn
Mooney, Gavin 291fn
Mossialos, Elias 252fn

National Council for Priority Setting in
    Health Care (Norway) 259
National Health Care Institute
    (Netherlands) 257fn
National Health Service (United Kingdom)
    253, 258, 276, 282
National Institute for Health and Care
    Excellence (United Kingdom) 250,

258, 264, 282, 287, 288, 290, 293fn,
    294, 300
National Model for Transparent
    Prioritisation in Swedish Health
    Care 259
naturalist approach 169, 170–173, 176, 178
Netherlands 254, 256, 259, 261, 265;
    and 2006 Health Insurance Act 254
Netten, Ann 292fn, 293
Neumann, Peter J. 282fn
New Zealand 253, 257
New Zealand Medicines System 257
Nielsen, Lasse 13fn, 17fn, 19fn, 20fn, 23fn,
    97fn, 101fn, 108fn, 104fn, 108fn, 110fn,
    113fn, 114fn, 115fn, 116fn, 141fn, 191fn
nonrelational approach 59, 60, 63
Nord, Erik 291fn, 300fn
Nordenfeldt, Lennart 147fn, 165fn, 173, 174,
    178, 183
Normand, Charles 291fn
normative approach 33, 148, 157, 158, 159,
    167, 169–170, 173–178, 182, 194, 250,
    265, 267, 268, 285
Norway 255, 258, 261, 265;
    and priority setting 261, 264
Norwegian Directorate of Health 259
Norwegian Knowledge Centre for the
    Health Services 259
Norwegian Medicines Agency 259
Norwegian Ministry of Finance 259fn
Nussbaum, Martha 8, 24fn, 31fn, 32,
    34fn, 39, 41fn, 108, 109, 112fn, 114,
    146, 149–150, 153, 157fn, 158–159, 162,
    174, 175fn, 186, 188–193, 190fn, 202,
    293fn, 294

Obama, Barack (United States
    President) 181
Oberlander, Jonathan 262fn
O'Connell, Thomas 268fn
Olsen, Jan A. 284fn
Oregon (state) 262, 264
Oregon Health Plan 262–263, 264
Oregon Medicaid 250, 262
O'Shea, Eamon 284fn

Otsuka, Michael 70fn
Ozar, David T. 43fn

Pacific (people) 257
paclitaxel 233, 235
Page, Edward 25fn, 74fn, 92fn, 93fn, 104fn,
    105fn, 132fn
palliative care 239, 292
Palmer, Stephen 284fn, 287fn
Panteli, Dimitra 265fn–266fn
Parfit, Derek 52, 58fn, 65, 75, 76fn, 132fn,
    154fn, 156
Parliamentary Priorities Commission
    (Sweden) 259
pattern pluralism 18–19, 22
Payne, Katherine 291fn
People Programme 47
personal responsibility 40, 51, 87, 97, 98,
    110, 129–130, 209, 231, 241, 248, 261
Pharmaceutical Management Agency
    (New Zealand) 257
Phend, Crystal 235fn
Pierson, Ransdell 233fn
Pigou-Dalton 57, 67
Pinchot, Gifford 125, 142
pluralist sufficiency 16, 18–19, 19fn, 21–22,
    21fn, 38, 86, 87, 97–99, 100, 191,
    203, 231;
  aspect pluralism 112–115, 118;
  dimension pluralism 191, 192, 193,
    201, 202;
  external pluralism 19, 19fn, 22, 191,
    192, 201;
  pattern pluralism 18–19, 19fn, 22,
    191–192;
  value pluralism 191, 192
polio 136
Ponthière, Gregory 125fn
Porter, Eduardo 221fn
poverty 93, 105, 276–279, 294–295
Powers, Madison 6, 19fn, 23, 24fn, 26fn,
    28fn, 31fn, 32fn, 33–35, 36, 188fn,
    189fn, 193, 206, 215–218, 219fn, 220,
    221, 236–241
preference satisfaction 72–73

President's Commission for the Study of
    Ethical Problems in Medicine and
    Biomedical and Behavioral Research
    (United States) 43fn
prioritarian 13, 14–15, 16, 25, 38, 40, 58, 60,
    63, 65, 69, 70, 71, 73–74, 75–79, 81–82,
    84, 88, 96, 103, 107, 109, 110, 144, 153,
    154–155, 156, 162, 165, 172, 176, 224, 225–
    226, 232, 258;
priority by age 6, 206, 213–214, 217–222,
    232, 258;
priority setting 260–262, 264–265
progressive universalism 269
protease inhibitors 231, 238, 240, 241

Qizilbash, Mozaffar 300fn
Quality of Well-Being Scale 262
quality-adjusted life-year (QALY) 8, 172fn,
    218fn, 233, 235, 258–259, 285, 287–294,
    299–300
Quiggin, John 292

race 123
Ram-Tiktin, Efrat 17fn, 19fn, 22fn, 32fn, 33,
    36–37, 43, 145fn, 147fn, 154fn, 155fn,
    156fn, 162fn, 166–168, 174, 176, 178, 183,
    189fn, 225fn, 226–227, 228, 236–237,
    238, 239, 240, 241, 292fn
Rawlins, Michael 265fn
Rawls, John 12, 41, 42fn, 83, 91fn, 92fn,
    131, 139, 145, 146fn, 166fn, 226fn,
    242, 276fn
Raz, Joseph 108fn
Rechel, Bernd 251fn, 252fn
Reed Johnson, F. 287fn
relational approach 58–60
renal dialysis 224
renal disease 224, 255, 270
reproduction 126
resources 85
responsibility 40, 51, 87, 97, 98, 110,
    129–130, 209, 215
rheumatoid arthritis 230
Rhodes, Rosamund 31fn
Rice, Thomas 255fn, 262fn, 271fn